The Modern Psychiatrist's Guide to Contemporary Practice

The Modern Psychiatrist's Guide to Contemporary Practice provides an overview of psychiatry, starting with the most fundamental question of all: why does psychiatry exist?

Key topics are covered, such as: diagnosing mental illness, controversial treatments, involuntary admission, human rights, suicide, and global inequality. The book incorporates history, medicine, neuroscience, service development, legislation, and service-user movements. It summarises key findings and discussions, provides opinions based on evidence, presents clear conclusions, and describes useful, radical directions for the future of this most contested of medical disciplines. Each chapter includes useful chapter summaries, and case studies are provided throughout.

This book is essential for mental health workers and trainees, academics, and those interested in what psychiatry is, why it exists, and its future potential.

The Open Access version of this book, available at http://www.taylorfrancis. com, has been made available under a Creative Commons Attribution (CC-BY) 4.0 International license.

Brendan Kelly is Professor of Psychiatry at Trinity College Dublin, Consultant Psychiatrist at Tallaght University Hospital, and Visiting Full Professor at University College Dublin. In addition to his medical degree (MB BCh BAO), he holds master's degrees in epidemiology (MSc), healthcare management (MA), Buddhist studies (MA), and mindfulness-based interventions (MSc); doctorates in medicine (MD), history (PhD), governance (DGov) and law (PhD); and a higher doctorate in history (DLitt). He has authored and co-authored over 300 peer-reviewed publications and 700 non-peer-reviewed publications.

T0384825

The Modern Psychiatrist's Guide to Contemporary Practice

Discussion, Dissent, and Debate in Mental Health Care

Brendan Kelly

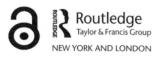
Routledge
Taylor & Francis Group
NEW YORK AND LONDON

Designed cover image: © Getty Images

First published 2025
by Routledge
605 Third Avenue, New York, NY 10158

and by Routledge
4 Park Square, Milton Park, Abingdon, Oxon, OX14 4RN

Routledge is an imprint of the Taylor & Francis Group, an informa business

© 2025 Brendan Kelly

ISBN: 978-1-032-45742-0 (hbk)
ISBN: 978-1-032-45740-6 (pbk)
ISBN: 978-1-003-37849-5 (ebk)

DOI: 10.4324/9781003378495

Typeset in Times New Roman
by Deanta Global Publishing Services, Chennai, India

The Open Access version of this book was funded by Trinity College Dublin.

This book is dedicated to Regina.

This book is dedicated to Regina.

Contents

About the Author

Brendan Kelly is Professor of Psychiatry at Trinity College Dublin, Consultant Psychiatrist at Tallaght University Hospital, Dublin, and UCD Visiting Full Professor at the School of Medicine at University College Dublin (UCD), Ireland.

In addition to his medical degree (MB BCh BAO), he holds master's degrees in epidemiology (MSc), healthcare management (MA), Buddhist studies (MA), mindfulness-based interventions (MSc), and an MA (*jure officii*) from Trinity College Dublin; doctorates in medicine (MD), history (PhD), governance (DGov), and law (PhD); and a higher doctorate in history (DLitt).

Professor Kelly has authored and co-authored over 300 publications in peer-reviewed journals, over 700 non-peer-reviewed publications, 25 book chapters and book contributions, and 20 books (including 13 as sole author). His recent books include 'Resilience: Lessons from Sir William Wilde on Life After Covid' (2023) and 'Asylum: Inside Grangegorman' (2023). In 2024, he co-edited, with Professor Mary Donnelly (University College Cork, Ireland), the first edition of the 'Routledge Handbook of Mental Health Law'.

Professor Kelly is a Fellow of the Royal College of Psychiatrists, Royal College of Physicians of Ireland, and Trinity College Dublin. In 2018, he became Editor-in-Chief of the *International Journal of Law and Psychiatry* and, in 2020, was elected as Dun's Librarian at the Royal College of Physicians of Ireland. In 2024, he was elected to membership of the Royal Irish Academy.

Disclaimer

This book is intended as general guidance only and does not in any way represent medical advice for individual persons. Readers are advised to attend their own healthcare professionals for advice and guidance appropriate to their particular needs. This book does not in any way replace the advice and guidance that your own doctor or other healthcare professional can give you. If you are concerned about any of the issues raised in this book, be sure to consult your doctor.

Clinical case histories and all patient names presented in this book are entirely fictional. They demonstrate common features of certain mental illnesses and their treatment, but do not correspond to specific individuals. Archival case histories have been anonymised.

While every effort has been made to ensure the accuracy of the information and material contained in this book, it is still possible that errors or omissions may occur in the content.

A Note on Language

Throughout this book, original language and terminology from the past and from various archives, reports, and publications have been maintained, except where explicitly indicated otherwise. This reflects an attempt to optimise fidelity to historical sources and does not reflect an endorsement of the broader use of such terminology in contemporary settings.

Content Advisory

This book discusses issues such as depression, suicide, self-harm, mental illness, and related matters in direct terms, in order to demystify, delineate, and understand them better. For this reason, certain readers might find certain sections distressing.

Permissions

- I am very grateful to the editors, publishers, authors, and copyright-holders who permitted the reuse of material in this book.

- Extracts from the *Guardian* and *Observer* are courtesy of *Guardian* News & Media Ltd.
- Anonymised clinical case histories and other material drawn from the archive of the 'Richmond District Lunatic Asylum' in Dublin, Ireland (later 'Grangegorman Mental Hospital') are used by kind permission of the Health Service Executive and the National Archives of Ireland.
- Some of the material in Chapter 10 is adapted and reused from: Kelly BD. AI in medicine – balancing prudence with possibility. *Medical Independent*, 23 January 2024 (https://www.medicalindependent.ie/comment/opinion/ai -in-medicine-balancing-prudence-with-possibility/) (accessed 24 January 2024), by kind permission of GreenCross Publishing.
- All reasonable efforts have been made to contact the copyright-holders for all material used. If any have been omitted, please contact the publisher. Many thanks.

Acknowledgements

Many people assisted and advised me as I wrote this book. I am deeply indebted to all the colleagues and friends who answered my emails and calls, and discussed various themes with me as the project progressed.

I am especially grateful to Dr Larkin Feeney, Dr John Bruzzi, Professor Aidan Collins, Professor Simon McCarthy-Jones, Ms Alison Collie, Ms Harriet Wheelock (Keeper of Collections at the Royal College of Physicians of Ireland), the National Archives of Ireland, Professor John Kelly, and my other extraordinary work colleagues at Trinity College Dublin, Tallaght University Hospital, and the Health Service Executive.

I owe a long-standing debt of gratitude to my teachers at Scoil Chaitríona, Renmore, Galway, Ireland; St Joseph's Patrician College, Nun's Island, Galway; and the School of Medicine at the University of Galway.

Above all else, I deeply appreciate the support of my wife, Regina, and children, Eoin and Isabel. I am also very grateful to my parents (Mary and Desmond), sisters (Sinéad and Niamh), and nieces (Aoife and Aisling).

Finally, I am deeply grateful to my patients, their families, and the many, many others who have helped and guided me along the way. Thank you, all.

Introduction

Aisha was 66 when she first showed symptoms of depression. Aisha had recently retired from her job as an engineer after a long career with the same company. She enjoyed her work for most of this time, but, over the previous decade, Aisha felt her job had become repetitive and less fulfilling. She completed her projects on time, but they no longer excited her as they once did. She did not feel a sense of fulfilment in her work. Aisha's job seemed meaningless to her at times. 'If I didn't do this', she said, 'the company could get someone else to do it better. What is the point?'

Aisha lived with her partner, who noticed a change in her too, especially since retirement. Aisha was less enthusiastic, less communicative, and less inclined to meet with their friends. Most surprisingly, Aisha stopped going to the swimming club that she had attended each week for more than twenty years. Aisha's partner did not think Aisha was depressed, but was worried about her, nonetheless. She just seemed so unhappy.

Immediately after Aisha retired from her job, she enjoyed a 'honeymoon period' with her new freedom. She took a holiday abroad with her partner, went for long walks, and even met with some of her old friends. Soon, however, Aisha began to isolate herself again, worried that she might have retired too early or that they might run out of money, despite Aisha's reasonable pension. Most of all, Aisha worried that she had 'wasted' her life. 'I should have been helping people', she said. 'I should have been a nurse or an aid worker or a social worker'. Aisha's partner spoke with her about the importance of her job as an engineer and the value of Aisha's relationships with other people, but Aisha was unconvinced: 'It just feels like a waste', she said: 'I could have done so much more'.

The situation deteriorated over the following months. Aisha's appetite declined, she had trouble sleeping, and she said that she had 'no energy for anything'. As she became increasingly morose, Aisha rarely left the house and spent long periods of time lying on her bed, staring into space. Aisha's partner was worried: this seemed like more than unhappiness. She asked Aisha to see her family doctor. Aisha agreed to this but was shocked when the doctor asked Aisha if she thought she might be depressed.

DOI: 10.4324/9781003378495-1

The possibility of 'depression' had never occurred to Aisha, although she admitted that she sometimes wondered if life was worth living. Even so, Aisha was angry with the doctor for suggesting she might have a 'mental illness'. Aisha would not consider talking therapy or other forms of treatment or support that the doctor suggested. She was even more surprised when the family doctor mentioned that Aisha might benefit from seeing a psychiatrist. 'A psychiatrist?' Aisha said, mystified: 'Why would I need one of those?'

Aisha's symptoms brought her into the realm of psychiatry, one of the most misunderstood and yet essential parts of medicine. Psychiatry is in a constant state of change and, for many people, is an entirely unknown quantity – at least until they or a family member experience problems that bring them into contact with psychiatrists or other mental health professionals.

Against this background, this book provides an overview of the contemporary state of psychiatry, explores key issues of discussion, dissent, and debate, and outlines likely directions for the future. For the purposes of the book, psychiatry is defined as 'the branch of medicine that is concerned with the study and treatment of disorders of mental function' (Clare, 1987; p. 868). While the understanding and management of disorders of mental function, psychological suffering, and mental illness extend into many fields outside psychiatry and, indeed, beyond medicine, this book focusses on the position and meaning of *psychiatry* within this broader landscape.

Consistent with this, a psychiatrist is a medical doctor who specialises in the understanding, prevention, diagnosis, and treatment of mental disorders. Again, there is usually a broad range of other people involved in these tasks, including patients, families, various health professionals, members of multi-disciplinary mental health teams, and others. This book, however, focusses on psychiatry and, therefore, on psychiatrists as specialist medical doctors working in this field.

Throughout this book, key issues of discussion, dissent, and debate are explored, and directions for the future are outlined. This is an evidence-based 'state of psychiatry' book, intended for both mental health professionals and general readers who are curious about the position of psychiatry in the world today and its prospects for the future. This is a broad task, which extends well beyond medical considerations and into the areas of physical health care, social support systems, criminal justice arrangements, political allocation of public resources, and the position of psychiatry in broader society.

The aim of this book is to summarise key evidence and discussions on major topics in psychiatry, express opinions based on evidence, present clear conclusions, and describe useful, logical directions for practice, policy, and research in the future. The book has a single author in order to provide consistency and a clear voice, which are often lacking in multi-author texts. This book takes a global view of psychiatry from clinical, scientific, policy, and legal perspectives, incorporating history, medicine, neuroscience, service development, legislation, human rights, and justice, among other themes, as they relate to contemporary debates within psychiatry.

It is not possible for a single book to cover every aspect of psychiatry and mental health, so this book focusses on adults (rather than children or adolescents) and does not probe specifically into certain subspecialties of psychiatry (e.g., intellectual disability, psychiatry of later life, forensic psychiatry).

Each chapter starts with an anonymised clinical case history illustrating key points which are explored later in the chapter, either directly or indirectly. Each chapter concludes with a bullet-pointed summary of the chapter's contents and key messages, which can be used as a handout or worksheet.

Overview of This Book

Chapter 1 of this book is titled 'Why Does Psychiatry Exist?' This chapter starts with an anonymised clinical case history and then explores definitions of 'psychiatry' and 'mental disorder' or 'mental illness'. It summarises the known epidemiology of mental illness globally and demonstrates that, notwithstanding cultural variations and changes in descriptive terminology, mental illness is common, complex, and costly. This leads to a discussion of how societies respond to mental illness, focussing on the nature and role of psychiatry in this context. This chapter sets the scene for the rest of the book and provides background about the rationale for psychiatry, the essential tasks of the discipline, and the fundamental nature of the problems it addresses.

Chapter 2 summarises 'The History of Psychiatry'. This chapter starts with an anonymised clinical case history from the nineteenth century, drawn from the archive of the 'Richmond District Lunatic Asylum' (later 'Grangegorman Mental Hospital'), a large, historic public asylum in Dublin, Ireland. This chapter explores accounts of apparent mental illness from religious texts and ancient literature, followed by a summary of the history of psychiatry as a medical discipline, including consideration of diverse treatments in the past, such as experimental surgical bacteriology, malaria therapy, insulin treatment, convulsive therapies, and lobotomy, which was the single greatest mistake in the history of psychiatry. This chapter also looks at historical critics of psychiatry in the 1960s, along with the work of psychiatrist Anthony Clare in the 1970s explaining the discipline, placing these diverse perspectives in the context of contemporary models of mental health care. Further case histories from the 'Richmond District Lunatic Asylum' in the early twentieth century are interspersed throughout the chapter and at the end, to illustrate relevant points.

Chapter 3 moves on to 'Diagnosing Mental Illness'. This chapter starts with an anonymised clinical case history focused on the diagnostic process, before exploring the purpose of diagnosis in psychiatry, the merits and demerits of diagnosis, and appropriate use of diagnostic systems. This discussion includes considerations of the American Psychiatric Association's *Diagnostic and Statistical Manual of Mental Disorders (Fifth Edition) (Text Revision)* (American Psychiatric Association, 2022), the World Health Organization's (WHO) *ICD-11: International Classification of Diseases (Eleventh Revision)* (World Health Organization, 2019), and general approaches to diagnosis in practice. The emphasis in this chapter is on skilful use of diagnosis as a tool for shared understanding and research, rather than dogmatic approaches to symptom-based syndromes in individual cases. Despite the limited role of biological tests in diagnosis in psychiatry, diagnosis remains essential in order to create a common language to talk about psychiatric conditions and human suffering; perform research into new treatments; hopefully identify the causes of mental illness, and protect human rights. Used wisely, diagnosis helps.

Chapter 4 focusses on 'Treating Symptoms and Disorders'. This chapter starts with an anonymised clinical case history of severe depression and its treatment. The chapter outlines the theory of the bio-psycho-social approach to care, and the evidence-bases for key treatments in psychiatry and their benefits; e.g., cognitive-behaviour therapy (CBT), interpersonal psychotherapy, certain mindfulness-based approaches, antidepressants, electro-convulsive therapy (ECT), antipsychotics, and some newer approaches (e.g., ketamine or psilocybin combined with psychotherapy). These summaries are based on systematic reviews, meta-analyses, and guidelines (where available). The overall approach is to describe the benefits of the main treatments, point to evidence to support their use, and note the need to balance adverse effects against therapeutic value in each individual case. Certain controversial topics require and receive particular attention; e.g., suicide and antidepressants, metabolic side-effects of antipsychotics, and ECT.

Chapter 5 moves on to the controversial topic of 'Treatment Without Consent'. Like the other chapters, this one starts with an anonymised clinical case history of involuntary admission and treatment. This chapter explores controversial legal issues associated with involuntary psychiatric admission and care. The discussion incorporates the United Nations' (UN) Convention on the Rights of Persons with Disabilities (United Nations, 2006) and other statements from UN committees and bodies, variously denouncing and supporting involuntary care. The chapter explores apparent variations in rates of involuntary admission across different jurisdictions, and concludes that treatment without consent should be possible, rare, and codified in law. Finally, this chapter discusses the idea that law and medicine are both fields that can deeply marginalise, or greatly assist, vulnerable members of society, so the interaction between law and medicine in psychiatry presents both significant risks and valuable opportunities that should not be missed.

Chapter 6 examines 'Neuroscience and Psychiatry', starting with an anonymised clinical case history of bipolar affective disorder (previously known as manic depression) before providing an account of the current position of neuroscience in psychiatry. While acknowledging the limited contributions that neuroscience has made to certain areas within this field, this chapter outlines the failure of neuroscience to substantially increase our understanding of the causes of common mental illnesses (such as depression, schizophrenia, and bipolar affective disorder) or to substantially inform new therapies. The chapter provides suggestions for a more focused, realistic, proportionate approach to neuroscience in psychiatry, optimising the promise of studies of imaging, genetics, inflammation, and new treatments, while remaining aware of the cost and opportunity cost of much neuroscience over past decades. This chapter concludes by outlining the need for a plurality of research methodologies in psychiatry – a true synthesis of techniques and understandings across neuroscience, medicine, law, history, spirituality, and other fields. Neuroscience needs to be contextualised as part of this broader search for knowledge and understanding, necessitating more radical, interdisciplinary approaches in the future, and wider, more inclusive frameworks for research and clinical care.

Chapter 7 is devoted to 'Psychiatry, Culture, and Society'. This chapter starts with an anonymised clinical case history that demonstrates the socially embedded nature of the lived experience of mental illness, with particular emphasis on culture, before exploring the relationship between psychiatry and culture, including public expectations of psychiatry, especially in terms of 'risk management'. This chapter explores professionalism in psychiatry and misuse of psychiatric diagnoses, practices, treatments, and institutions, both in history and today. There is a particular focus on cultural psychiatry and issues related to discrimination, including sexism, racism, and LGBTQIA+ (lesbian, gay, bisexual, transgender, queer, questioning, intersex, and asexual) issues, as well as ways to improve matters. Key steps include teaching and modelling professionalism within psychiatry; deepening awareness of cultural factors; addressing sexism, racism, and discrimination; and realising psychiatry's potential to act as a vehicle for empowerment, especially for people who experience several kinds of discrimination and marginalisation at the same time.

Chapter 8 examines issues relating to 'Self-Harm and Suicide', starting with an anonymised clinical case history. It explores definitions of self-harm and suicide; suicide in the history of psychiatry; global rates of suicide over recent decades; and the impact of the Covid-19 pandemic. This chapter pays particular attention to the limited value of 'risk assessment', the use of evidence-based approaches to suicide prevention, and the broader social context in which self-harm and suicide occur and are managed around the world. Issues relating to suicide and the law are explored, including the decriminalisation of suicide and attempted suicide in various jurisdictions (e.g., in India's Mental Healthcare Act, 2017), the use of 'risk' of suicide in mental health legislation (commonly as part of criteria for admission or treatment without consent), and some of the issues surrounding physician-assisted suicide, which is a topic that commands increasing attention around the world. The chapter concludes with a consideration of useful directions for future research and service developments in this area.

Chapter 9 explores 'Global Injustice in Mental Health Care'. This chapter starts with an anonymised clinical case history demonstrating a lack of care for complex social exclusion, substance misuse, and mental illness. The chapter uses evidence from the WHO and other sources to demonstrate and describe global inequity in mental health care. Particular attention is given to the relationships between mental illness and poverty, unemployment, homelessness, imprisonment, reduced rates of marriage, and issues relating to migration. The concept of 'structural violence' is used to explore the political, economic, and social circumstances that shape the landscape of risk for mental illness, the likelihood of receiving care, and contrasting outcomes for people with mental illness around the world. The chapter starts with evidence on this topic, summarises responses at the international level, emphasises the centrality of dignity, and concludes with an outspoken manifesto for culturally informed change.

Chapter 10 is devoted to 'The Future of Psychiatry: Person-Centred Care and System-Level Change'. This chapter starts with an anonymised clinical case history of anorexia nervosa. It goes on to explore specific themes of relevance to psychiatry and mental health care over the decades to come, including the future of diagnosis in psychiatry; the right to mental health care; the future of mental health legislation (including consideration of the 'Geneva impasse'); potential roles and risks of artificial intelligence (AI) in psychiatry; global mental health policy (including environmental sustainability in the provision and expansion of services); and the overall future of psychiatry both as a discipline within medicine and as a transformative movement to protect and promote the rights of people with mental illness and their families. Throughout the chapter, emphasis is placed on blending compassionate, person-centred, evidence-based care at the level of individuals and families with global pronouncements, national policies, and system-level change, with the aims of alleviating suffering, promoting rights, and improving mental health for all.

Finally, the book's 'Epilogue' starts with an anonymised clinical case history and provides further reflection on key themes discussed throughout earlier chapters, including the further potential and possibilities of psychiatry for the future, focused on preventing mental illness, alleviating suffering, and promoting the rights of people with mental illness and their families. The key message is that psychiatry offers a reasoned and reasonable path forward, once it is approached and practised with knowledge, awareness, humility, and compassion. The greatest challenge that psychiatry currently faces is global injustice in the distribution of preventive measures, treatment options, social support, and protection of rights. These are political matters as well as medical ones, requiring broad-based, inter-disciplinary action to address the challenges presented by mental illness across all communities and in all societies around the world.

Aisha, the retired woman with symptoms of depression whom we met at the start of this chapter, agreed to see a psychiatrist. The meeting was not what she expected. The psychiatrist asked Aisha how she felt and what was troubling her. The psychiatrist invited Aisha to speak at some length about her career as an engineer, her recent retirement, her problems sleeping, her lack of energy, and her withdrawal from her usual activities and relationships. The psychiatrist listened, asked for clarification of one or two points, and made some notes. He was unhurried, interested in details, and keen to know more about Aisha's current state of mind.

When Aisha finished her story, the psychiatrist asked Aisha what she thought about it all. Did Aisha feel that she needed to see someone like a doctor, a psychiatrist, or a therapist? What was her view? Aisha said she was unhappy, but did not think she was depressed, although she admitted that she did not really know what depression looked like. 'Am I depressed?', Aisha asked, looking a little bewildered.

The psychiatrist put down his pen, took off his glasses, and said: 'Let's see if we can figure this out'. The psychiatrist went on to explain the key symptoms of depression: low mood, lack of enjoyment, poor energy, reduced appetite, problems sleeping. There is also sometimes a sense of worthlessness, hopelessness, and doubts about whether life is worth living. 'Are the negative thoughts that you describe enough to be called depression?', he wondered aloud. 'Are your symptoms more than unhappiness?', he said, looking at Aisha as she, too, thought it through.

The psychiatrist explained that many of the symptoms of depression are also features of day-to-day life and features of unhappiness, but they tend to be more severe in depression, more persistent, and more disabling. Sometimes, the presence of even some of the symptoms of depression, if severe enough, can make it logical and useful to diagnose 'depression', and then use some of the treatments that are proven to help: talking therapies, medication, or other forms of support.

In Aisha's case, the psychiatrist said, it seemed to him that, regardless of whether they felt she met all of the official criteria for depression, some of the treatments for depression might help. Specifically, he recommended that she see a clinical psychologist with a view to cognitive-behaviour therapy, a type of talking therapy that helps many people with different kinds of problems, including symptoms of depression. The psychiatrist was happy not to reach a definitive position on 'diagnosing' or 'not diagnosing' depression, and focused more on Aisha and him agreeing a path forward that made sense to her. 'Diagnosis is important in research and in many other settings, but sometimes, in the clinic, diagnosis matters less than doing something useful', he said.

Aisha was happy with this, preferring to avoid labels, but also keen to feel better. She left the consultation with a referral to a clinical psychologist and another appointment with the psychiatrist for two months' time. 'Come back sooner if you want', he said. 'Sometimes antidepressant medication helps, too. And it's always good to re-consider how things are going. Also, do your best to get back to swimming if you can. Swimming is magic'.

References

American Psychiatric Association. *Diagnostic and Statistical Manual of Mental Disorders* (Fifth Edn, Text Revision). Washington, DC: American Psychiatric Association Publishing, 2022.

Clare AW. Psychological medicine. In: Kumar PJ, Clark ML (eds), *Clinical Medicine: A Textbook for Medical Students and Doctors* (pp. 868–-900). London: Ballière Tindall, 1987.

United Nations. *Convention on the Rights of Persons with Disabilities.* New York: United Nations, 2006.

World Health Organization. *ICD-11: International Classification of Diseases (Eleventh Revision).* Geneva: World Health Organization, 2019.

1 Why Does Psychiatry Exist?

Pablo was a happy child. He did well in school, played with his brother and sister, and had a good number of friends during his childhood and teenage years. He was healthy and, for the most part, happy.

From early on, Pablo's parents noticed that Pablo had a tendency to count things. Pablo counted his fingers, his toes, his toys, his books, and his family members. He counted his friends, the rows of seats at school, the number of rooms in his school, and the number of stones in the wall around the school. Sometimes, it was not clear what Pablo was counting, but he could be heard muttering numbers under his breath, counting something.

Pablo seemed to enjoy counting. If anyone commented about it, Pablo would laugh and stop counting, although he often came back later to finish counting on his own. Pablo did not seem distressed by this, but it was a habit that people sometimes noticed.

Pablo's parents mentioned Pablo's counting to their family doctor when Pablo was a child. The doctor said that children often count things or show other repetitive behaviours, and this generally stops as the child grows up. Many children count things, touch objects in a particular way, or perform the same actions again and again in a repetitive and often soothing manner. It usually just fades away, the doctor said. Pablo's parents were reassured by the conversation. After all, Pablo's counting did not disable him, he was not teased about it at school, and he seemed to have some control over it – at least to a certain extent.

Pablo's counting diminished significantly during his teenage years, but never went away fully. It seemed more prominent when Pablo was upset or under pressure or doing his end-of-school examinations. It eased in the summer when Pablo was out of school and when he was away on holiday with his family. Pablo's counting seemed like an eccentricity, rather than a major problem in his life. Pablo did not complain or comment about it in any way.

Pablo moved away from his family home in his early twenties to attend university. He lived alone in student accommodation for several years. At this point, Pablo's counting behaviour intensified. He started counting cars parked on each street he walked along, counting people on the bus, and counting books on the shelves in the library. Pablo became slightly upset when his counting was interrupted and often had to start again. On some occasions, while walking along

DOI: 10.4324/9781003378495-2

the street counting parked cars, a car would drive away, and Pablo would feel a
need to start counting again from the top of the street.

At this point, Pablo began to wonder if his counting was a problem. Walking
to university used to take 20 minutes, but now took more than an hour. Pablo
might feel a need to count the cars on the street three or four times, to be certain
he had counted them correctly. Also, people looked at Pablo strangely from time
to time as he walked up and down the street, counting cars. On one occasion,
Pablo made five efforts to count the cars on the street but still did not feel he got
it right. He went back to his apartment and skipped classes for the day. This was
not a regular occurrence, but it made Pablo worried about his counting.

Pablo did some Internet searches and began to wonder if he was mentally
ill. The thought of 'mental illness' or 'mental disorder' frightened him. One
website suggested seeing a psychiatrist and this unnerved him even more. What
was a psychiatrist? Pablo had only seen them in films and on television, and the
portrayals were frequently strange and often negative. Most of all, Pablo won-
dered: 'Am I losing my mind?'

Introduction

Pablo's experience is a common one: a person experiences a gradual build-up of
specific behaviours, thoughts, or symptoms. Eventually they (or someone else)
wonder if they need professional help for their mood, their negative thoughts,
their unusual experiences, or – as in Pablo's case – their excessive and now
disabling compulsive behaviour. Just when does eccentric behaviour become a
'mental disorder' or 'mental illness'? At what point does someone need to see
a mental health professional, such as a psychiatrist? These questions eventually
troubled Pablo and, at times, his family as Pablo's symptoms intensified and his
life was more and more affected. What should Pablo do?

This chapter explores some of the issues relevant to Pablo's dilemma. What is
psychiatry? Why does it exist? What are 'mental disorders' or 'mental illnesses',
and how common are they? What are society's responses to mental disorder and
mental illness? And what is the role of psychiatry in this context?

It is, perhaps, useful to start with definitions of 'psychiatry' and 'mental disorder' or 'mental illness' and then see how these might apply in Pablo's case.
Then, we can consider broader issues related to the prevalence of mental illness
around the world, the nature and role of psychiatry, the rationale for psychiatry,
the tasks of the discipline, and the state of psychiatry today. These are big questions about issues which are foundational for the discipline of psychiatry and
are, therefore, central to this book.

First, let's focus on a definition of psychiatry that both reflects the state of the
discipline today and provides the basis for the rest of this chapter.

Psychiatry is best defined as 'the branch of medicine that is concerned with
the study and treatment of disorders of mental function' (Clare, 1987; p. 868).

This is a broad definition, articulated in the 1980s by Irish psychiatrist Anthony Clare, who was a leading figure at that time and an innovative thinker about the nature and meaning of psychiatry (Kelly & Houston, 2020). Clare's 1976 book *Psychiatry in Dissent: Controversial Issues in Thought and Practice* both defended and critiqued contemporary psychiatry at a time when fierce debates raged about the discipline (Clare, 1976). Clare demystified psychiatry, analysed its problems, and argued that psychiatry, for all its flaws, offered a reasoned and reasonable path forward for understanding and treating mental illness (Kelly, 2023). His arguments remain highly relevant today, sometimes eerily so.

Clare's definition of psychiatry is consistent with most mainstream definitions both then and now, but – like virtually all definitions – it leaves considerable room for discussion, dissent, and debate. In other words, Clare's definition is probably as good as any definition can be, but it is still imperfect. In this way, it is not unlike psychiatry itself: serviceable but imperfect, useful but in need of development, adequate but likely to change over time, hopefully.

The issues raised by definitions of psychiatry, including Clare's one, are myriad and long-standing. Psychiatry might be concerned with 'disorders of mental function', but what are 'disorders of mental function'? Is forgetfulness a disorder of mental function and does it, therefore, fall within the remit of psychiatry? What about dyslexia? Or confusion? The division between 'psychiatric' and 'neurological' disorders has always been poorly defined and likely always will be, at least as long as diagnoses of mental illness are based solely on symptoms rather than biological tests.

There are even definitional questions about conditions which are generally considered to lie at the very heart of psychiatry. Is depression, which is routinely seen as coming within the ambit of psychiatry, really a disorder of 'mental function'? Is depression not better described as a disorder of emotions and bodily function, as well as mental function? If this is so, and if depression still comes under the heading of 'psychiatry', should unhappiness come within the purview of psychiatry too? And mild irritation? Are emotions part of 'mental function', or something else? Is mental function a constituent part of physical function, albeit incompletely understood (for now)? There are many questions.

Despite these issues – or possibly because of some of them – Clare's definition of psychiatry is still as relevant, useful, and specific as is possible at present. The phrase 'disorders of mental function' is as close to a consensus phrase as can be found, and the definition wisely specifies that psychiatry involves the 'study' of these disorders, as well as 'treatment', thus admitting the possibility that 'study' of such conditions might change matters as more information comes to light. Psychiatry is, then, by very definition, an evolving, changing field that incorporates 'study', as well as concerning itself with treating 'disorders of mental function'. Implicit uncertainty is built into the definition.

These definitional issues, with all their contingencies, are not unique to psychiatry. They reflect broader definitional challenges across medicine, not least of which is the understanding of 'medicine' itself, a term which arguably encompasses everything from specific interventions at the level of the individual patient to political decisions about the allocation of public resources at the level of countries or even internationally. That is a very broad scope for any defini-tion of anything. Such a definition is almost infinite and, as a result, medicine is almost infinite too. The same can be said of psychiatry to an even greater degree: 'mental function' underlies virtually everything we think, feel, and do, so this makes the field of psychiatry essentially infinite too. Psychiatry is the impossible discipline. It has no horizon.

The net result is that, while definitions matter to a significant degree, they are always imperfect, usually contested, inevitably evolving, and invariably in need of interrogation with a view to refinement. In addition, most definitions of high-level concepts such as 'medicine' or 'psychiatry' incorporate other definitions within them, such as 'illness', 'mental disorder', or 'mental illness'. While Clare used the term 'disorders of mental function' in his definition of psychiatry, the terms 'mental disorder' and 'mental illness' have become more common over recent decades, so these are discussed in the next section.

For the moment, we will take Clare's definition of psychiatry as the basic operational definition for the remainder of this chapter and for much of this book. Later in this chapter, we will expand the definition to include the pre-vention of mental illness, and in subsequent chapters we will expand it further when considering the broader landscapes in which mental illness develops (or does not develop), is recognised (or not), is treated (or not), and is followed by recovery (or not). We will broaden to an even wider lens when considering the role of social, economic, and political contexts in relation to mental illness and (especially) access to treatment and support (e.g., Chapter 9: 'Global Injustice in Mental Health Care').

For now, however, we will take Clare's definition as it stands and move on to ask another foundational question for this book: What is mental illness?

What Is Mental Disorder or Mental Illness?

Definitions of 'mental disorder' and 'mental illness' have changed considerably over time and across cultures. Today, the terms 'mental disorder' and 'mental illness' are generally used interchangeably, except in certain legal contexts, so both terms will be used here, especially 'mental illness'.

To begin to explore definitions, it is helpful to start with current consensus statements before taking a historical perspective and examining early accounts of apparent mental illness in ancient literature, religious texts, and other his-torical sources (in Chapter 2: 'The History of Psychiatry'). The move towards consensus definitions, such as those currently provided by the World Health Organisation (WHO) and American Psychiatric Association (APA), is a rela-tively recent development. It was driven by a desire to standardise diagnostic practice as much as feasible and provide a reasonably firm basis for research into causes, treatments, and – hopefully – prevention of mental illness (see Chapter 3: 'Diagnosing Mental Illness').

The central problem with defining 'mental disorder' or 'mental illness' is that psychiatric diagnoses are based almost exclusively on symptoms and signs, rather than biological tests. This means that diagnostic systems are fundamentally rooted in judgements about the severity and impact of specific symptoms, rather than the results of blood tests or brain imaging. These tests can be used to rule out other diagnoses, but not to confirm the presence of mental illnesses such as schizophrenia, bipolar disorder, depression, obsessive-compulsive disorder (OCD), or other psychiatric conditions. As far as biological tests are concerned, most mental illnesses remain diagnoses of exclusion: if characteristic symptoms of mental illness are present at the required severity for a specified period of time, and if relevant biological tests (if any) rule out potential 'non-psychiatric' explanations, then mental illness is diagnosed.

While this paradigm leaves no alternative to relying on symptoms for diagnosis, it is problematic. To return to the case of Pablo outlined at the start of this chapter, it is apparent that Pablo's long-term habit of counting things has intensified in recent times. He is now significantly slowed down by counting parked cars and his obsession with ensuring that he has counted them comprehensively and correctly. But this was a feature of Pablo's personality since early childhood, so at what point might this behaviour be deemed to have become a symptom of 'mental disorder' or 'mental illness'? And who decides this? Pablo is worried that he might be mentally ill. Is he?

According to the WHO's *ICD-11: International Classification of Diseases (Eleventh Revision)*, 'mental, behavioural or neurodevelopmental disorders' are 'syndromes characterised by clinically significant disturbance in an individual's cognition [thinking process], emotional regulation, or behaviour that reflects a dysfunction in the psychological, biological, or developmental processes that underlie mental and behavioural functioning' (World Health Organization, 2019). The ICD adds that these conditions are generally associated with impairment or distress involving 'personal, family, social, educational, occupational, or other important areas of functioning'.

This is an interesting, useful definition of 'mental, behavioural, or neurodevelopmental disorders', but, like Clare's definition of psychiatry, it is imperfect. There are two key issues with the ICD definition.

First, this definition includes three arguably similar but somewhat different types of 'disorders' in the same category: 'mental', 'behavioural', and 'neurodevelopmental disorders'. The borderlines between these categories are sometimes clear and sometimes blurred. Schizophrenia, for example, can be conceived as all three kinds of disorder at the same time: 'mental', 'behavioural', and 'neurodevelopmental'. Which language we use to describe schizophrenia is a matter of choice and perspective: some people see schizophrenia as essentially neurodevelopmental, but others emphasise the behavioural aspect. Other conditions, such as OCD, appear to have stronger mental and behavioural components, but are not without neurodevelopmental dimensions. In other words, the fundamental category of 'mental, behavioural, or neurodevelopmental disorders' outlined in the ICD is hugely variegated and internally diverse. While the resultant definition is somewhat understandable and operationally useful to a degree, it is not clear that it maps onto any identifiable clinical or biological reality, or even a logical aggregation of such realities. It is simply too broad.

The second key issue with the high-level ICD definition is its reliance not on the symptoms of illness itself, but on (a) a 'clinically significant disturbance', and (b) the 'dysfunction' that underpins it. In its own words, the ICD definition requires (a) a 'clinically significant disturbance' in a person's 'cognition, emotional regulation, or behaviour', and (b) a 'dysfunction in the psychological, biological, or developmental processes that underlie mental and behavioural functioning'. This definition is slightly circular and conceptually confused although it is not without merit. Let's return to Pablo.

In Pablo's case, his obsessional counting is a long-standing feature of his personality since childhood, but has now intensified to the point that it likely fulfils criterion (a) of the ICD definition; i.e., Pablo's counting now causes 'clinically significant disturbance' to his 'cognition, emotional regulation, [and] behaviour', owing to the frequency and extent of his counting, its impact on his day-to-day activities, and his growing concerns about it. Pablo's behaviour also now likely fulfils criterion (b) of the ICD definition, i.e., his counting stems from an underlying 'dysfunction' in the psychological processes that underpin 'mental and behavioural functioning'. More specifically, Pablo appears to have developed an obsession about counting correctly and a compulsive behaviour linked with this.

As a result, Pablo now likely has a mental disorder according to the ICD. While this is relatively clear, it is substantially less apparent when Pablo's counting ceased being a feature of his personality or an eccentricity and became a mental disorder. Was it when the behaviour intensified, or only when it started to impair his life? If it is the latter, then social context becomes central to diagnosis: perhaps if Pablo still lived with his family rather than living alone, his symptoms might not have intensified to the point that he fulfils criteria for mental disorder. This presents a dilemma to conceptualisations of mental disorder and research about its causes: if social circumstances shape diagnostic thresholds, how likely are we to find a biological cause for symptom-based syndromes, such as mental illnesses?

Similar issues are raised by the other main consensus-based definition of 'mental disorder', which is provided by the APA in its *Diagnostic and Statistical Manual of Mental Disorders (Fifth Edition) (Text Revision)* (DSM) (American Psychiatric Association, 2022). The DSM defines a 'mental disorder' as 'a syndrome characterised by clinically significant disturbance in an individual's cognition, emotion regulation, or behaviour that reflects a dysfunction in the psychological, biological, or developmental processes underlying mental functioning'. The DSM adds that these 'disorders are usually associated with significant distress or disability in social, occupational, or other important activities'. The DSM specifies that 'an expectable or culturally approved response to a common stressor or loss, such as the death of a loved one, is not a mental disorder'. In addition, 'socially deviant behavior (e.g. political, religious, or sexual) and conflicts that are primarily between the individual and society are not mental disorders', unless they stem from 'a dysfunction in the individual', as already outlined.

Like the ICD definition, this one relies on both (a) a 'clinically significant disturbance' and (b) an underpinning 'dysfunction' in 'psychological, biological, or developmental processes'. Also like in the ICD, this definition is slightly circular but still moderately useful. And, again like the ICD, the DSM notes that social distress and disability are often associated with a mental disorder, acknowledging the functional or social dimension to these conditions. According to both the ICD and DSM, Pablo has a 'mental disorder' or, to use the more common term, 'mental illness'.

Epidemiology of Mental Illness

Mental illness is common, complex, and costly. The WHO states that one person in every eight, a total of 970 million people live with a mental disorder, although most people do not have access to effective care (World Health Organization, 2022a). Anxiety and depressive disorders are recognisably the most common conditions, notwithstanding cultural variations in descriptive terminology across communities, societies, and countries. In other words, mental illness is common around the world, with almost one billion people affected directly and many others impacted indirectly: family, friends, colleagues, and wider communities.

Much research has been devoted to understanding the prevalence of mental illness in more detail in order to clarify and refine these headline figures. In 2008, the WHO World Mental Health Survey Initiative reported in some detail about the 12-month prevalence of mental disorders (Kessler et al., 2008). Twelve-month prevalence is the proportion of a population that has suffered from a mental disorder within the past 12 months. In the WHO research, the 12-month prevalence of any mental disorder varied considerably between countries, ranging from 6% in Nigeria to 27% in the United States (US). The interquartile range (IQR, which is the range after excluding the highest and lowest surveys) was 9.8% to 19.1%, suggesting that between 1 person in 10 and 1 person in 5 has a mental disorder in any given year.

Global surveys are difficult to perform with consistency for many reasons, including the sheer scale of such projects, local variations in language and customs, and differing understandings of psychological suffering. Even so, the

WHO World Mental Health Survey Initiative and similar studies provide fascinating information about the occurrence and prevalence of mental illness, even if their data should be interpreted with care and an understanding of the intrinsic limitations of these methodologies.

In terms of severity, the WHO results show not only differences in the prevalence of mental disorders across countries but also a wide range of severity: 28.0% of mental disorders in Israel were classified as 'mild', compared to 74.7% in Nigeria (Kessler et al., 2008). Severity estimations were not strongly related to region or development status and so remain largely unexplained.

Despite these variations, there were notable points of consistency in the WHO survey. For example, relative prevalence estimates were generally similar across countries, even when overall prevalence and severity varied. This means that the relative frequencies of specific disorders were reasonably constant across borders, although overall rates of mental disorder differed. Anxiety disorders were the most common conditions in most countries studied, with prevalence estimates ranging between 3.0% and 19.0% (IQR: 6.5%–12.2%). Mood disorders were the next most common mental illnesses in most places, with prevalence estimates between 1.1% and 9.7% (IQR: 3.4%–6.8%).

More recent data and results from other studies generally support the WHO figures, including research from individual countries. In 2016, for example, a report based on the National Psychiatric Morbidity Surveys of common mental disorders in England from 1993 to 2007 explored the frequency of these conditions, service contact, and treatment received (Spiers et al., 2016). This analysis found that the prevalence of common mental disorders in England was relatively consistent, at 14.3% in 1993, 16.0% in 2000, and 16.0% in 2007. This is broadly similar to the WHO figures (9.8%–19.1%), suggesting that this is a reliable estimate overall.

The English surveys also reported consistent results for contact with primary care physicians (general practitioners or family doctors) for psychological problems over the past year, at 11.3% in 1993, 12.0% in 2000, and 11.7% in 2007. Antidepressant receipt in people with common mental disorders more than doubled over this period (from 5.7% in 1993 to 15.9% in 2007) and use of psychological treatments increased among men with common mental disorders (from 4.8% in 1993 to 10.4% in 2007). Even so, many people with common mental disorders still received no treatment, even in England. This, too, is consistent with WHO findings from around the globe.

Most of these figures refer to common mental disorders, chiefly anxiety and depression, which are often managed and treated by primary care physicians, counsellors, psychotherapists, or other forms of local care, including self-management and family care. The term 'serious mental illness' (SMI), by contrast, is used for conditions that frequently require interventions from specialist mental health services and psychiatrists. These conditions commonly include moderate or severe depression, schizophrenia, bipolar disorder, panic disorder, post-traumatic stress disorder (PTSD), OCD, and certain personality disorders, among other mental disorders.

In the US, the National Institute of Mental Health (NIMH) states that 5.5% of all US adults (an estimated 14.1 million people) have SMI (National Institute of Mental Health, 2023). The prevalence is higher among females (7.0%) than males (4.0%), and among young adults aged 18 to 25 years (11.4%) compared to those aged 26 to 49 years (7.1%) or 50 years and older (2.5%). The NIMH reports that the prevalence of SMI in the US is highest among American Indian/ Alaskan Native adults (9.3%), followed by adults reporting two or more races (8.2%), and is lowest among Asian adults (2.8%). While more data are needed to develop clearer estimates, especially in low-income and middle-income countries, figures from elsewhere are broadly similar to the US; e.g., in Australia, an estimated 3.3% of adults experience SMI each year (Whiteford et al., 2017).

Overall, accumulated data paint a clear picture. Mental illness is common around the world, especially anxiety and depression, but also SMI. It should be noted that anxiety and depression, too, can be serious and enduring, but most cases are either mild or moderate, and while they require intervention and support, they do not necessarily require specialist mental health services in the way that schizophrenia and bipolar disorder usually do. Everyone is different, and so is every case of mental illness.

Is mental illness increasing or decreasing over time? There is continual speculation on this point. What, if anything, do prevalence surveys tell us about this?

The English survey suggests stability (Spiers et al., 2016; above), but it can be difficult to identify changes over time. The reasons for this include continual revisions of diagnostic systems such as the ICD and DSM, and shifts in diagnostic practices, some of which are positive and some of which are questionable. These issues are explored in some detail in Chapter 3 of this book, which is devoted to 'Diagnosing Mental Illness'. Overall, however, the picture appears to be generally stable, notwithstanding occasional changes such as during the Covid-19 pandemic, which is discussed in Chapter 8 in the context of 'Self-Harm and Suicide'.

The Costs of Mental Illness

The costs of mental illness can be truly described only in terms of human suffering, loss of opportunity, and impact on psychological wellbeing and social flourishing. For Pablo, the idea of 'mental illness' came to mind only when his behaviour began to command an identifiable cost in his life: missing classes at the university and attracting glances and comments from strangers on the street. In this case, it was the escalating impact on Pablo's life and the cost to his social wellbeing that prompted Pablo to seek information, advice, and care.

The human cost of mental illness is also apparent among the families and friends of people affected. Pablo's parents spent many nights worrying about him when he was a child and his symptoms were at a milder level: As parents, what should they do? Was their child ill or just slightly unusual? Did Pablo need specialist assessment and care? Even when Pablo became an adult, it is likely that his symptoms continued to cause concern among family and friends, who are often profoundly affected by psychological suffering and mental illness in other family members or friends.

With this in mind, it is difficult to assess the 'cost' of mental illness to society, but it is nonetheless a worthwhile task. The best efforts in this direction acknowledge the difficult-to-measure costs to the individual and their family and friends, but also do their best to estimate economic costs in the broadest sense, often with a view to focussing public attention and galvanising policymakers into positive action.

In 2011, the World Economic Forum published a report titled *The Global Economic Burden of Non-communicable Diseases* which included a summary estimate of the costs of all mental health conditions around the world (Bloom et al., 2011). This study estimated that the global cost of mental health conditions in 2010 was US $2.5 trillion, with this cost projected to reach US $6.0 trillion annually by 2030. Approximately two-thirds of this cost comes from the indirect costs of mental illness (such as reduced productivity) and the remainder from direct costs (such as costs of care). This total exceeds the cost of heart disease, is more than the costs of diabetes, cancer, and respiratory disease combined, and is deeply disturbing by any standards (Insel et al., 2015). In essence, the financial and economic costs of mental illness are vast and getting vaster.

A 2020 editorial in *The Lancet Global Health* drew additional attention to these issues and noted that the costs of mental illness are spread across social services as well as primary, secondary, and tertiary care (Lancet Global Health, 2020). The editorial emphasised the economic case for investing in mental health: every US $1 spent on improved treatment for depression and anxiety results in a US $4 return in better health and productivity. Investing in mental health makes sense at every level: personal, inter-personal, and economic.

In September 2022, a further study confirmed these findings and underlined the need for effective interventions (Arias et al., 2022). This research estimated that 418 million disability-adjusted life years (DALYs) could be attributable to mental disorders each year. A DALY is the loss of the equivalent of one year of full health. As a result, mental illness potentially accounts for 16% of global DALYs. The economic burden associated with this is now estimated at approximately US $5 trillion annually (consistent with World Economic Forum figures). At the regional level, the resultant losses could account for between 4% of the gross domestic product in Eastern sub-Saharan Africa and as much as 8% in high-income North America. That is an enormous impact on any country.

Studies and policy documents from individual countries confirm the scale of the problem and its substantial, disseminated impact. In May 2022, the US President's Council of Economic Advisors published a briefing titled *Reducing the Economic Burden of Unmet Mental Health Needs* (Council of Economic Advisors, 2022). The Council noted that 'the [US] Federal Government covers some of the costs of treating mental health disorders. Around $280 billion was spent on mental health services in 2020, about a quarter of which came from the US Medicaid program':

> Society also bears many of the costs of mental health disorders through public disability programs that pay for income support for those who cannot work. People with psychiatric disabilities were the largest contributor to growth in Social Security Disability Insurance (SSDI) rolls in the early 2000s. As of 2020, 18 percent of SSDI beneficiaries, or 1.4 million individuals in current payment status, suffered from depression, bipolar, or psychotic disorders.[1] Overall, the mental disorder category accounted for 29 percent of beneficiaries in 2020, or 2.4 million people – a share larger than beneficiaries who cannot work due to injuries, cancer, or diseases of the circulatory and nervous system, combined. While these supports are important and necessary, too many people fall through the cracks and do not receive the treatment that could both improve their livelihoods and reduce their reliance on disability insurance.

These issues are by no means unique to the US: people with mental illness fall through the cracks in most countries around the world, amplifying social exclusion, diminishing access to care, increasing symptoms, and snowballing costs. In consequence, the Council of Economic Advisors notes that 'additional costs to society of inadequately treated mental illness include increased homelessness and incarceration':

> The homeless population has significantly higher rates of mental illness than the population as a whole, and lifelong mental illness is associated with higher rates of incarceration. Both homelessness and incarceration are likely to be exacerbated by difficulties maintaining work or close relationships due to mental illness. In addition to the severe economic consequences for those affected, supportive services for the homeless impose large societal costs, and incarceration leads to millions of dollars of direct and indirect costs on society. Other societal costs include increased co-occurring mental health problems, loss of earnings, and premature death.

While the Council of Economic Advisors and other groups and researchers do their best with available data to produce vital estimates of economic cost, it is important to remember that it is essentially impossible to quantify the 'cost' of disabling symptoms, loss of potential, social marginalisation, and premature death associated with mental illness. While the economic costs are vast, they are estimable to a significant degree and are now approximately US $5 trillion per year (Arias et al., 2022). The personal costs, however, cannot be measured fully and will always be infinite.

The 'Crisis' in Mental Health

In light of the high prevalence of mental illness and its human and economic costs, efforts to support and help those affected are a feature of all societies. The history of psychiatry, as one part of that societal response, is explored in Chapter 2 of this book ('The History of Psychiatry'). But looking beyond psychiatry, there is also a broader social or public response to mental illness which evolves over time, sometimes in response to changes in society, sometimes as a result of shifts in understandings or interpretations of mental illness, and sometimes for reasons that are considerably less clear and not always useful or productive.

One of the most common positions both now and in the past is to describe the prevalence of mental illness as a 'crisis' that is continually getting worse and requires an emergency response by governments and societies. This 'crisis' narrative is ubiquitous across politics, media, and public discourse (e.g., Shackle, 2019). Following Covid-19, the US President's Council of Economic Advisors placed particular emphasis on this 'crisis' terminology in *Reducing the Economic Burden of Unmet Mental Health Needs*:

> It is vital to understand the full costs of the mental health crisis affecting our nation. Left untreated, mental health disorders affect the well-being of children, adults, families, and communities - both because of the emotional costs as well as the economic ramifications. These disorders were already too common before the COVID-19 pandemic, and the pandemic magnified the crisis by simultaneously increasing the need for care and diminishing access to it.
>
> (Council of Economic Advisors, 2022)

We will see in Chapter 2 that the idea of a 'crisis' in mental health is an old one which contributed directly to the emergence of vast networks of public 'asylums' around the world during the nineteenth century. While declaring a 'crisis' has always indicated concern and might command short-term attention, the precise meaning of words matters deeply in the longer-term. Words such as 'crisis' can generate attitudes and actions that fail to engage with the true complexity of problems like mental illness and fail to produce effective, sustainable solutions after the 'crisis' rhetoric has faded or another, unrelated 'crisis' comes along. As psychiatry knows to its detriment, the rush to ill-considered, short-term, emergency action in an apparent 'crisis' can have profoundly negative results and perpetuate the very problems it seeks to address.

Moreover, the notion of a 'crisis' in mental health is poorly supported by reliable, peer-reviewed, systematic evidence. Mental illness is indeed common and must be addressed better and more, but rates of mental illness appear generally stable over time, with any perceived increase likely attributable to changed diagnostic practices and the lowering of diagnostic thresholds across all areas of medicine, not just psychiatry. The role of diagnosis in psychiatry, along with its merits and demerits, are explored in Chapter 3 of this book ('Diagnosing Mental Illness').

And, as we will see in Chapter 8 ('Self-Harm and Suicide'), there is clear evidence of progress rather than deterioration in at least one important indicator of mental health, rates of suicide, although there is (of course) still considerable work to be done. Yet, even during Covid-19, rates of suicide were either stable or declined in many countries (e.g., Yan et al., 2023), and there was more resilience apparent than most people might have anticipated in such circumstances. There were certainly mental health problems during the pandemic and after it, but there was no surge of mental illness, notwithstanding the 'crisis' narrative adopted by the Council of Economic Advisors and others now and in the past.

The language of 'crisis' in mental health is largely impervious to facts and statistics which might moderate, modulate, or otherwise refine the terminology, and might help identify reasonable, proportionate solutions to the enduring problems of mental illness. The desire to describe 'mental illness' (or even, on occasion, 'mental health') as a 'crisis' is clearly rooted in a desire to help, but it also demonstrates a degree of virtue signalling rather than pragmatic, level-headed determination to delineate problems, generate sustainable solutions, and follow them up into the future.

The 'crisis' narrative is also motivated by fear of being seen as ignoring the problems presented by mental illness or not recognising the suffering involved. After all, we have discussed how mental illness is common and costly, so there is a strong and understandable impulse to help and to be seen as concerned. Using the word 'crisis' at least indicates the intention to take mental illness seriously, so is there any real harm in 'crisis' terminology?

The problem is that continual talk of a 'crisis' in mental health is poorly supported by reliable evidence and rarely leads to planned, sustained action that is effective in the longer term. Crisis solutions are inappropriate for an enduring health challenge such as mental illness. In a 'crisis', politicians rush to make announcements about short-term measures in response to 'crisis' headlines, but their emergency promises occupy the space that should be filled with moderate, sustainable, effective plans. In other words, continual talk of 'crisis' undermines credible action and allows the issue of mental illness to appear on political agendas in bursts and starts, rather than in a sustained, impactful way. Mental illness (or even 'mental health') becomes just one more 'crisis' rolled up in short-term, crisis-driven news cycles, rather than landing on the long-term agenda for health and social care.

It is important to be absolutely clear that mental illness is common, costly, and presents an enormous challenge to individuals, families, and societies, as discussed throughout this book. The problem with the continual 'crisis' narrative lies not with the *impulse* to describe the situation as a 'crisis' or to act, but with the *effect* of the 'crisis' framing of the problem, which is often – ironically – precisely the opposite of the effect intended. Constant talk of a 'crisis' in mental health impairs long-term planning and has no discernible short-term benefit. It fails to remind the public about the real, enduring problems that mental illness presents, as opposed to being a passing 'crisis'.

The Rationale for Psychiatry

This chapter is titled: 'Why Does Psychiatry Exist?' So far, we have explored definitions of 'psychiatry' and 'mental disorder' or 'mental illness', and established that mental illness is common, affecting one person in every eight, or a total of 970 million people globally, at any given time (World Health Organization, 2022a). We have noted that mental illness is costly in terms of human impact, social exclusion, missed life opportunities, and economic burden for societies, which is currently estimated at approximately US $5 trillion annually (Arias et al., 2022). We have explored the 'crisis' narrative that is commonly applied to 'mental health' which, while not without a certain justification, is not the most supported, reasonable, or effective way to frame the challenges presented by mental illness, which require a sustained long-term response, not a short-term 'crisis' one.

These discussions go some way towards addressing the question that lies at the heart of this chapter: 'Why Does Psychiatry Exist?' Psychiatry exists to address these needs and hopefully prevent some of the problems occurring in the first place, or, at least, prevent them from deteriorating over time. How does this work in practice?

If we return to Pablo, the man with counting obsessions and compulsions whom we met at the start of this chapter, it is clear that Pablo initially did not realise that he was becoming mentally ill and did not appreciate that assistance might be available. Psychiatry has many potential roles in this situation.

First, it is possible that enhanced baseline awareness of the nature of mental illness and psychiatric symptoms might have informed and hopefully reassured Pablo and his family at an earlier stage in the development of his problems. Perhaps they might have understood sooner that these behaviours can be perfectly normal to a degree but can sometimes escalate to the extent that psychiatric referral or mental health care is helpful. This is, perhaps, the first therapeutic role of psychiatry: increasing public education about psychiatric symptoms, providing reassurance about variations on normal anxieties, and indicating at what point referral for assessment, support, and treatment can be useful.

The second role of psychiatry, as outlined in Clare's definition, is the treatment of these conditions. Therapies can include reassurance, guided self-care, and enhanced family or community support. Treatment can also involve counselling and more structured supports in addition to what is offered by family and friends, but still outside a formal mental health framework; e.g., various psychotherapies, bibliotherapy, or different social interventions. For other people, treatment can involve mental health care in primary care settings, provided by primary care physicians and other members of multi-disciplinary primary care teams: nurses, therapists, and various others. Finally, treatment can involve specialist mental health care and psychiatric interventions with psychiatrists, clinical psychologists, mental health nurses, social workers, occupational therapists, speech and language therapists, and various other mental health professionals. Support should also be offered to families, who commonly experience significant anxiety, even when their family member is attending mental health services.

The third role of psychiatry, again suggested in Clare's definition, is to study mental illnesses so as to better understand how they are caused, how they are best treated, and how they can be prevented. This is a complex task given that most mental illnesses are currently defined by symptoms rather than biological tests and are thus likely to evade detailed biological explanation based on current conceptualisations. The broader challenges presented by symptom-based diagnoses are explored in Chapter 3 of this book ('Diagnosing Mental Illness') and some of the issues with biological research into causation are examined in Chapter 6 ('Neuroscience and Psychiatry').

Despite this lack of knowledge about the causes of mental illness, a significant degree of prevention is still likely to be possible. The role of psychiatry in preventing these conditions does not receive sufficient attention at present. Despite the many unknowns, much can be done in the areas of primary, secondary, and tertiary prevention of certain conditions.

Primary prevention refers to preventing mental illness developing in the first place. Possibilities here range from general advice about diet, exercise, and lifestyle (in the hope of preventing mild depression and anxiety) to more specific guidance about particular exposures linked with various conditions. Cannabis is a good example. A multitude of studies support a link between cannabis and increased risk of SMI such as schizophrenia (e.g., Vaucher et al., 2018; Godin & Shehata, 2022). In 2017, the US National Academies of Sciences, Engineering, and Medicine reviewed the evidence pertaining to possible links between cannabis and psychosis, and concluded that the higher the cannabis use, the greater the risk of schizophrenia and other psychoses (National Academies of Sciences, Engineering, and Medicine, 2017). While the issue of legalising cannabis is controversial and involves many medical and non-medical considerations, the medical evidence is clear: cannabis presents a risk to mental health (regardless of whether it is illegal, decriminalised, or legal).

Secondary prevention refers to reducing the impact of a condition by detecting and treating it as soon as possible to prevent its progression. In Pablo's case, this might mean earlier assessment by a mental health professional and practical advice about preventing obsessional thoughts and compulsive behaviours becoming more deeply embedded. This might help reduce distress, increase Pablo's sense of control, and alleviate the condition to a greater degree at an earlier stage, even if formal treatment is still required at some point.

Finally, tertiary prevention means reducing the impact of an existing condition by helping people to manage their persisting symptoms, find ways to minimise disability, and hopefully prevent any further complications developing. Tertiary prevention can play a vital role in long-term conditions such as schizophrenia by helping to improve social function, optimise quality of life, and even preserve or enhance life-expectancy (see Chapter 4: 'Treating Symptoms and Disorders').

These, then, are the three key tasks of psychiatry: (a) increasing awareness of the symptoms of mental illness (in order to reassure most people that they are not mentally ill and to facilitate early assessment for those who might be); (b) providing treatment and support to people with mental illness and their families (including biological, psychological, and social approaches, combined to meet the needs of individual patients and families), and (c) study of mental illnesses so as to better understand causation, treatment, and prevention, and thereby enhance care.

Finally, it is essential that protection of human rights forms part of all of these tasks. Issues relating to rights are further explored elsewhere in this book, including Chapters 5 ('Treatment Without Consent') and 9 ('Global Injustice in Mental Health Care'). It is vital that human rights are a consideration in all psychiatric treatment owing to the unique ability of mental illness to affect an individual's judgement and the distinctly mixed history of psychiatry in relation to human rights. This issue is further explored in the next chapter, Chapter 2, which is devoted to 'The History of Psychiatry'.

The State of Psychiatry Today

So, how is psychiatry faring with the three key tasks it faces: increasing awareness, treating mental illness, and studying the causation, treatment, and prevention of psychiatric conditions?

In June 2022, the WHO published its largest review of mental health since the turn of the century: *World Mental Health Report: Transforming Mental Health for All* (World Health Organization, 2022b). The WHO notes that almost one billion people live with a mental disorder, and suicide still accounts for more than 1 in 100 deaths (World Health Organization, 2022c). Despite this, 71% of people with psychosis worldwide do not receive mental health care. Even in high-income countries, only one third of people with depression access formal treatment. This is not an inspiring picture.

To complicate matters, the failure to deliver care to a sufficient number of people is compounded by the failure of neuroscience to transform psychiatry the way it has transformed other areas of medicine over the past decades. Since the 1970s, it was hoped that brain imaging and psychiatric genetics would have a substantial impact on clinical psychiatry, but this has not happened for most mental illnesses. Despite billions of dollars of research, advances in treatment have been minor and incremental, rather than substantial and transformative (Kelly, 2022). The scientific literature increasingly recognises that the enormous data generated by sophisticated, costly neuroscience has failed to impact significantly on the treatment of common conditions such as schizophrenia and bipolar disorder. The journey from bench to bedside in psychiatry is very long indeed. This topic is further explored in Chapter 6 of this book ('Neuroscience and Psychiatry'), along with suggestions for change.

Notwithstanding this failure to deliver care in much of the world, and despite the extremely limited impact of neuroscience to date, treatments such as antidepressants, antipsychotics, and psychological therapies are effective for many mental illnesses. This too is explored later in this book, in Chapter 4 ('Treating Symptoms and Disorders'). In summary, there is much that we can do now, but there is even more that we should do in the future.

These facts place psychiatry in a unique and complicated position: necessary but poorly understood, effective but limited in practice, and demonstrating much progress in all three tasks (increasing understanding, delivering treatments, and studying mental illness), but not nearly enough advancement for anyone to be satisfied with the current state of affairs. We have further to travel on this road, but at least we are on the way.

These three tasks have faced psychiatry for many decades now, and most overall assessments (like this one) have been mixed, ranging from Clare's classic, critical *Psychiatry in Dissent: Controversial Issues in Thought and Practice* in the 1970s (Clare, 1976) to Tom Burns's more recent, essential contribution, *Our Necessary Shadow: The Nature and Meaning of Psychiatry* (Burns, 2013). Many of the key issues have remained the same over these decades, but some of the context has changed, including, but not limited to, increased globalisation, deeper recognition of the need to protect rights, incrementally improved treatments, certain (very limited) advances in understanding the genesis of specific conditions, and (arguably) the perceived impact of the Covid-19 pandemic on mental health.

What has not changed is the dominance of a 'crisis' narrative in mental health, and the tendency of media to focus on specific issues for short periods of time, rather than maintaining attention in order to stimulate considered debate, look deeply under the surface of psychiatric treatments or alternative suggestions, and identify balanced, sustainable solutions. This is not a flaw with either the media or psychiatry: it is simply a reflection of the nature of modern communication and the speed of contemporary news cycles.

Thankfully, not all media coverage takes a short-term 'crisis' position. Some is both critical and reflective. In the *Guardian* in 2023, an anonymous 'NHS [National Health Service] psychiatrist in a city in England' wrote that some 'young people' who 'need help' wait 'many months' before seeing someone:

Waiting times for care are what worries me the most because these young people need timely care so their condition doesn't get any worse. Mental healthcare for under-18s at the moment is clearly inadequate. As a country we are letting young people and their families down by having such inadequate mental health care. I'm not a parent. But if I had a child and were seeking mental health support for my son or daughter, I would be very worried.

(Campbell, 2023)

Media contributions such as this play a vital role in public education and increasing pressure for better services. But it is important to differentiate between different kinds of critical commentaries: those that identify problems with mental health service delivery, and those that outline problems with the content of services when they are delivered. Commentaries in the former category are extremely helpful provided they move beyond a simple 'crisis' narrative, interrogate services in detail, and suggest practical pathways to better care. These voices are vital.

Commentaries in the latter category are also essential, especially when they eschew ideological bias, focus on evidence, and ideally avoid extremely vague suggestions that are supported by substantially less evidence than the mainstream psychiatric interventions that they critique. Too often, such commentaries and books present no systematic evidence whatsoever, preferring to rely on highly selected accounts (with no effort at representativeness), arbitrary assortments of 'experts' (selected for no apparent reason), or narratives that recount the author 'discovering' facts that are already firmly established in the psychiatric literature for decades, such as the social correlates of depression, the importance of economics and politics in shaping suffering (and our responses to it), and the imperfections of current treatments. All of this is already known: psychiatry is far from perfect, but its task is important, and its systematic evidence base is open to the public to interrogate. (For further discussion of some of these arguments, see: Kelly, 2022.)

The fact is that, given the sheer scale of suffering involved in mental illness and the numbers affected, effective interventions are always needed, and nobody has come up with a system that is even faintly as evidence-based as psychiatry is. In other words, we have psychiatry in the absence of anything superior; psychiatry is much better at treating mental illness than it is given credit for, and psychiatry will seamlessly absorb any 'non-psychiatric' interventions *that are supported by systematic evidence*. Some of these issues are further explored later in this book, with particular reference to psychiatric medications (Chapter 4: 'Treating Symptoms and Disorders').

All told, psychiatry is moderately effective overall, and sometimes very effective. One of the growing risks in this field, however, is that focus will shift away from supporting and treating patients and their families, and towards addressing the perceived 'crisis' as primarily a social or economic problem. In the US, the President's Council of Economic Advisors was clear in 2022 that 'improving people's mental health' is vital for 'increasing the productive capacity of the economy':

> The mental health crisis facing Americans imposes significant costs to the well-being of affected individuals, their loved ones, and society as a whole. This crisis took hold long before the onset of the COVID 19 pandemic, but its effects were amplified as the pandemic resulted in the loss of lives and livelihoods and unprecedented social isolation. Increasing the productive capacity of the economy going forward requires improving people's mental health, which can be done by improving the affordability of mental health treatment, expanding the behavioral health workforce, and removing barriers to seeking care.
>
> (Council of Economic Advisors, 2022)

Yes, 'increasing the productive capacity of the economy going forward requires improving people's mental health', but improving mental health is a goal in itself – the economic benefits are substantial but secondary. People matter most. And that is why psychiatry exists.

Pablo, the man with counting obsessions and compulsions whom we met at the start of this chapter, did some Internet searches and began to wonder if he was mentally ill. Filled with trepidation,he read about 'mental disorders', 'psychiatrists', and 'obsessive compulsive disorder' (OCD). He recognised descriptions of repetitive behaviours, intrusive thoughts, a preoccupation with counting, and general anxiety. Based on what he found, Pablo spoke with his father, who agreed that Pablo should reach out for help. Pablo went to see his primary care physician (family doctor or general practitioner) who listened carefully and felt that Pablo had many of the features of OCD. 'If this is becoming a problem in your life', he said, 'I suggest you see a clinical psychologist' (i.e., a non-medical mental health professional who is qualified in psychology).

Pablo attended a clinical psychologist who provided cognitive behaviour therapy, a type of talking therapy that helped Pablo considerably. Pablo managed to identify his obsessional thoughts and behaviours, devise alternative coping strategies, and reduce his distress considerably. He made real progress over subsequent months, but his counting habit remained, albeit at a lower level. Pablo returned to his primary care physician to see if anything further could be done, so the physician arranged for Pablo to see a psychiatrist (i.e., a medical doctor who specialises in the treatment of mental illness).

Pablo read online that antidepressant medication can sometimes help in OCD. The psychiatrist agreed that antidepressants can be useful for some people but felt that Pablo should give the psychological therapy some more time. Three months later, they discussed the matter again, at which point Pablo still felt that more could be done. He remained quite distressed by his symptoms. The psychiatrist prescribed an antidepressant which provided additional benefit that enabled Pablo to use his psychological strategies to a greater extent. He began to feel much better. Or, as Pablo put it: 'I'm back'.

After nine months, Pablo and his psychiatrist agreed that the antidepressant could be carefully stopped, provided Pablo continued to apply the lessons from cognitive behaviour therapy. Pablo still had appointments with the clinical psychologist to help sustain progress. Happily, Pablo's symptoms remained very diminished after stopping the medication, although, as Pablo said: 'I still count things sometimes. I guess that's just me'.

Key Messages

- Psychiatry is the branch of medicine that is primarily concerned with the study and treatment of disorders of mental function or, to use more current terminology, 'mental disorder' or 'mental illness'.
- A 'mental illness' is a syndrome that is characterised by a clinically significant disturbance of thinking, emotional regulation, or behaviour, which reflects an underlying dysfunction in psychological, biological, or developmental processes relevant to mental and behavioural function. This slightly awkward, somewhat circular definition is the current one; it might change.
- Mental illness is common: 1 person in every 8, a total of 970 million people, lives with a mental disorder, although most do not have access to effective care, according to the World Health Organization. Anxiety and depressive disorders are the most common conditions.
- Mental illness is costly: in addition to the profound human costs, social exclusion, and missed life opportunities, the economic burden is estimated at approximately US $5 trillion annually.
- The key tasks of psychiatry are to (a) increase awareness of the symptoms of mental illness (in order to reassure most people that they are not mentally ill and to facilitate early assessment for those who might be); (b) provide treatment and support to people with mental illness and their families (including biological, psychological, and social approaches), and (c) study mental illnesses so as to better understand causation, treatment, and prevention, and to better protect human rights.
- Psychiatry is in a unique and complicated position: necessary but poorly understood, effective but limited in practice, and demonstrating much progress in all three key tasks (increasing understanding, delivering treatments, and studying mental illness), but not nearly enough advancement for anyone to be satisfied with the current state of affairs. We have further to travel on this road, but we are on the way.

Note

1 A 'psychotic disorder' is a condition involving 'psychosis', which is a state of mind in which the person loses contact with reality in at least one important respect for a period of time (e.g., has paranoid delusions or hallucinations), while they are not intoxicated with alcohol or drugs, and while they are not affected by an acute physical illness that better explains their symptoms (e.g., having a fever or high temperature). Psychosis can be associated with schizophrenia, severe depression, mania, certain other conditions, and, more rarely, the period following childbirth (i.e., postpartum).

References

American Psychiatric Association. *Diagnostic and Statistical Manual of Mental Disorders* (Fifth Edn, Text Revision). Washington, DC: American Psychiatric Association Publishing, 2022.

Arias D, Saxena S, Verguet S. Quantifying the global burden of mental disorders and their economic value. *eClinicalMedicine* 2022; 54: 101675 (https://doi.org/10.1016/j .eclinm.2022.101675).

Bloom DE, Cafiero ET, Jané-Llopis E, Abrahams-Gessel S, Bloom LR, Fathima S, Feigl AB, Gaziano T, Mowafi M, Pandya A, Prettner K, Rosenberg L, Seligman B, Stein AZ, Weinstein C. *The Global Economic Burden of Noncommunicable Diseases*. Geneva: World Economic Forum, 2011 (http://www3.weforum.org/docs/WEF_Harvard_HE _GlobalEconomicBurdenNonCommunicableDiseases_2011.pdf) (accessed 4 May 2023).

Burns T. *Our Necessary Shadow: The Nature and Meaning of Psychiatry*. London: Allen Lane, 2013.

Campbell D. 'We are letting young people down': the secret psychiatrist on NHS mental health delays. *Guardian*, 9 February 2023 (https://www.theguardian.com/society /2023/feb/09/waiting-is-damaging-how-nhs-england-fails-young-mental-health -patients) (accessed 5 May 2023) (Courtesy of *Guardian* News & Media Ltd.).

Clare AW. *Psychiatry in Dissent: Controversial Issues in Thought and Practice*. London: Tavistock Publications Limited, 1976.

Clare AW. Psychological medicine. In: Kumar PJ, Clark ML (eds), *Clinical Medicine: A Textbook for Medical Students and Doctors* (pp. 868–900). London: Ballière Tindall, 1987.

Council of Economic Advisors. *Reducing the Economic Burden of Unmet Mental Health Needs*. Washington, DC: The White House, 2022 (https://www.whitehouse.gov/ cea/written-materials/2022/05/31/reducing-the-economic-burden-of-unmet-mental -health-needs/). (Link to licence: https://creativecommons.org/licenses/by/3.0/us/) (accessed 1 May 2023).

Godin SL, Shehata S. Adolescent cannabis use and later development of schizophrenia: an updated systematic review of longitudinal studies. *Journal of Clinical Psychology* 2022; 78: 1331–40 (https://doi.org/10.1002/jclp.23312).

Insel TR, Collins PY, Hyman SE. Darkness invisible: the hidden global costs of mental illness. *Foreign Affairs* 2015; 94: 127–35 (https://www.foreignaffairs.com/articles/ africa/darkness-invisible; https://www.jstor.org/stable/24483225).

Kelly BD. *In Search of Madness: A Psychiatrist's Travels Through the History of Mental Illness*. Dublin: Gill Books, 2022.

Kelly BD. *Psychiatry in Dissent*: Anthony Clare's critique, defence and reinvigoration of psychiatry. *BJPsych Advances* 2023; 29: 426–7 (https://doi.org/10.1192/bja.2023.29). (Link to licence: https://creativecommons.org/licenses/by/4.0/) (accessed 26 January 2024).

Kelly BD, Houston M. *Psychiatrist in the Chair: The Official Biography of Anthony Clare*. Newbridge, County Kildare: Merrion Press, 2020.

Kessler RC, Aguilar-Gaxiola S, Alonso J, Angermeyer MC, Anthony JC, Brugha TS, Chatterji S, de Girolamo G, Demyttenaere K, Gluzman SF, Gureje O, Haro JM, Heeringa SG, Hwang I, Karam EG, Kikkawa T, Lee S, Lépine J-P, Medina-Mora ME, Merikangas KR, Ormel J, Pennell B-E, Posada-Villa J, Üstün TB, Von Korff MR, Wang PS, Zaslavsky AM, Zhang M. Prevalence and severity of mental disorders in the World Mental Health Survey Initiative. In: Kessler RC, Üstün TB (eds), *The WHO World Mental Health Surveys: Global Perspectives on the Epidemiology of Mental Disorders* (pp. 534–40). Cambridge: Cambridge University Press, 2008.

Lancet Global Health. Mental health matters. *Lancet Global Health* 2020; 8: e1352 (https://doi.org/10.1016/S2214-109X(20)30432-0).

National Academies of Sciences, Engineering, and Medicine. *The Health Effects of Cannabis and Cannabinoids. The Current State of Evidence and Recommendations for Research.* Washington, DC: The National Academies Press, 2017 (https://www.nap.edu/catalog/24625/the-health-effects-of-cannabis-and-cannabinoids-the-current-state) (Accessed 5 May 2023).

National Institute of Mental Health. *Mental Illness.* Bethesda, MD: National Institute of Mental Health, 2023 (https://www.nimh.nih.gov/health/statistics/mental-illness#part_2538) (accessed 30 April 2023).

Shackle S. 'The way universities are run is making us ill': inside the student mental health crisis. *Guardian*, 27 September 2019 (https://www.theguardian.com/society/2019/sep/27/anxiety-mental-breakdowns-depression-uk-students) (accessed 5 May 2023) (Courtesy of *Guardian* News & Media Ltd.).

Spiers N, Qassem T, Bebbington P, McManus S, King M, Jenkins R, Meltzer H, Brugha TS. Prevalence and treatment of common mental disorders in the English national population, 1993–2007. *British Journal of Psychiatry* 2016; 209: 150–6 (https://doi.org/10.1192/bjp.bp.115.174979).

Vaucher J, Keating BJ, Lasserre AM, Gan W, Lyall DM, Ward J, Smith DJ, Pell JP, Sattar N, Paré G, Holmes MV. Cannabis use and risk of schizophrenia: a Mendelian randomization study. *Molecular Psychiatry* 2018; 23: 1287–92 (https://doi.org/10.1038/mp.2016.252).

Whiteford H, Buckingham B, Harris M, Diminic S, Stockings E, Degenhardt L. Estimating the number of adults with severe and persistent mental illness who have complex, multi-agency needs. *Australian and New Zealand Journal of Psychiatry* 2017; 51: 799–809 (https://doi.org/10.1177/0004867416683814).

World Health Organization. *ICD-11: International Classification of Diseases (Eleventh Revision)*. Geneva: World Health Organization, 2019 (https://icd.who.int/en) (accessed 6 May 2023).

World Health Organization. *Mental Disorders.* Geneva: World Health Organization, 2022a (https://www.who.int/news-room/fact-sheets/detail/mental-disorders) (accessed 30 April 2023).

World Health Organization. *World Mental Health Report: Transforming Mental Health for All.* Geneva: World Health Organization, 2022b (https://www.who.int/publications /i/item/9789240049338) (accessed 6 May 2023).

World Health Organization. *WHO Highlights Urgent Need to Transform Mental Health and Mental Health Care.* Geneva: World Health Organization, 2022c (https://www .who.int/news/item/17-06-2022-who-highlights-urgent-need-to-transform-mental -health-and-mental-health-care) (accessed 6 May 2023).

Yan Y, Hou J, Li Q, Yu NX. Suicide before and during the COVID-19 pandemic: a systematic review with meta-analysis. *International Journal of Environmental Research and Public Health* 2023; 20: 3346 (https://doi.org/10.3390/ijerph20043346).

2 The History of Psychiatry

Ellen was a 28-year-old woman committed to the Richmond District Lunatic Asylum in Dublin, Ireland in mid-1908. The Richmond was a large, public asylum for the mentally ill that opened almost a century earlier, in 1814. By the start of the twentieth century, when Ellen was admitted, the institution had expanded considerably but was still grossly overcrowded, housing some 1,600 patients in premises designed for far fewer.

This was not Ellen's first admission. Ellen had been committed to the asylum three years earlier when, according to medical notes, she had 'given birth to a child' and on the 'following evening was very violent and difficult'. Ellen spent several months in the Richmond on that occasion before her family 'removed her from [the] asylum against the wishes of the Medical Superintendent'. Ellen 'was very poorly for [the] first five or six months' after leaving, but 'eventually she improved'.

Three years later, in 1908, Ellen was re-admitted to the Richmond with 'auditory hallucinations' (hearing voices that were not there) and refusing to eat. The medical file summarises her presentation:

> *She has been in a dull state since her removal from here, but did her household work. When her husband came into the room, she would always walk out of it. Depressed for past fortnight. Refused food for few days [...] Says she is brought back for not taking her food. Didn't consider it right to take it. Thought she was offending God by taking it. Heard the voice of God and of the Blessed Virgin.*

One week after admission, Ellen was 'in a state of confusion', according to medical notes:

> *Quietly depressed and confused. Up and dressed but sits with her head down and looks miserable. Says she did not eat on account of God being displeased with her. Did not sleep with her husband 'because she was not married to him'. Asked what made her think that, says, 'I was <u>dead</u>'. Does not now think she is dead and admits that she is married 'or supposes so'.*

DOI: 10.4324/9781003378495-3

Two weeks after admission, Ellen had 'various ideas about her soul' and 'thinks she has not repented properly'. One month after admission, she was 'dull and tearful and depressed':

> *Says she is not properly married and that she __died__ since she was married and came to life again and will not live with her husband now as it is wrong. Sits all day with head bent. Does no work.*

Patients often worked in the asylum. Cleaning, knitting, and needlework were common among female patients, although Ellen did not participate initially. Taking part in 'work' was considered both a form of treatment and a sign of improvement.

Two months after admission, Ellen believed 'it would be a sin to live with her husband now, but is anxious to go out and live with his mother'. Three months after admission, she was 'apathetic but I think a trifle brighter than she was'. One year after admission, Ellen was still in the asylum, and when 'pressed, admits hearing holy voices which sometimes tell her not to take her food'. After two years, Ellen was described as 'dull, stupid, uncommunicative. Speaks in a whisper. Hears holy voices'.

Four years after admission, medical notes describe Ellen as 'most restive and troublesome [...] will not speak [...] constantly attempting to get through windows [...] sleeps badly'. Soon, Ellen was 'the most restive patient in the house. Often has to be carried to bed'. This situation persisted and, in her sixth year in the institution, Ellen was still 'very restive', according to medical notes.

> *Has to be led by force in and out of dining hall. Violent. Attempts to kick anyone near her. Uncommunicative. Semi-stuperose condition. Appetite voracious. Sleeps badly.*

Ellen's condition continued to deteriorate, and she died in the asylum the following year. Ellen's cause of death is recorded as 'phthisis' or tuberculosis, which was common in the unhygienic, overcrowded institutions of the early twentieth century. Ellen had spent the last seven years of her life in the Richmond Asylum in a distressed, disturbed, deteriorating state, eventually dying there at the age of 35 years.

Introduction

Ellen's story reflects the state of institutional care for mental illness in Ireland at the start of the twentieth century, which was a time of enormous psychiatric institutions in many parts of the world. How did matters reach a point at which large numbers of people with mental illness were forcibly confined in gargantuan institutions such as Richmond District Lunatic Asylum in Dublin? Over time, how did the focus shift from care and cure of mental illness to custody and control of the mentally ill? And how has the situation changed since then?

This chapter starts by exploring early accounts of apparent mental illness from religious texts and ancient literature, followed by a summary of the history of psychiatry as a medical discipline, with consideration of diverse treatments in the past, including experimental surgical bacteriology, malaria therapy, insulin treatment, convulsive therapies, and lobotomy, which was the single greatest mistake in the history of psychiatry. This chapter also looks at historical critics of psychiatry in the 1960s, along with the work of psychiatrist Anthony Clare in the 1970s, placing these diverse perspectives in the context of contemporary models of mental health care.

Case histories from the Richmond District Lunatic Asylum (later 'Grangegorman Mental Hospital') in the early twentieth century are interspersed throughout the chapter to illustrate relevant points and give voice to the forgotten asylum patients of the past. Not everyone had the same experience as Ellen, whom we met at the start of this chapter, although familiar patterns emerge across many patient stories in Ireland and elsewhere. Like all institutions, the Richmond in Dublin was a complex place with many different tales to tell (Reynolds, 1992). The case of Richard is a good example of another experience of psychiatric institutionalisation that was briefer than Ellen's, less negative, and possibly even helpful, at least to a degree.

Richard was a 35-year-old plumber who was admitted to the Richmond as a 'dangerous lunatic' in mid-1907 after being 'about three weeks violent' and threatening his father (Kelly, 2023a). Richard was 'addicted' to alcohol. He had two previous head injuries while drunk and had been discharged from the Richmond just three months earlier.

On this occasion, Richard's father told asylum staff that Richard's 'mother, soon after marriage, became very much given to drink. All of their family were so and died from its effects. I did not know this in time'. Richard's father described Richard as 'always peculiar':

> We have often seen him wash his hands ten times in half a hour, dry each time, then wash water tap and pipe down to trap. He has treated me as his greatest enemy, smashed windows, delph and glass jugs, and other missiles he has repeatedly thrown at me. I have three pocket-knives we wrenched from him in these fits of dangerous conduct, with detestable language. An hour after, he is lying on his bed in fits of grimacing or laughing.

On admission to the Richmond, Richard's liver was 'enlarged', owing to alcohol misuse. He told the doctor that 'he had a row with his brother and father over some work they were all engaged in':

> They had a fight which he 'got the worst of' and then because he was in the 'Richmond' before, they got him in easily. He is a very plausible person and answers all my questions intelligently. His memory is good. He admits he has

been drinking since his discharge three months ago. He always had quarrels with his family when he was drunk.

One week after admission, Richard was described as 'somewhat dull. Complains about family quarrels. They are all against him and want to get rid of him'. After two weeks, however, Richard was 'very bright' and said 'that his drinking has been the whole cause of it'. After three months in the Richmond, Richard was 'quite rational and tranquil'. He was 'discharged, recovered'.

Early Accounts of Mental Illness

Mental illness, often termed 'madness', appears in some form in every cultural and religious tradition in history, along with descriptions of symptoms, signs, and emotions that are often consistent with what are now regarded as 'mental disorders' but were interpreted or patterned differently at the time (Kelly, 2016a).

In the Bible, the Book of Deuteronomy specifies 'madness' and 'confusion of mind' among the punishments threatened 'if you do not obey the Lord your God and do not carefully follow all his commands and decrees':

> The Lord will send on you curses, confusion and rebuke in everything you put your hand to, until you are destroyed and come to sudden ruin because of the evil you have done in forsaking him. The Lord will plague you with diseases until he has destroyed you from the land you are entering to possess. The Lord will strike you with wasting disease, with fever and inflammation, with scorching heat and drought, with blight and mildew, which will plague you until you perish [...] The Lord will afflict you with the boils of Egypt and with tumours, festering sores and the itch, from which you cannot be cured. The Lord will afflict you with madness, blindness and confusion of mind.
>
> (Deuteronomy 28: 15, 20-22; 27, 28)

In the Book of Kings, the prophet Elijah experiences suicidal despair in response to difficult events:

> Now Ahab told Jezebel everything Elijah had done and how he had killed all the prophets with the sword. So Jezebel sent a messenger to Elijah to say, 'May the gods deal with me, be it ever so severely, if by this time tomorrow I do not make your life like that of one of them'. Elijah was afraid and ran for his life. When he came to Beersheba in Judah, he left his servant there, while he himself went a day's journey into the wilderness. He came to a broom bush, sat down under it and prayed that he might die. 'I have had enough, Lord,' he said. 'Take my life; I am no better than my ancestors'.
>
> (1 Kings 19)

In the Book of Psalms, King David describes despondency, despair, and hopelessness:

> I am worn out from my groaning.
> All night long I flood my bed with weeping
> and drench my couch with tears.
> My eyes grow weak with sorrow;
> they fail because of all my foes.
>
> (Psalm 6: 6–7)

Texts from other religious traditions provide similar descriptions of mental distress, as well as words about healing. The Quran, for example, the central religious text of Islam, refers to the resolution of grief:

> They will say, 'All praise belongs to Allah, who has removed all grief from us. Indeed Our Lord is all-forgiving, all-appreciative, who has settled us in the everlasting abode by His grace. In it we are untouched by toil, and untouched therein by fatigue'.
>
> (Chapter 35: 34–5)

The Quran also explores the idea that people with apparent 'madness' might be tellers of difficult truths:

> Is it that they do not recognize their apostle, and so they deny him? Do they say, 'There is madness in him'? Rather he has brought them the truth, and most of them are averse to the truth.
>
> (Chapter 23: 69–70)

The idea of 'divine madness' is common across many traditions, including Christianity, in which saints experienced visions and other unusual experiences that might today be seen as symptoms of mental illness. Similarly in Hindu tradition, various gods and saints are often described or portrayed as if 'mad' (Kinsley, 1974).

These portrayals are not confined to early religious texts. Apparent mental illness also features in the *Iliad* and *Odyssey*, the oldest surviving works of Western literature (Scull, 2015). In the *Iliad*, Homer describes Greek warrior Achilles as 'mad':

> So, then, you would all be on the side of mad Achilles, who knows neither right nor ruth? He is like some savage lion that in the pride of his great strength and daring springs upon men's flocks and gorges on them. Even so has Achilles flung aside all pity, and all that conscience which at once so greatly banes yet greatly boons him that will heed it. A man may lose one

far dearer than Achilles has lost - a son, it may be, or a brother born from his own mother's womb; yet when he has mourned him and wept over him he will let him bide, for it takes much sorrow to kill a man; whereas Achilles, now that he has slain noble Hector, drags him behind his chariot round the tomb of his comrade. It were better of him, and for him, that he should not do so, for brave though he be, we gods may take it ill that he should vent his fury upon dead clay.

(Book XXIV)

In the *Odyssey*, Homer links alcohol with becoming 'mad':

It was wine that inflamed the Centaur Eurytion when he was staying with Peirithous among the Lapithae. When the wine had got into his head, he went mad and did ill deeds about the house of Peirithous; this angered the heroes who were there assembled, so they rushed at him and cut off his ears and nostrils; then they dragged him through the doorway out of the house, so he went away crazed, and bore the burden of his crime, bereft of understanding.

(Book XXI)

Herodotus, a Greek historian and geographer in the fifth century BC, linked disrespect for custom with being 'mad', in the *History of Herodotus*:

It is clear to me therefore by every kind of proof that Cambyses was mad exceedingly; for otherwise he would not have attempted to deride religious rites and customary observances. For if one should propose to all men a choice, bidding them select the best customs from all the customs that there are, each race of men, after examining them all, would select those of his own people; thus all think that their own customs are by far the best: and so it is not likely that any but a madman would make a jest of such things.

(Book 3: 38)

The terminology used in these texts has been replaced by different language today, but some of the underpinning issues are remarkably constant, especially interpreting unusual experiences or behaviours as being, variously, religious manifestations, social disobedience, criminal acts, or evidence of 'madness' or 'mental disorder'. As we will see throughout this book, these issues remain pertinent and often unresolved today, but have a history as long as humanity itself.

The History of Psychiatry as a Medical Discipline

The emergence of psychiatry as a medical discipline was a gradual process. Texts written in the tradition of Hippocrates (c.460–c.370 BCE), a Greek physician, accorded the brain a central role in generating emotions, knowledge, and perceptions:

> Men ought to know that from nothing else but thence [the brain] come joys, despondency and lamentations. And by this, in an especial manner, we acquire wisdom, and knowledge, and see and hear, and know what are foul and what are fair, what are bad and what are good, what are sweet, and what unsavoury; some we discriminate by habit, and some we perceive by their utility. By this we distinguish objects of relish and disrelish, according to the seasons; and the same things do not always please us.

In addition, the brain was responsible for 'madness':

> And by the same organ we become mad and delirious, and fears and terrors assail us, some by night and some by day; and dreams and untimely wanderings, and cares that are not suitable, and ignorance of present circumstances, desuetude and unskilfulness. All these things we endure from the brain when it is not healthy, but is more hot, more cold, more moist, or more dry, than natural, or when it suffers any other preternatural and unusual affection.
>
> And we become mad from humidity [of the brain]. For when it is more moist than natural, it is necessarily put into motion, and the affected part being moved, neither the sight nor hearing can be at rest, and the tongue speaks in accordance with the sight and hearing.

For Hippocrates, the secret lay in maintaining a balance between 'rest' and activity of the brain, as well as an overall balance of the four 'humours': black bile, yellow bile, phlegm, and blood. Balance produced health, including mental health.

With 'madness' increasingly located in the body rather than the heavens or the spiritual sphere, various societies began to medicalise 'madness'. In China, demonic possession and disturbances to cosmic forces were commonly invoked to explain 'madness' but were increasingly joined by physical considerations such as cold, damp, and wind (Kelly, 2022). In Islamic tradition, folkloric tales and supernatural therapies persisted in popular culture, but the Islamic hospitals in the eighth century also made specific 'medical' provision for the 'insane'. The first psychiatric hospital was reputedly built in Baghdad in 705. Treatments included baths, music, and occupational therapy, often alongside bloodletting, vomiting, purging, opium, and herbs (to expel noxious 'humours'), as well as physical restraint and beating, seeking to quell furious 'insanity'.

By the start of the nineteenth century, the management of mental illness was still conducted, for the most part, outside of dedicated institutions. Some people with mental illness were in prisons or confined in private dwellings, but many were homeless, destitute, and in states of poor physical and mental health. As psychiatric institutions emerged in the nineteenth century, some countries developed models of state medicine which were controlled centrally (e.g., France) while decentralised models evolved elsewhere (e.g., Germany, Great Britain) (Shorter, 1997). For many, however, the impulse was the same: to care for, and ideally cure, the 'insane' in large institutions designed and operated for this purpose. This was underlined by the idea that mental illness was on the increase, apparently presenting a new and urgent crisis to society.

Many early asylums were based on the idea of 'moral management' which meant treating each patient as an individual and using reason, discussion, occupation, and exercise as active therapies, rather than mere restraint. This idea was highly progressive, but the unstoppable growth of the new institutions soon shifted focus from the treatment of individuals to the management of the institutions themselves. Quickly, the act of admission became the solution, and everything else was secondary.

An emergent class of asylum doctors were aware of both the risks and potential benefits of institutional care. One English doctor, John Conolly, wrote at length about this in his 1830 book *An Inquiry Concerning the Indications of Insanity with Suggestions for the Better Protection and Care of the Insane* (Conolly, 1830). Conolly drew particular attention to the cruelty of certain institutional regimes:

> When an unruly patient enters a common lunatic house, he is bled, dressed in a strait waistcoat, has his head shaved, is subjected to the shower bath, put upon low diet, kept in darkness, and compelled to swallow some active purgative medicine. If measures of this kind, which may be well enough suited to active delirium, do not effect any amendment, the medical resources of the establishment are at an end. Starvation, imprisonment, loneliness, and threats are then resorted to; or if the proprietor of the house happens to be very alert, some desperate, or some unjustifiable experiment is tried; whirling round upon an horizontal wheel, intoxication, or some strange method of astonishing the patient; such as leading him blindfold and headlong into a cold bath. At last peace is effected. The patient is exhausted; or his excitement is succeeded by what is called the low state; or he has learned cunning, and moderates his actions.
>
> (Conolly, 1830; pp. 15–16)

For some patients, he said, improvement followed these alarming and deeply inhumane measures:

> In a few cases, the disease is soon at an end, and it is possible the amendment may be perceived, and the patient restored to his family: *possible*, but not as a general fact, *probable*; for the patient is seldom seen by those who are judges of his amendment: a few minutes every two or three days seeming to be the

maximum of medical attendance in the best circumstances; and many weeks, or months, passing over in other cases, without the patient being seen by any medical man [sic] at all.

(p. 16)

Conolly warned, however, that 'too often, the low state, considered but a continuance of the malady in another form, is succeeded by another paroxysm of excitement, and the rest of a miserable life is passed in hopeless alternations between the two' (p. 16).

Conolly was 'well acquainted with the guardians of several lunatic houses, who are men [sic] of intelligence and of great humanity, but it is impossible for them, under the present system, to prevent many of these evils from being incurred in their own establishments' (p. 31). To remedy these problems, Conolly did not propose the abolition of institutions, but government control and changes to how they operated:

- 'Medical men [sic], by enjoying better opportunities of acquiring practical knowledge in cases of insanity, should be assisted in devising improved methods of treatment'.
- 'All persons of unsound mind should become the care of the State; and should continue so until recovery'.
- 'Every Lunatic Asylum should be the property of the State, and be controlled by public officers'.
- 'Every Lunatic Asylum should be a School of Instruction for Medical Students, and a place of education for male and female keepers'.
- 'No patient should be confined in a Lunatic Asylum, except on the particular representation of the relatives or friends, that he [sic] could not have proper care and attention out of it'.
- 'There should be attached to every Asylum a certain number of medical officers and keepers [...] ready, at all times, to attend to insane patients at their own houses' (p. 481).

The core belief in public institutions was deeply ingrained in the asylum doctors of the times, even as they exposed the misuse of existing establishments and highlighted the desperate plight of many patients within them.

Asylums, Infections, and Diagnoses

By the early twentieth century, this belief in asylum care was accompanied by increased awareness that the institutions were overcrowded and extremely unhygienic. Infectious diseases were a particular problem, especially tuberculosis (Kelly, 2016a). The case of Ellen at the start of this chapter is a good example of someone who was admitted to a large public asylum for several years, before dying there of tuberculosis at the age of 35 years.

Similarly, Mary, a 30-year-old woman, was admitted to the Richmond as a 'dangerous lunatic' in 1907. Mary was 'violent at times', having 'assaulted her sister and uncle'. Admission notes record that this 'patient is a case of congenital mental deficiency' [likely intellectual disability], adding that her 'mother got a fright in the early months of the pregnancy'. Mary 'took "weaknesses" from 12-years old'. It was not possible to examine Mary on admission:

Patient was very excited and jumping about in the bed to such an extent that I was not able to examine her heart and lungs. As far as I could make out, she had no ribs broken. Patient appears to be tongue tied [...] When asked her name, she made no reply and in fact never spoke a word the whole time I was examining her.

In the asylum, Mary was 'very restless and troublesome', suffered from regular epileptic seizures, and was frequently incontinent. Over the following months, she remained 'speechless, but doesn't seem to be deaf'. Mary continued in this state for more than two years, after which she died of 'broncho-pneumonia', a lung infection that was common in the crowded asylums of the nineteenth and early twentieth centuries.

While patients like Ellen and Mary were admitted to and died in psychiatric institutions, other patients came and went, often for social reasons or problems with addiction, rather than mental illness. Patrick, for example, was a 45-year-old butcher admitted to the Richmond in early 1908 because he 'did threaten to kill' his wife. Patrick had a history of 'intemperance' (misuse of alcohol) and *delirium tremens* (acute withdrawal from alcohol). He had 'lately complained very much of his head and nerves'. Admission notes record that Patrick's 'youngest sister and brother died of consumption' (tuberculosis) and his aunt was 'in the Richmond Asylum some years ago'.

Patrick had 'very romantic, flighty ideas from boyhood, but later years morose'. Now, he was 'appearing naked before his children and very lustful in his habits'. On admission, the doctor described Patrick as 'a rather frail man' with 'the appearance of an alcoholic':

He is very plausible answering all my questions with great tact. He denies assaulting his wife and states it is a trumped up charge because he would not bring her in money. He states he had a lot of drink taken and was looking for work but could find none.

After two weeks in the Richmond, Patrick had 'improved':

Admits drinking but so did his wife. She drank more than he did. She would be drunk every second night and retch all over the place. 'I would have to wipe it up myself'. He does not believe she has been unfaithful to him.

One month after admission, Patrick told the doctor that 'there was nothing wrong with me only that I took drink on an empty stomach. I broke about ten shillings worth of furniture and then the wife got me charged'. After seven weeks in the asylum, Patrick was 'discharged, recovered'.

As this case demonstrates, the boundaries between mental wellness, mental illness, addiction, and social problems were not clearly defined and were, perhaps, indefinable in certain cases. Nevertheless, one of the great historic shifts in diagnostic practices occurred at around the time that Ellen, Mary, and Patrick were in the Richmond, and centred on the work of Emil Kraepelin (1856–1926), an asylum doctor in Germany (Anonymous, 1968). Kraepelin is often regarded as the founder of modern psychiatry and arguably did more than anyone else to delineate the diagnosis of manic depression or bipolar affective disorder (as it is now known) (Kelly 2022).

Kraepelin studied thousands of cases of severe mental illness in an effort to identify different 'psychotic' disorders based on symptoms (Shepherd, 1995). In 1899, he proposed two key patterns: in one, 'manic depression', patients had an intermittent disorder and were reasonably symptom-free between episodes, while in the other, 'dementia praecox' (later schizophrenia), there were fewer intervals between episodes and the condition often ran a more deteriorating course (Kraepelin, 1899). Kraepelin acknowledged considerable overlap between the symptoms of both disorders, but still felt that the distinction was merited, especially in terms of outcomes.

In 1904, Kraepelin emphasised that the episodic course of 'maniacal-depressive insanity' best characterised the condition, noting that 'this disease generally runs its course in *a series* of *isolated attacks,* which are not uniform, but present either states of depression […] or characteristic states of excitement […] The isolated attacks are generally separated by longer or shorter intervals of freedom' (Kraepelin, 1904; p. 13). This, he argued, distinguished it from schizophrenia.

Over the course of his career, Kraepelin practised, researched, and wrote extensively on this and other themes (e.g., Kraepelin, 1921). Like many of his contemporaries, Kraepelin also, regrettably, supported the eugenics movement that featured in psychiatric circles (and beyond) around this time. While Kraepelin's diagnostic ideas were not uniformly accepted during his lifetime (Drapes, 1909), and while Kraepelin later felt that his efforts had not been a success, he remained of the view that different disease entities existed (Shepherd, 1995). Today, Kraepelin's work still resonates in psychiatry, which generally recognises bipolar disorder and schizophrenia as different entities, albeit with certain overlaps in terms of possible causes, common symptoms, and treatments. Kraepelin's distinction between the two conditions was not fully right, but neither was it fully wrong.

Experimental Surgical Bacteriology and Malaria Therapy

At the time when Kraepelin was performing his research, around the end of the nineteenth century and the start of the twentieth, the asylums continued to expand in many countries, apparently unstoppably. This was partly owing to the persisting belief that admission was a treatment in itself, even when admission appeared to be related to social problems rather than an identifiable illness or medical condition. This was as true in Ireland as it was elsewhere.

Brendan, for example, was a 23-year-old, single waiter admitted to the Richmond District Lunatic Asylum in Dublin in early 1908. Brendan had attempted 'to commit suicide', according to medical notes. Brendan had been unemployed for six months:

> His sister turned him out of her house and would not keep him any longer. 'I thought then that everyone and everything was going against me and that cutting my throat was the only thing'. He was sorry for it afterwards and does not believe he would do it again. He has several small scratches on the front of his throat, none of them of any importance. His health seems good.

Brendan 'slept well and took food' in the Richmond. After a week, he was 'much less depressed. Would not attempt suicide again'. After a month, Brendan was 'cheerful and intelligent and very quiet in manner. Quite lucid'. He was 'discharged, recovered' after six weeks in the Richmond.

In this case, Brendan's treatment was admission to the institution, food, sleep, and letting a certain amount of time pass, before discharging him back to (presumably) precisely the same situation from which he had been admitted. The core belief here was in the value of *the institution* as a response to mental or social distress. While this appears relatively benign in Brendan's case, it had the overall effect of overcrowding the mental hospitals in many countries. As a result, conditions were often poor: large numbers of patients slept and ate together, infectious diseases swept through the buildings, and rigid institutional practices replaced the idealistic 'moral management' idea which had inspired the original institutions.

Dismayed at the size of the mental hospitals and problems with discharging patients, asylum doctors turned to a series of novel treatments that reflected both therapeutic optimism and a desperate need to discharge people. One of the most disturbing examples of this trend was 'experimental surgical bacteriology', pioneered by American psychiatrist Henry Andrews Cotton (1876–1933). Cotton served as medical director of New Jersey State Hospital in Trenton from 1907 to 1930. Cotton developed the view that mental illness resulted from untreated infections in the body, so he and his staff removed some or all of their patients' teeth, tonsils, spleens, colons, ovaries, or other organs (Scull, 2005). Despite Cotton's resultant popularity and his claim of an 85 per cent success rate, an investigation was ordered by the New Jersey State Senate in 1925 (Kelly, 2022). A horrific picture emerged: up to 45 per cent of patients had died, many more were disabled, and the surgeries were eventually stopped.

The story of 'experimental surgical bacteriology' is a terrifying tale of therapeutic zeal that went too far, even in a doctor who was otherwise humane: Cotton made countless positive changes at Trenton, including removing mechanical restraints, establishing a nursing school, introducing occupational therapy, hiring social workers, and installing fire alarms (Wessely, 2009). Even so, Cotton's therapeutic enthusiasm went unchecked for too long, with devastating consequences. Lessons should have been learnt but, largely, were not. Similar problems followed later in the twentieth century.

First, however, another hugely unlikely treatment emerged in the asylums, with apparently surprising results: giving patients malaria to treat advanced syphilis or 'general paralysis of the insane'. General paralysis of the insane, now known as neurosyphilis, was a common problem in nineteenth- and twentieth-century asylums, including the Richmond. The case of Daniel is a good example.

In early 1908, Daniel, a 36-year-old bricklayer, was transferred to the Richmond from a local prison. Prison staff described Daniel as violent and placed his hands in 'muffs' (restraints). On arrival at the Richmond, Daniel was 'in a state of acute mania', according to medical notes:

> Patient is very excited and noisy. He is a millionaire. 'Has millions beyond counting'. He is Lord Daniel. He will be sitting in a gold chair. He got his money by giving a false name.

Daniel said that 'he had syphilis a great many years ago'. Advanced syphilis that affected the brain (general paralysis of the insane or neurosyphilis) is now rare, but it also affected the eyes, resulting in small pupils that did not constrict in the normal fashion when exposed to bright light, but constricted when focused on a nearby object. Admission notes initially recorded that Daniel's 'pupils are small, but the right, I think, is a little larger. They respond to light'.

Two weeks after admission, Daniel remained grandiose and paranoid:

> Still in the same excited state and at present in a single room [...] Offers to make me a Lord if I allow him out of the asylum. States the attendants are always trying to throttle him.

One month after admission, Daniel's pupils was 'contracted and responding to light badly if at all', suggesting advancing neurosyphilis. Two months after admission, Daniel's behaviour were more disturbed, also consistent with the condition:

> Has sudden outbursts of passion and pugilistic tendencies. Today he is in a bad humour, pouring torrents of abuse and blasphemy on me when I attempt to speak to him.

Matters deteriorated rapidly. The following month, Daniel 'tore up all his mattress' and lost a considerable amount of weight. Fewer than four months after admission, Daniel died in the Richmond, presumably from advanced neuro-syphilis. Had Daniel been admitted two decades later, he might well have been treated with malaria therapy, which was commenced at the hospital in the 1920s (Dunne, 1926).

Malaria treatment was developed by Julius Wagner-Jauregg (1857–1940), an Austrian physician whose main interest was pyrotherapy, which was the treatment of mental illness by causing the patient to develop a fever or high temperature (Kelly, 2022). In 1917, Wagner-Jauregg tried injecting malaria parasites into patients with general paralysis of the insane, a condition which was usually fatal, as it was in Daniel's case. Initial outcomes appeared positive. In 1927, Wagner-Jauregg won a Nobel Prize in Medicine for his innovation. Malaria therapy seemed to result not only in decreased deaths, but also increased discharges, with remission rates of up to 46 per cent reported from some sources (Stafford-Clark, 1952). The subsequent decline in the condition was also related to the fall in new cases, as early treatment of syphilis improved. Later assessments of malaria therapy were more nuanced, and the treatment went into decline (Sargant and Slater, 1946; Scull, 2015).

Insulin Treatment, Convulsive Therapy, and Lobotomy

Insulin therapy was developed in the 1920s and 1930s by Austrian psychiatrist Manfred Sakel (1900–1957). Sakel was interested in the use of insulin (a hormone usually produced in the pancreas) to induce coma and convulsions, and noted that producing comas in this way appeared to help in cases of psychosis or drug addiction. The resultant therapy involved administering insulin to induce a coma five or six mornings per week until such time as either 50 to 60 comas had been achieved or there was sufficient improvement (Kelly, 2022). The patient spent up to 15 minutes in a coma on each occasion and the coma was terminated with glucose.

Insulin therapy became popular in the 1940s and 1950s. Initial results often appeared positive (Dunne and O'Brien, 1939), but it was soon clear that there were substantial risks, including intellectual impairment and death due to hypoglycemic encephalopathy, heart failure, or pneumonia (Sargant and Slater, 1946). The nature of these adverse effects became clearer over time and ranged from obesity to brain damage that could prove permanent. Eventually, the mortality rate was estimated at between 1 and 5 per cent but might have been higher. Insulin therapy went into decline in the late 1950s and early 1960s owing to its poor outcomes and the emergence of safer, more effective treatments for schizophrenia, such as antipsychotic medication.

Convulsive therapy was another treatment that soon emerged, even though the relationship between convulsions and mental illness was always complex. Epilepsy appeared to be associated with mental illness, but, on the other hand, convulsions were thought to be curative in some cases. This was an ironic and somewhat unlikely position for psychiatry to hold, not least because convulsive conditions such as epilepsy presented substantial management problems in the asylums. The case of Eileen is a good example.

Eileen was a 48-year-old woman admitted to the Richmond District Lunatic Asylum in late 1908. Medical notes record that Eileen 'says she is damned. Appears to wish to destroy herself [...] Has had previous attacks like the present but not so violent'. Eileen had previously 'injured her head in one of these attacks by falling on the floor'. Her husband told asylum staff that the current 'attack' started four weeks earlier 'after working hard'.

Eileen had five children, the youngest being 19 years of age. Two of Eileen's brothers and two of her sisters 'died of consumption' (tuberculosis), although her 'parents lived to be a good old age'. The family had 'no history of insanity', but admission notes record that Eileen was tormented:

> She says that this is hell and I am the devil's mother. Hears devils [...] Asked why she thinks this is hell, says because she never praised God. These girls (the nurses) never praised God and are going fast to hell with her.

A week after admission, Eileen was 'at present quiet', but 'says she feels very weak. Asked if anything distresses her, says 'Nothing that I know'. Does not know the name of the place'. After a month, Eileen was largely unchanged: she 'had an epileptic fit' which 'did not affect her mental condition', but she could not remember the doctor's name or where she was. After two months, epileptic seizures ('fits') were a frequent occurrence:

> She is at present getting fits which are of a slight kind and in which the face only is involved. She is now asleep and I did not wake her.

After three months in the Richmond, Eileen was still having 'these fits periodically' but was now also 'most incoherent'. The situation deteriorated and soon Eileen was 'very excitable and noisy – gets into paroxysms of crying and rambles incoherently and it is impossible to stop her while she is in one of these fits of excitement'. After five months in the Richmond, Eileen died of 'status epilepticus' – a sustained epileptic seizure without recovery.

Notwithstanding cases like that of Eileen, and the clear problems that epilepsy presented, the idea that convulsions were therapeutic continued to grow. Formal programmes of convulsive therapy were introduced in 1934 by Hungarian psychiatrist Ladislas Meduna (1896-1964), who induced epileptic-type seizures using chemicals such as pentamethylene tetrazol, a camphor-like compound (Kelly, 2022). At Rome University Psychiatric Clinic, Italian neurologist Ugo Cerletti (1877–1963) used electricity to produce convulsions in a man with schizophrenia found in the train station suffering from delusions, hallucinations, and confusion. Cerletti's initial results appeared encouraging, and electroconvulsive therapy (ECT) soon came into widespread use (Shorter and Healy, 2007). The treatment was introduced at the Richmond District Lunatic Asylum (or Grangegorman Mental Hospital, as it was then known) in the early 1940s, and good results were reported in patients with depression there and elsewhere (Sargant and Slater, 1946; Dunne, 1950; Kelly, 2023b).

Over the following decades, ECT was commonly administered excessively and inappropriately, but its use changed over time, as rates of application were rationalised, and 'straight' ECT (i.e., without anaesthetic) was replaced by 'modified' ECT (i.e., with anaesthetic), making the treatment more focused, effective, and safer. ECT use declined in many countries during the 1970s but, in 2010, a definitive assessment was published by the UK's National Institute for Clinical Excellence, recommending ECT for rapid, short-term improvement of severe symptoms after a trial of other treatments had been ineffective and/ or when the condition was potentially life-threatening, in people with severe depressive illness, catatonia, or severe or prolonged mania (National Institute for Clinical Excellence, 2010).

ECT is, therefore, the only one of this group of novel biological treatments to remain in use into the twenty-first century, as experimental surgical bacteriology, malaria therapy, and insulin treatment were all consigned to history. Perhaps the most notorious of these treatments, however, and the final one to be considered here, is lobotomy, which was also abandoned before the start of the twenty-first century, but still merits attention as another example of relatively uncritical therapeutic enthusiasm in the history of psychiatry.

Frontal lobotomy or leucotomy involves surgery on the frontal part of the brain. The operation was developed as a treatment for mental disorder in the early 1930s by Portuguese neurologist António Egas Moniz (1874–1955), who shared a Nobel Prize for his work in 1949 (Kelly, 2016b). Lobotomy was a controversial, contested treatment from the start, but the practice was adopted enthusiastically in the US by Walter Freeman, who organised and performed up to 3,500 lobotomies over the course of his career. Along with James W. Watts, Freeman's patients included Rosemary Kennedy, sister of US president John F. Kennedy; she underwent lobotomy at age 23, with tragic consequences (El-Hai, 2005).

Lobotomy was introduced to patients of Grangegorman Mental Hospital in April 1946 (Kelly, 2022). In 1950, detailed outcome data from Grangegorman showed that, out of 63 patients with schizophrenia and poor prognosis who underwent lobotomy, 19 recovered sufficiently to be discharged; 19 showed considerable improvements in behaviour; 18 showed no change; four disimproved markedly; and three died (Dunne, 1950). Even among those who were discharged, problems remained, and lobotomy went into decline during the 1950s, owing largely to its adverse effects and lack of efficacy for many patients (Sargant & Slater, 1946). In addition, better, safer treatments became available at this time, including antipsychotic medication for schizophrenia.

Lobotomy was the single greatest mistake in the history of psychiatry, a disturbing story of therapeutic enthusiasm that went unchecked for too long. It stemmed from a deep desire to discharge people from large, overcrowded mental hospitals, but the procedure was untested, and was used too widely and for too long, often with fatal results. Today, psychosurgical intervention is rare in psychiatry, and radical psychosurgery for mental disorder is an exclusively historical phenomenon in most parts of the world.

Varied Practices and Perspectives

It is not possible, in a single chapter, to summarise the development of psychiatry in every country and culture. While certain themes recur, there are significant variations on this history around the world. In the US, for example, asylums developed along broadly similar lines to parts of Europe, with many US states passing complex mental health legislation during the nineteenth century (Clouston and Folsom, 1884).

In India, ancient traditions linked disease with diet, and Unani medicine included *Ilaj-I-Nafsani* as a form of psychotherapy (Nizamie and Goyal, 2010). Other practices offered different kinds of assistance in various parts of India, and there were early hospitals for people with mental illness during the reign of King Asoka (268–232 BCE). Later, colonisation resulted in the building of asylums to cater primarily for European people who developed mental illness in India, and this system of Indian asylums soon became a complex but integral part of the colonial enterprise (Kelly, 2022).

Notwithstanding these variations in the pace of change and in the combinations of measures outlined, certain general patterns emerged in many countries: neglect of the mentally ill, medicalisation of their management, the emergence of asylums, and the transition of these institutions from places primarily aimed at cure to places primarily aimed at control. Against this background of overcrowded mental hospitals and a desperate desire to empty them, the novel physical treatments of the twentieth century emerged one after the other: experimental surgical bacteriology, malaria therapy for neurosyphilis, insulin treatment, convulsive therapy, and lobotomy.

In parallel with these events, psychoanalysis gained significant sway over psychiatric practice in some but not all countries as the twentieth century progressed. Sigmund Freud's creation migrated especially successfully to the United States, where it came to dominate psychiatry for several decades (Hays, 1971; Shorter, 2007). In other places, such as Ireland, psychoanalysis had minimal impact on mainstream psychiatry, owing to both cultural factors and the traditional dominance of institutions (Kelly, 2017). In time, psychoanalysis was largely eclipsed in most countries by other forms of 'talking therapies', most notably cognitive-behaviour therapy (CBT). The arrival of effective antipsychotic medication in the 1950s brought further changes to psychiatry and arguably facilitated widespread de-institutionalisation (Kelly, 2022). Antipsychotic medication is considered further in Chapter 4 of this book, which is concerned with 'Treating Symptoms and Disorders'.

For the present discussion, it is sufficient to note that psychiatric institutions emerged in the nineteenth century, continued to expand in the first half of the twentieth century, and proved difficult to dismantle for a host of medical, social, and political reasons. The perils of institutions were well recognised by psychiatrists and others, as well as the various limitations of psychiatry as it was practised at the time. Even so, the 1960s brought a fresh wave of criticism of the psychiatric enterprise, some of which was merited and some of which reflected the counter-cultural impulses of the era more than psychiatry itself.

In 1961, Canadian-American sociologist Erving Goffman (1922–1982) published a now classic book titled *Asylums: Essays on the Social Situation of Mental Patients and Other Inmates*, drawing much-needed attention to the dehumanising nature of institutions (Goffman, 1961). Also in 1961, Hungarian-American psychiatrist Thomas Szasz (1920–2012) published *The Myth of Mental Illness: Foundations of a Theory of Personal Conduct* questioning current understandings of mental disorder (Szasz, 1961). Scottish psychiatrist R. D. Laing (1927-1989) published a series of books during this period, including *The Divided Self: An Existential Study in Sanity and Madness* (Laing, 1960) and *The Self and Others* (Laing, 1961), generally critical of psychiatry as it was being practised.

French philosopher Michel Foucault (1926–1984) was another significant voice at this time. In April 1965, Laing provided a 'Reader's Report' about Foucault's book *Madness and Civilisation* for Tavistock Publications (Foucault, 2006). Laing described Foucault's mammoth volume of philosophy as 'quite an exceptional book of very high calibre. Brilliantly written, intellectually rigorous, and with a thesis that thoroughly shakes the assumptions of traditional psychiatry'. Laing was colourful, incisive, and wrong.

Foucault developed the idea of the 'medical gaze' by which doctors allegedly focused biomedical elements of patients' problems only, and filtered out all other aspects of the person's life story (for a discussion, see: O'Callaghan, 2022). This was an oversimplification at best, as the history of psychiatry is replete with doctors who were seized by the personal and social problems of their patients. As a result, Foucault's relevance to psychiatry, if he had any, is greatly diminished. The creation of a 'biomedical' strawman is always a favourite rhetorical technique, but the foundations of 'traditional psychiatry' remain distinctly unshaken by Foucault's thoughts.

Despite this, Foucault's work created a seductive intellectual empire of its own, beloved of academics but oddly divorced from the world of psychiatric practice. There are many reasons for this. Often, philosophical discussions of psychiatry, such as Foucault's, are pitched in an obscurantist style that deters engagement by practitioners but not theoreticians. This problem is more than rhetorical. By disappearing into an otherworld of abstraction, various commentators end up proceeding in parallel with psychiatry, rather than in dialogue with it. As a result, their impact is limited, their potential unrealised, and mainstream psychiatry does not benefit from their critical insights. This is a pity. Psychiatry needs criticism that is clear, cogent and, if necessary, coruscating.

Any allure that Foucault's baroque theorising still holds is based on its internal architecture rather than logic or relevance. Foucault's grasp of history was selective at best and sometimes just plain wrong (Scull, 2015). Despite this, his ideas remain oddly attractive to philosophers, artists, and theoreticians who value elegance over accuracy. Clinicians do not enjoy this luxury, and neither do those who suffer with mental illness or their families.

One of the most comprehensive responses to such critics appeared in 1976 in the form of Irish psychiatrist Anthony Clare's book *Psychiatry in Dissent: Controversial Issues in Thought and Practice* (Clare, 1976). Clare's text appeared at a time when psychiatry was under fire from many angles: the existence of 'mental illness' was continually questioned, the efficacy of treatments widely debated, and the legitimacy of psychiatry as a branch of medicine was the topic of endless, agonised discussion (Kelly & Houston, 2020).

Into this arena, *Psychiatry in Dissent* brought engagement, reasonableness, and respect for diverse perspectives (Kelly, 2023c). Most importantly, Clare knew that different audiences had different needs: the public deserved an honest account of the true state of psychiatry as a branch of medicine, and people working in mental health services needed a robust intellectual framework that inspired their confidence. *Psychiatry in Dissent* provided both, combined with a lively intellectual approach and a careful, compassionate tone that fostered unity and collaboration rather than division and despair. Five decades later, Clare's book remains fiercely relevant, as key themes and arguments remain valid today, sometimes eerily so.

Psychiatry in Dissent started with a clear, open-minded exploration of the concept of mental illness, arguing that it was probably an error to conceptualise mental health and mental illness as dichotomous, and better to see them as opposite ends of a continuum – a position which was richly validated over subsequent decades (Kelly & Feeney, 2006). Clare also discussed different models of mental illness and noted that, when the diagnostic process was used in a rational, competent manner, the results compared favourably with other fields of medicine.

Clare considered a range of key issues including the nature of schizophrenia, which, he argued, might be one condition or several grouped together – another view that remains vital, relevant, and debated today, many decades later (Murray, 2017). Clare also explored ECT, psychosurgery, issues pertaining to responsibility and involuntary hospitalisation, and the realities of psychiatric services. Most of all, he offered compelling arguments that things could be better, that psychiatry offered a reasonable and reasoned path forward, and that honest public discussion was an important part of this process. Clare defended contemporary

psychiatry, explored its flaws, restored public confidence, and inspired a generation of doctors to enter psychiatry with confidence, enthusiasm, and self-belief.

More recent considerations of psychiatry include psychiatrist Tom Burns's
superb *Our Necessary Shadow: The Nature and Meaning of Psychiatry* (Burns,
2013) and a number of books by sociologist Andrew Scull, including his magis-
terial *Madness in Civilization: A Cultural History of Insanity from the Bible to
Freud, from the Madhouse to Modern Medicine* (Scull, 2015). A more detailed
consideration of Scull's work is beyond the scope of the present chapter but
suffice it to say that Scull provides a more cogent, if still critical, account of the
development of the field, compared to most critics.

Perhaps the greatest deficit across all the critical literature, however, is a
reluctance to engage with the evidence-base for current psychiatric interventions, which is often implicitly presented as a continuation of discredited practices of the past. The evidence-base for contemporary psychiatric treatments is
equal to, or better than, the evidence-base for treatments in other areas of medicine, such as cardiology. This, however, is often ignored in books about contemporary psychiatry, so this evidence is explored further in this book, especially in
Chapter 4, titled 'Treating Symptoms and Disorders'.

Psychiatry, Institutions, Stories

The history of psychiatry is a history of therapeutic enthusiasm, with all the
triumph and tragedy, hubris and humility that such enthusiasm inevitably brings
(Kelly, 2016a). It is in many ways a deeply disturbing story, filled with sadness
and missed opportunities, good intentions frustrated, and genuine progress at
various points.

Certain themes recur, especially the idea that mental illness is on the increase.
This idea fuelled the emergence of psychiatry as a medical discipline in the first
place and has now become a staple of mental health discourse. As recently as
May 2022, the US President's Council of Economic Advisors referred to 'the
mental health crisis affecting our nation' (Council of Economic Advisors, 2022).
They stated that there were 'several indications that Americans were experiencing a mental health crisis prior to the [Covid-19] pandemic', and that 'its effects
were amplified as the pandemic resulted in the loss of lives and livelihoods and
unprecedented social isolation'. For a full discussion of this long-standing idea
of a mental health 'crisis' that is always getting worse, see Chapter 1, titled
'Why Does Psychiatry Exist?'

Another recurring (and linked) feature in the history of psychiatry is the
emergence and persistence of institutions. The stories of those who lived and
died in these vast 'mental hospitals' are the real history of this discipline. Too
often, these stories have been forgotten, although they are now being re-dis-
covered in various ways, such as in Colin Murphy's play about the Richmond
District Lunatic Asylum in Dublin, titled *The Asylum Workshop* (Murphy,

2023). To finish this chapter and its account of the emergence of psychiatry, it is fitting that we, too, return to the Richmond with another case history from its archive.

Catherine was admitted to the Richmond District Lunatic Asylum from the North Dublin Union (workhouse for the poor) in late 1908. She gave her age as 57 years but, according to medical notes, was 'obviously more'. Catherine had 'a delusion as to being pursued by the Irish in America who want to ruin her and have done so'. She was 'extremely and persistently voluble':

> *Rattles on unceasingly about the Irish being robbers and scoundrels [...] says she is followed from country to country, 'it is by the fall of their bodies' they do it.*

One week after admission, Catherine was 'incoherent and hard to follow'. After a month in the asylum, she continued 'to abuse the Irish' and, when 'asked what they do to her, says it would take her a week to tell me and she won't go into details'. After three months in the Richmond, Catherine was unchanged, saying 'she was kidnapped in here by someone who is the head of this place and who has a thousand agents. He has pursued her for years.'

Two years after admission, Catherine was 'depressed. Silent. Hardly ever speaks to anybody'. After four years, medical notes record that her 'depression becomes more marked [...] when she is spoken to. Believes her food is poisoned'. The following year, Catherine was 'in bed', 'quiet', 'depressed', and 'continually talking to herself'. Two months later, after more than five years in the asylum, Catherine died. No cause of death is recorded in her file.

Key Messages

- Mental illness, often termed 'madness' in the past, appears in some form in every cultural and religious tradition in history, along with descriptions of symptoms, signs, and emotions that are often consistent with what are now regarded as 'mental disorders' but were interpreted or patterned differently at the time.
- The emergence of psychiatry as a medical discipline was a gradual process that started, arguably, when Hippocrates (c.460–c.370 BCE), a Greek physician, accorded the brain a central role in generating emotions, knowledge, and perceptions.
- The nineteenth and twentieth centuries saw the emergence and dominance of psychiatric institutions ('mental hospitals') in many countries around the world, along with increased medicalisation of the management of mental illness.
- Given the overcrowded, unhygienic nature of many psychiatric institutions at the start of the twentieth century, a succession of 'biological treatments'

emerged, rooted in a desire to empty the hospitals; these included experimental surgical bacteriology, malaria therapy, insulin treatment, convulsive therapies, and lobotomy (which was the single greatest mistake in the history of psychiatry).
- There were variations on this history in different countries around the world, and vocal critics of psychiatry emerged with particular energy in the 1960s, including Erving Goffman, Thomas Szasz, R. D. Laing, and Michel Foucault.
- More recent decades saw renewed emphasis on evidence-based care, although certain patterns from the history of psychiatry persist today.
- There is much to be learnt from the history of psychiatry, and more to be done to give voice to the forgotten asylum patients of the past.

References

Anonymous. Emil Kraepelin (1856–1926): psychiatric nosographer. *JAMA* 1968; 203: 978–9 (https://doi.org/10.1001/jama.1968.03140110070018).

Burns T. *Our Necessary Shadow: The Nature and Meaning of Psychiatry.* London: Allen Lane, 2013.

Clare AW. *Psychiatry in Dissent: Controversial Issues in Thought and Practice.* London: Tavistock Publications Limited, 1976.

Clouston TS, Folsom CF. *Clinical Lectures on Mental Diseases to Which is Added an Abstract of the Statutes of the United States and of the Several States and Territories Relating to the Custody of the Insane.* Philadelphia: Henry C. Lea's Son and Co., 1884.

Conolly J. *An Inquiry Concerning the Indications of Insanity with Suggestions for the Better Protection and Care of the Insane.* London: John Taylor, 1830.

Council of Economic Advisors. *Reducing the Economic Burden of Unmet Mental Health Needs.* Washington, DC: The White House, 2022 (https://www.whitehouse.gov/cea/written-materials/2022/05/31/reducing-the-economic-burden-of-unmet-mental-health-needs/). (Link to licence: https://creativecommons.org/licenses/by/3.0/us/) (accessed 1 May 2023).

Drapes T. On the maniacal-depressive insanity of Kraepelin. *Journal of Mental Science* 1909; 55: 58–64 (https://doi.org/10.1192/bjp.55.228.58).

Dunne J. The malarial treatment of general paralysis. *Journal of Mental Science* 1926; 72: 343–6 (https://doi.org/10.1192/bjp.72.298.343).

Dunne J. Survey of modern physical methods of treatment for mental illness carried out in Grangegorman Mental Hospital. *Journal of the Medical Association of Eire* 1950; 27: 4–9.

Dunne J, O'Brien E. Insulin therapy: a short review of the work done in Grangegorman Mental Hospital. *Journal of Mental Science* 1939; 85: 498–504 (https://doi.org/10.1192/bjp.85.356.498).

El-Hai J. *The Lobotomist: A Maverick Medical Genius and His Tragic Quest to Rid the World of Mental Illness.* Hoboken, NJ: John Wiley and Sons, Inc., 2005.

Foucault M. *History of Madness*. London and New York: Routledge, 2006 (first published as: Foucault M. *Folie et Déraison: Histoire de la Folie à l'Âge Classique*. Paris: Librarie Plon, 1961).

Goffman E. *Asylums: Essays on the Social Situation of Mental Patients and Other Inmates*. New York: Anchor Books, Doubleday & Co., 1961.

Hays P. *New Horizons in Psychiatry* (Second Edn). Harmondsworth: Penguin, 1971.

Kelly BD. *Hearing Voices: The History of Psychiatry in Ireland*. Dublin: Irish Academic Press, 2016a.

Kelly BD. Lobotomy in Ireland: single greatest mistake in the history of psychiatry. *Irish Medical Times*, 11 November 2016b (https://www.imt.ie/features-opinion/lobotomy-in-ireland-the-single-greatest-mistake-in-the-history-of-psychiatry-09-11-2016/) (accessed 17 June 2023).

Kelly BD. Ego, id, and Ireland. *Lancet Psychiatry* 2017; 4: 281–2 (https://doi.org/10.1016/S2215-0366(17)30085-8).

Kelly BD. *In Search of Madness: A Psychiatrist's Travels Through the History of Mental Illness*. Dublin: Gill Books, 2022.

Kelly BD. Modern approaches to an age-old problem. *Forum* 2023a; 40: 31–2.

Kelly BD. *Asylum: Inside Grangegorman*. Dublin: Royal Irish Academy, 2023b.

Kelly BD. *Psychiatry in Dissent*: Anthony Clare's critique, defence and reinvigoration of psychiatry. *BJPsych Advances* 2023c; 29: 426–7 (https://doi.org/10.1192/bja.2023.29). (Link to licence: https://creativecommons.org/licenses/by/4.0/) (accessed 26 January 2024).

Kelly BD, Feeney L (2006) Psychiatry: no longer in dissent? *Psychiatric Bulletin* 2006; 30: 344–5 (https://doi.org/10.1192/pb.30.9.344).

Kelly BD, Houston M. *Psychiatrist in the Chair: The Official Biography of Anthony Clare*. Newbridge, County Kildare: Merrion Press, 2020.

Kinsley D. 'Through the looking glass': divine madness in the Hindu religious tradition. *History of Religions* 1974; 13: 270–305 (https://doi.org/10.1086/462707).

Kraepelin E. *Psychiatrie*. Ein Lehrbuch für Studirende und Aerzte (Sixth Edn). Leipzig: Verlag von Johann Ambrosius Barth, 1899.

Kraepelin E. *Lectures on Clinical Psychiatry*. New York: William Wood and Company, 1904.

Kraepelin E. *Manic-Depressive Insanity and Paranoia*. Edinburgh: E. & S. Livingstone, 1921.

Laing RD. *The Divided Self: An Existential Study in Sanity and Madness*. Harmondsworth: Penguin, 1960.

Laing RD. *The Self and Others*. London: Tavistock Publications, 1961.

Murphy C. *The Asylum Workshop*. London: Methuen, 2023.

Murray RM. Mistakes I have made in my research career. *Schizophrenia Bulletin* 2017; 43: 253–6 (https://doi.org/10.1093/schbul/sbw165).

National Institute for Clinical Excellence. *The Use of Electroconvulsive Therapy (Update: May 2010)*. London: National Institute for Clinical Excellence, 2010 (https://www.nice.org.uk/guidance/ta59/resources/the-use-of-electroconvulsive-therapy-pdf-371522989) (accessed 17 June 2023).

Nizamie SH, Goyal N. History of psychiatry in India. *Indian Journal of Psychiatry* 2010; 52 (Suppl.1): S7–S12 (https://doi.org/10.4103%2F0019-5545.69195).

O'Callaghan AK. 'The medical gaze': Foucault, anthropology and contemporary psychiatry in Ireland. *Irish Journal of Medical Science* 2022; 191: 1795–7 (https://doi .org/10.1007/s11845-021-02725-w).

Reynolds J. *Grangegorman: Psychiatric Care in Dublin since 1815.* Dublin: Institute of Public Administration in Association with Eastern Health Board, 1992.

Sargant W, Slater E. *An Introduction to Physical Methods of Treatment in Psychiatry.* Edinburgh: E. S. Livingstone Ltd., 1946.

Scull A. *Madhouse: A Tragic Tale of Megalomania and Modern Medicine.* New Haven and London: Yale University Press, 2005.

Scull A. *Madness in Civilization: A Cultural History of Insanity from the Bible to Freud, from the Madhouse to Modern Medicine.* London: Thames Hudson, Ltd., 2015.

Shepherd M. Kraepelin and modern psychiatry. *European Archives of Psychiatry and Clinical Neuroscience* 1995; 245: 189–95 (https://doi.org/10.1007/BF02191796).

Shorter E. *A History of Psychiatry: From the Era of the Asylum to the Age of Prozac.* New York: John Wiley and Sons, 1997.

Shorter E, Healy D. *Shock Therapy: A History of Electroconvulsive Treatment in Mental Illness.* New Brunswick, NJ and London: Rutgers University Press, 2007.

Stafford-Clark D. *Psychiatry To-day.* Harmondsworth: Penguin Books Ltd., 1952.

Szasz T. *The Myth of Mental Illness: Foundations of a Theory of Personal Conduct.* New York: Harper and Row, 1961.

Wessely S. Surgery for the treatment of psychiatric illness: the need to test untested theories. *Journal of the Royal Society of Medicine* 2009; *102:* 445–51 (https://doi.org /10.1258/jrsm.2009.09k038).

3   Diagnosing Mental Illness

Kate was 16 when she first felt the urge to harm herself. Two years earlier, such a thought would have been unimaginable to her. But now, Kate felt that she wanted to cut herself in an effort to release 'tension' and feel less 'empty'. She wanted to see how it would feel to harm herself, or if she would feel anything at all.

Kate was a soft-spoken, high-achieving girl. She was not very sociable but had a small number of close friends at school. Her family was stable and supportive. They lived in a quiet suburb and had no financial problems. There were no significant arguments in the house. Kate had one older brother and a younger sister. They generally got on well together, but were not very close.

When Kate was 15, one of her best friends moved to another country, and they soon lost touch. Kate was upset at the time, but seemed to get over it. She continued to do well at school and meet her other friends at the weekends to go to the cinema or just hang out.

But Kate felt lonely. She kept a journal in which she wrote that she was 'empty'. She felt bad that she could not explain this feeling in any more detail. She wrote: 'I don't have any problems, but everything seems empty to me'. Despite these concerns, Kate continued to attend school. Her energy, appetite, and sleep were normal. As far as anyone could see, Kate was fine.

One day at school, Kate wrote an essay about 'The Future'. Towards the end of the essay, she wrote that the world was 'empty of everything, and getting emptier'. Kate's teacher was concerned and arranged a counselling appointment. Kate told the counsellor that she was not depressed, just uncertain about the future. The counsellor listened to Kate, reassured her as best she could, and arranged to see Kate again the following week. Kate agreed to this, but wrote in her journal later that night: 'I was right. The counsellor had nothing to say'.

Two evenings later, Kate confided to her journal that 'the emptiness is everywhere. I feel nothing'. Kate was on her own in the house, sitting in her room. At this point, the idea of harming herself came into Kate's mind. Perhaps if I cut myself, she thought, I will feel something? Anything? Perhaps that will fill the emptiness, and take this tension away, she told herself. After an hour or so, Kate decided to cut her wrists.

DOI: 10.4324/9781003378495-4

Introduction

This case scenario is not unusual. Kate feels upset and 'empty'. She does not know how to cope or even what she needs to cope with, exactly. She decides to harm herself to 'relieve tension'. There is little doubt that Kate is distressed and in need of support, but is she 'mentally ill'? Does she require 'treatment'? And, if so, for which mental illness, exactly?

The fundamental question is: at what point does it become useful, logical, and evidence-based to describe Kate's upsetting feelings and experiences as a 'mental illness' or 'mental disorder' rather than unhappiness? At what stage is it reasonable to decide that Kate would benefit from seeing a mental health professional and considering psychiatric care, rather than relying solely on her own coping mechanisms and the support of family and friends?

These are issues and dilemmas which have troubled and shaped psychiatry since the discipline first emerged. Who is 'mentally ill'? Who is not? Who decides? And who decides who decides? If a person is mentally ill, is their mental illness entirely unique to them, or is there a defined number of mental illnesses that different people develop? Or is there only one 'mental illness', which includes everyone who is deemed not 'mentally well'?

Against the background of these issues, this chapter is devoted to 'Diagnosing Mental Illness'. The chapter explores the purpose of diagnosis in psychiatry, the merits and demerits of diagnosis, and the appropriate use of diagnostic systems. The discussion includes considerations of the American Psychiatric Association's (APA) *Diagnostic and Statistical Manual of Mental Disorders (Fifth Edition) (Text Revision)* (DSM) (American Psychiatric Association, 2022), the World Health Organization's (WHO) *ICD-11: International Classification of Diseases (Eleventh Revision)* (ICD) (World Health Organization, 2019), and general approaches to diagnosis in clinical practice. The focus in this chapter is on the skilful use of diagnosis as a tool for shared understanding and research, rather than dogmatic approaches to symptom-based syndromes in individual cases. The chapter concludes by returning to Kate's story, looking at skilful use or judicious non-use of diagnosis in her case. Diagnosis can be very helpful and, at times, essential, but one size does not fit all – and that includes the very idea of diagnosing in the first place.

The fundamental message of this chapter is that diagnosis in psychiatry, like diagnosis in many areas of medicine, is generally provisional and imperfect, rather than permanent and definitive. No diagnosis encompasses all aspects of a person's experience and no diagnosis fits anyone perfectly. Diagnoses are links between symptoms and signs on the one hand, and understanding and treatment on the other. They are tools and guides, rather than ends in themselves, and they can always change.

The Purpose and Nature of Diagnosis in Psychiatry

The idea of diagnosing mental illness is a controversial one. We discussed the fundamental concept of 'mental illness' or 'mental disorder' in Chapter 1, which asked: 'Why Does Psychiatry Exist?' The current chapter focusses not on the issue of whether or not a person has a 'mental illness' in the first instance, but rather on the idea of diagnosing a *specific* mental illness, as opposed to simply concluding that a person is 'mentally ill' in the very broad sense of not possessing full mental health at a given point in time.

The issues here hinge on the threshold for diagnosis in the first place and then the boundaries of specific conditions. Are various mental illnesses truly distinct from each other, in the way they are described in the DSM and ICD? Are they really stand-alone entities with their own criteria, albeit that these criteria often overlap? Or should everyone who does not enjoy complete 'mental health' automatically be considered 'mentally ill' by exclusion? If the latter is the case, this creates a very broad, undifferentiated category of 'mental illness' which likely includes most people most of the time. Given the intrinsic diversity of human experience and the ups and downs of everyday life, a category of 'mental illness' this broad would be essentially meaningless.

The *Constitution of the WHO* intimates a difference between the absence of health and the presence of illness. The WHO states that 'health is a state of complete physical, mental, and social well-being and not merely the absence of disease or infirmity. The enjoyment of the highest attainable standard of health is one of the fundamental rights of every human being without distinction of race, religion, political belief, economic or social condition' (World Health Organization, 2020). This is a rather utopian definition of health which most people do not fulfil most of the time, so it is not useful, reasonable, or realistic to suggest that everyone who lacks 'complete […] mental […] well-being' is mentally ill.

In terms of an overall approach, it makes sense to note the WHO definition of 'health' as a utopian ideal; accept that most people fall short of this description most of the time *without being ill*; define what mental illness is (as outlined in Chapter 1), and then specify sub-types of mental illness if (and only if) common patterns recur and sub-categorising appears useful for understanding or treatment. This is a more reasoned and reasonable approach to the matter, rather than making 'mental illness' a condition that automatically includes everybody whose mental health falls short of the WHO definition of health. Essentially, that would be everyone.

With this in mind, the issue of diagnosis is clearly a fluid one which changes over time, owing largely to the fact that most diagnoses in psychiatry are based on symptoms or clinical signs, rather than biological tests (Kelly, 2022). Critics of psychiatry have long pointed to this as a particular weakness in the field, despite long-standing acknowledgement that when the diagnostic process is used in a rational, competent manner, the results in psychiatry compare favourably with other fields of medicine (Clare, 1976; Kelly, 2023). Biological tests in areas such as cardiology or endocrinology are not always as definitive as they appear, not least because cut-offs for many medical conditions such as hypertension (high blood pressure) change over time, just as thresholds for diagnoses in psychiatry shift. Across all of medicine, diagnostic thresholds are falling, and more people are being diagnosed with more conditions (Burns, 2013). Psychiatry is by no means unique in this regard.

Against this background, it is useful to consider the two main diagnostic systems in use in psychiatry today: the DSM (American Psychiatric Publishing, 2022) and the ICD (World Health Organization, 2019). Both the DSM and ICD present lists of symptoms which need to be present to a specified degree of severity over a particular period of time for a given diagnosis to be made (Kelly, 2017). Depression is a good example. A DSM diagnosis of 'major depressive disorder' requires the existence of five or more symptoms out of nine key symptoms for more than a fortnight, and this must represent a change from previous functioning. The nine key symptoms are:

- Generally depressed mood.
- Reduced pleasure or interest.
- Significant weight change (loss or gain).
- Insomnia (poor sleep) or hypersomnia (too much sleep) almost daily.
- Psychomotor agitation or retardation (i.e., physical agitation or slowing down) almost daily.
- Loss of energy or fatigue almost daily.
- Feelings of worthlessness or excessive guilt.
- Reduced decisiveness or diminished concentration.
- Recurring thoughts of death, self-harm, or suicide, or related acts.

For a DSM diagnosis of major depressive disorder, at least one of the five symptoms must be either generally depressed mood or reduced pleasure or interest; symptoms must result in significant distress or impairment in functioning; symptoms must not be attributable to a substance (e.g., alcohol), a medical condition, or another mental illness; and there must not have been an episode of mania or hypomania which might indicate a diagnosis of bipolar affective disorder ('manic depression'), instead of major depressive disorder.

The ICD criteria for a 'depressive disorder' are quite similar to the DSM (World Health Organization, 2019). They include a period of depressed mood or diminished interest in activities for most of the day, almost every day during a period lasting for a minimum of two weeks, as well as other symptoms such as problems concentrating, feelings of worthlessness or inappropriate or excessive guilt, hopelessness, recurring thoughts of death or suicide, alterations in sleep or appetite, psychomotor retardation or agitation, and diminished energy or fatigue. Like the DSM, there must have never been manic, hypomanic, or mixed episodes previously, which would suggest the presence of bipolar affective disorder. *Recurrent* depressive disorder, according to the ICD, requires a history of at least two depressive episodes which are separated by at least several months without significant mood disturbance.

Both the DSM and ICD go on to define many more conditions in this highly ordered fashion, sometimes in astonishing detail. But while these diagnostic classification systems are clearly pragmatic and, to a degree, atheoretical (Pietikainen, 2015), they have both merits and demerits, and a great deal depends on how they are used in practice, if they are applied at all. These matters are considered next.

Merits and Demerits of Diagnostic Systems

Diagnostic systems such as the DSM and ICD raise many issues, ranging from their cultural appropriateness (or inappropriateness) in different settings (Watters, 2010) to their exclusion of specific conditions that were described over the course of history but were dropped from current classifications (Shorter, 2015). For the present discussion, it is useful to adopt a clinical perspective and outline some of the benefits and risks of diagnosis in day-to-day psychiatric practice, rather than considering the matter from purely philosophical, theoretical, or political viewpoints.

One of the primary and most important roles of diagnostic systems is to create a common language for sharing experiences of mental illness, psychiatric symptoms, and psychological suffering (Kelly, 2017). Because diagnosis of most mental illnesses is based primarily on history, symptoms, and clinical signs, rather than biological tests (which are generally used to exclude other disorders), it is necessary to identify clusters of psychiatric symptoms which commonly occur together in order to ensure some consistency in care. If mental disorders are ever to be understood, it is important that when someone in Australia mentions 'depression', they know that they are talking about roughly the same thing as someone in Brazil, Nigeria, or Vietnam.

This does not mean that any individual case of depression in Australia is identical to any individual case in Brazil, Nigeria, or Vietnam. Clearly, each case is different in many ways, even within countries and within cultures. This is equally true in other areas of medicine: no two people have precisely the same heart attack (myocardial infarction) or stroke (cerebrovascular event). Everyone is different to a significant degree, but articulating diagnostic entities reflects the fact that certain common features tend to occur together in, for example, 'depression', no matter where you are in the world.

Recognising this means that we are all *generally* talking about the same *general* thing when we mention 'depression', even if there are cultural variations in the expression and interpretation of symptoms. This means that we can, at least to an extent, create and share a common language when we talk about mental illness, psychological suffering, and human distress. This is essential: a great deal of human experience is shared to a substantial degree, so we should be able to talk about it. We have more in common than we think, especially when we suffer.

That is not to say that the DSM or ICD are used (or should be used) by all mental health professionals all the time, everywhere in the world. There is inevitably a great deal of variation in practice. In 2022, Vrigkou and colleagues studied the literature on the 'frequency of diagnostic classification systems' usage by mental health professionals in day-to-day clinical practice' and identified interesting differences between professions and across world regions (Vrigkou et al., 2022). Overall, they report that 69% of mental health professionals use diagnostic classification systems 'often, almost always or always' in day-to-day practice, mostly 'for administrative/billing purposes and assigning a diagnosis'. More specifically, 68% of psychiatrists who were studied and 74% of psychologists use such systems 'often, almost always or always'. This level of use was reported among 75.3% of mental health professionals in the Americas, 73.5% in the African region, 71.6% in the western Pacific, 69.4% in Europe, 66.8% in south-east Asia, and 57.1% in the eastern Mediterranean.

These interesting statistics suggest that a majority of mental health professionals use diagnostic systems commonly, although by no means universally or inevitably. There is flexibility in their use for clinical care, as there should be. These systems are helpful but not always essential. They are tools for description and understanding, not rigid, inflexible codes that must be applied every time. Everyone is different. Diagnostic systems highlight both what we have in common and how we differ. This is a valuable role.

Judicious use of diagnosis is also important for helping ensure that pharmaceutical companies or others do not 'create' new 'mental illnesses' which are not rooted in lived experience, in order to promote new products or services. The DSM and ICD offer important protections in this regard: evidence-based revisions of these classification systems can defend against manipulation by vested interests and foster opportunities for open, ethical engagement of patients, families, carers, mental health professionals, voluntary agencies, health care providers, and governmental bodies in refining classification systems, improving services, and advancing shared understanding.

This is important if the search for new treatments for mental illness is to proceed in a rational, evidence-based fashion. When people present to mental health services, professionals need some kind of guide as to which treatments work best to address commonly occurring clusters of symptoms (Kelly, 2016). Diagnosis and classification are required to perform research studies and conduct clinical trials that collect evidence about the best treatments for particular collections of symptoms or mental illnesses. This is the only way that interventions can be proven to work and not cause harm.

The importance of randomised controlled trials of treatments for specific conditions is supported by a knowledge of the darkest periods in the history of psychiatry. These include the eras of experimental surgical bacteriology, insulin treatment, and lobotomy (see Chapter 2: 'The History of Psychiatry'). We need to know which treatments work, and for whom, if we are to avoid these errors again. This involves careful diagnosis as a first step in designing and testing specific interventions (e.g., psychotherapies, medications, etc.), and then knowing how to carry these interventions into clinical practice, and for whom. Not every treatment helps everyone. A certain amount of classification, once it is performed flexibly, can better target interventions and better alleviate different kinds of suffering. Again, one size does not fit all.

In a similar fashion, careful diagnosis facilitates study of the causes of mental illness and different patterns of psychological distress. For example, there is long-established evidence that people are more likely to develop schizophrenia if they have a first-degree relative (e.g., mother, father, sister, or brother) with that same constellation of symptoms (Kelly, 2017; Jauhar et al., 2022). While the precise underpinnings of this fact are not established, the pattern is clear, not least because diagnostic systems such as the DSM and ICD facilitated research into patterns of occurrence of schizophrenia. The same argument applies to other conditions and states of psychological distress; e.g., establishing the role of life trauma in depression is only possible if there is broad agreement on certain core features of 'depression' in the first place. We need to know what we are talking about, even in general terms.

Each individual case will always be different from every other case in certain ways, so it is important that diagnostic classifications are not taken too literally or used inflexibly (Garfinkel, 2014). But there is also significant commonality in how we suffer. Recognising this should not deny anyone their individuality, but rather help with understanding, identifying treatments, and searching for causes. Used wisely, diagnosis helps.

Psychiatric Diagnosis and Human Rights

Diagnostic systems such as the DSM and ICD help to protect human rights. Clear, published diagnostic guidelines can bring clarity and accountability to the diagnosis of mental illness and its treatment. This is profoundly important: terms such as 'mental disorder', 'depression', and 'schizophrenia' carry enormous weight and should only be used in certain, specific circumstances. In many societies, these diagnostic terms carry not only personal meaning, but also social stigma and certain legal implications, depending on the person's circumstances. Diagnostic terminology is uniquely powerful in this regard, so its use should be judicious, circumspect, evidence-based, and accountable.

This is especially important given that virtually every country has mental health laws that can have a significant impact on the lives of some people diagnosed with mental illness. Most mental health legislation permits involuntary admission and treatment of people with a severe mental disorder who fulfil various criteria, often including a lack of understanding of their condition, impaired decision-making capacity, and/or apparent risk to themselves or to other people (see Chapter 5: 'Treatment Without Consent'). Admission and treatment without consent under such legislation is an exceptionally serious intrusion into someone's life. It involves limiting a person's rights to liberty and bodily integrity for a period of time, in the interests of protecting their rights to health care, health, and – on occasion – life. This is a difficult balance to achieve, usually in deeply challenging circumstances, but it is an essential one.

Mental health laws affect only a minority of people with mental illness. Among those who access formal mental health care, most avail of voluntary treatment in primary care settings, provided by family doctors and other health professionals such as nurses or counsellors (i.e., treatment to which they consent). Among the minority of people with mental illness who are referred to secondary care (e.g., psychiatry outpatient clinics or other specialist mental health services), most are treated with their consent, outside of psychiatric hospitals (Kelly, 2017). Finally, among those admitted to inpatient psychiatric care, approximately 90% are treated on a voluntary basis with their informed consent. Only a minority ever require involuntary admission or treatment under mental health legislation.

Nonetheless, for people who become subject to involuntary care for a period of time, there is a strong need for as much clarity as possible about diagnosis in order to ensure that appropriate interventions are provided, treatment meets their demonstrated needs, and there is accountability at all times. In other words, doctors and other mental health professionals must explain clearly why *this* person is being admitted and treated in *this* way without their consent or against their wishes at *this* time. Diagnosis is an essential element in ensuring such accountability. While each individual case will differ, certain key elements must be present if a person is to be diagnosed with a specific mental illness, especially if that diagnosis forms part of the basis for admission and treatment without consent.

Inevitably, both the DSM and ICD are imperfect systems, and they change continually, but they are still the best way to optimise clarity and accountability. Or, at the very least, nobody has come up with anything better. The evolutionary nature of these systems simply reflects the facts that the biological basis of most mental disorders is largely unknown (see Chapter 6: 'Neuroscience and Psychiatry') and societal expectations of mental health care change continually (see Chapter 7: 'Psychiatry, Culture, and Society'), chiefly in the direction of seeking more professional help for symptoms that were previously managed within families or communities. Despite these changes and revisions, diagnostic classification systems still facilitate accountability during periods when people are at their most distressed, vulnerable, and disempowered. For this reason, they are essential.

The history of psychiatry strongly supports the need for this accountability. The historical misuse of psychiatric concepts and institutions relates not only to the overuse of asylums in many countries during the nineteenth and twentieth centuries (see Chapter 2: 'The History of Psychiatry'), but also the alleged labelling of political dissidents as psychiatrically ill in, for example, the former

Soviet Union during the twentieth century (Clare, 1976). Psychiatry is uniquely prone to such overuse, misuse, and abuse. There are lessons here.

There are especially well-documented allegations of political and state abuse of psychiatry in Russia. In 1977, Sidney Bloch (a psychiatrist) and Peter Reddaway (a political scientist) published a hard-hitting book titled *Russia's Political Hospitals: The Abuse of Psychiatry in the Soviet Union* (Bloch and Reddaway, 1977), which they followed, in 1985, with another volume, *Soviet Psychiatric Abuse: The Shadow Over World Psychiatry* (Bloch & Reddaway, 1985). The situation that Bloch and Reddaway described was distressing in the extreme: political dissent diagnosed as mental illness; psychiatry used by the state for the oppression of some of its people; and many cases of involuntary psychiatric hospitalisation and 'treatment' of political dissidents. Their assessment is consistent with detailed accounts of the Soviet psychiatric system in personal memoirs from the 1970s and 1980s (Kelly, 2022).

While many countries have updated their mental health legislation and policies since that era, concerns persist about practices in certain jurisdictions today. In 2006, Robin Munro published a harrowing book looking at these issues in China, titled *China's Psychiatric Inquisition: Dissent, Psychiatry and the Law in Post-1949 China* (Munro, 2006). Based on detailed study and many case histories, Munro concluded that psychiatric abuse of dissidents and specific groups not only occurred in China, but was more widespread than in the Soviet Union. This is immensely discouraging in an era of human rights and growing awareness of the profound social injustices perpetrated against people with mental illness (see Chapter 9: 'Global Injustice in Mental Health Care').

Clearly, the temptation for governments to misuse psychiatry for political reasons simply will not go away, so ceaseless vigilance is needed. Many of the alleged abuses of psychiatry centre on the misuse of diagnoses to label and control people who are seen as different, dissonant, or challenging the *status quo*. Describing such individuals or groups as mentally ill is one way to marginalise or silence them. This problem needs to be approached from many angles, but correct, accountable use of internationally recognised diagnostic systems can help greatly. Provided that the DSM and ICD are used with care and an awareness of their limitations, they bring openness and accountability to diagnosis and to external oversight by mental health tribunals, review boards, inspectors, and courts. These mechanisms are essential to protect rights.

With this in mind, some countries have added specific diagnostic obligations to their mental health laws. India's Mental Healthcare Act 2017, for example, includes a requirement for clear, accountable diagnosis that is in accordance with international standards and not based on political, social, religious, or various other factors:

(1) Mental illness shall be determined in accordance with such nationally or internationally accepted medical standards (including the latest edition of

the International Classification of Disease of the World Health Organisation) as may be notified by the Central Government.

(2) No person or authority shall classify a person as a person with mental illness, except for purposes directly relating to the treatment of the mental illness or in other matters as covered under this Act or any other law for the time being in force.

(3) Mental illness of a person shall not be determined on the basis of (a) political, economic or social status or membership of a cultural, racial or religious group, or for any other reason not directly relevant to mental health status of the person; (b) non-conformity with moral, social, cultural, work or political values or religious beliefs prevailing in a person's community.

(4) Past treatment or hospitalisation in a mental health establishment, though relevant, shall not by itself justify any present or future determination of the person's mental illness.

(5) The determination of a person's mental illness shall alone not imply or be taken to mean that the person is of unsound mind unless he has been declared as such by a competent court (Mental Healthcare Act 2017; Section 3).

Legislation in other countries often contains similar provisions. Ireland's Mental Health Act 2001, for example, specifies that nothing 'shall be construed as authorising the involuntary admission of a person [...] by reason only of the fact that the person [...] is socially deviant' (Section 8(2)). Few countries go into as much detail as India, however, especially with its explicit mention of the ICD and detailed list of factors which are *not* relevant to a diagnosis of mental illness. This kind of clarity optimises accountability in both law and practice.

Stigma, Critiques, and the Social Context of Diagnosis

In addition to describing symptoms that frequently co-occur, creating a common language for psychiatric suffering, facilitating research about causes and treatments, and protecting human rights, careful diagnosis can also bring various other benefits to patients and families alike. These additional advantages include addressing stigma, alleviating the blame or guilt that people sometimes feel about mental illness, facilitating the establishment of networks of people affected by similar problems, and crafting treatment and management plans in an open, collaborative, accountable way in individual cases.

In the first instance, judicious diagnosis can help to reduce the stigma that is often wrongly associated with mental illness and its treatment. Too often, people are given the message that their problems are 'all in your head' or, more recently, are entirely 'psycho-social' in origin. The latter interpretation recognises important social factors but also commonly, if inadvertently, downplays the power and agency of the individual (presenting their experiences as entirely the product of social circumstance), diminishes or denies the reality of their impairment (implying that their problems are solely psychologically or socially constructed), and intimates that if social circumstances were different their problems would not only be lessened (which is likely true for many people) but would be entirely eliminated (which is regrettably untrue for most people who attend mental health services).

The careful, judicious, and compassionate use of clear diagnostic systems can help to address some of these issues, legitimise a person's suffering, draw attention to their strengths, and start to build a shared understanding of a path forward. A broader formulation of the person's problems is another necessary step to address stigma and achieve these goals. This means contextualising any diagnosis using psychiatry's broad bio-psycho-social approach. This encompasses not only 'psycho-social' dimensions of the person's situation, but also biological considerations which will apply to varying degrees in different people. Any truly holistic approach will consider *all* relevant biological, psychological, *and* social factors in the particular circumstances of the individual, rather than being limited to a reductive 'psycho-social' model that diminishes or denies biological dimensions. Thoughtful use of classification systems can play an important role throughout this process and help destigmatise mental illness and its treatment, provided diagnoses are explored carefully, flexibly, humbly, and with a broad, multi-dimensional awareness of context.

Diagnostic systems can also help to alleviate the disproportionate blame or guilt that individuals or families sometimes feel when a person develops psychiatric symptoms or a mental illness. Given that the root causes of many psychiatric conditions remain resolutely obscure, there is a tendency to assign significance to circumstances or events in people's lives, some of which might be relevant (e.g., traumatic experiences), but some of which might not have contributed. In this process, family members or others can feel that they are being held responsible to a degree that is not always justified, with resultant blame and guilt among family, friends, co-workers, or other people who play significant roles in the person's life.

This search for causes reflects a very human desire to understand why people develop particular psychological states or mental illnesses at specific points in time. But it can also prove harmful and hurtful to the very individuals that the person needs now more than ever. Using a diagnostic system like the DSM or ICD demonstrates that a person's condition has (in general terms) been experienced by other people in the past and broadly maps onto a certain pattern of human suffering that has been described before. This sharing of experience immediately alleviates some of the disproportionate guilt and blame that can be felt in these situations, affirming that this person's experience, although unique in certain respects, is not entirely unprecedented. As a result, and in the absence of other factors (such as abuse), family members and others (including the patient) should not feel uniquely or solely responsible for the situation.

This sense of commonality and community leads to another one of the benefits of classification systems that describe psychiatric symptoms in detail, which is assisting with the creation of networks of people and families affected by similar conditions. Psychological distress can be an isolating experience owing to the presence of unusual symptoms that the person has never had before: hearing voices, feeling that thoughts are being inserted into their head, or developing an impulse to self-harm (as with Kate in the vignette at the start of this chapter). These are all upsetting, frightening occurrences which can leave a person feeling distressed, confused, and, sometimes, unable to find the words for what they are going through.

Symptom-based diagnostic systems help by outlining shared experiences such as these and suggesting language for particular patterns of symptoms. Reading these lists can help to relieve some of the loneliness, recognising one's own experiences in some (but rarely all) of the features of a given condition outlined in the DSM or ICD. Or, alternatively, identifying with specific symptoms that are described under different diagnostic headings, indicating that this person's individual experiences are not entirely unique, even if their particular combination of them is. All of this facilitates self-awareness, sharing, discussion, and reaching out to people who can use the same language to describe their experiences. Nobody needs to suffer alone. No matter how imperfect, a common language helps us to connect. Used well, the DSM and ICD can provide that language.

Finally, clear diagnostic systems help to guide patients, families, and clinicians in choosing the best treatments for mental illnesses or for particular combinations of psychiatric symptoms. Evidence-based care lies at the heart of mental health services and is integral to these decisions. Before deciding which treatment to offer, it is important that randomised clinical trials provide robust information to guide choices about interventions that are proven to help with particular collections of symptoms. Clear diagnosis is essential to perform these research studies.

Careful diagnosis is also required if the information from such research is to be applied correctly in clinical practice. In other words, open, accountable diagnosis can link specific problems with particular interventions that are proven to help in these situations. In this way, diagnostic systems like the DSM and ICD play a central role in crafting treatment and management plans in an open, collaborative, effective fashion. After a treatment is given to a particular person, only one clinical trial matters: how does *this* person benefit from *this* treatment at *this* time? But to get to that point, diagnosis is essential to ensure that the likelihood of benefit is as high as possible, by informing both research studies and individual care decisions with careful, flexible diagnosis.

Risks of Diagnosis, Perils of a 'Tick Box' Approach, and Diagnostic Acceleration

Despite the many benefits and potential advantages of diagnostic systems such as the DSM and ICD, there are risks and perils associated with these approaches, especially their overuse, misuse, and abuse. At all times, it is important to remember that the DSM and ICD are symptom-based systems. In consequence, diagnoses based on these classifications do not necessarily map onto discrete biological entities. More research will hopefully clarify this matter further in the future, and possibly change diagnostic understandings dramatically, but progress has been very slow (see Chapter 6: 'Neuroscience and Psychiatry'). For now, it is wise to bear in mind that most diagnoses in psychiatry remain primarily based on symptoms and clinical signs, rather than biological tests, and this means that the categories outlined in the DSM and ICD are syndromic rather than biological in nature.

It is also useful to remember that while diagnostic systems appear to locate pathology within the individual, the social landscape is clearly relevant to many if not all conditions, including, but by no means limited to, depression (Brown & Harris, 1978; Blazer, 2005). The DSM and ICD do not deny this, so, when using their tools, it is important to remain aware that a variety of factors, such as social and cultural issues, are relevant to diagnosis, and possibly more relevant to certain diagnostic categories than others (Horowitz, 2002; Bhugra et al., 2010). While distress is experienced at the level of the individual, it is also shaped at the level of communities, societies, counties, and even globally. Everything has a context, including mental illness and its diagnosis.

Perhaps the greatest concern about diagnostic classification systems is their potential for misuse in a 'tick box' fashion in order to simplify complex scenarios or avoid engaging with the many dimensions of human suffering. This is an understandable temptation in situations of deep distress, confusion, and uncertainty. The apparent fixity of diagnostic criteria can seem like the only steady point in a very fluid world, a lifeboat in a sea of troubles. This can lead to over-estimation of the reassurance provided by lists of symptoms and over-reliance on diagnostic classifications to supply structure and meaning at times when both are scarce. This is a very human response, but it risks misuse or overuse of diagnostic systems and provides excessive reassurance which will not prove helpful in the end. The DSM and ICD are useful tools, but they have their limits.

Diagnostic systems can indeed help in situations of acute distress and uncertainty, but only if they are used judiciously and flexibly, and applied in the particular context of each individual's life and social situation. Nobody's suffering or distress can be understood solely in terms of a list of symptoms, no one fits any category perfectly, and many people will have features of several mental illnesses at the same time, but fulfil all of the criteria for none. This is especially true in emergency situations, when people often experience an array of symptoms and emotions at the same time, and it is difficult to clarify what is happening.

In view of all of these factors, a rigid, 'tick box' approach to diagnosis is wrong, unhelpful, and potentially harmful. The DSM contains a stern warning against using the manual in such a mechanistic fashion. The story of the individual person always takes precedence over any diagnostic paradigm. The

DSM and ICD present outline guidance only. Using them rigidly or literally accords them a weight and importance that is inappropriate. The DSM and ICD have specific uses, especially in guiding research and ensuring accountability in services, but they are neither complete nor perfect. They are always trumped by each person's individual circumstances and life story. Using these systems without acknowledging this fact is futile, impossible, and potentially harmful.

Owing to these issues, and despite the many advantages of diagnostic systems, their impact in clinical practice has been distinctly mixed (Garfinkel, 2014). On the one hand, they can bring clarity and a sense of understanding to complex situations of distress and unusual experiences, but they can also create an illusion of certainty if they are accorded more weight than they merit. The emphasis in this chapter is on skilful use of diagnosis as a tool for shared understanding and research, rather than dogmatic approaches to symptom-based syndromes. A flexible attitude is vital if the positive potential of diagnosis is to be harnessed for the benefit of patients, their families, and society as a whole.

It must be noted, however, that the process of diagnosis can have unintended effects, including its misuse for non-psychiatric purposes, overuse of specific diagnoses to access services, and escalating rates of diagnosis of certain conditions without clear evidence that incidence is increasing or that a legacy of under-diagnosis fully justifies a recent rush to diagnose. These are often system-level problems that relate to misuse of diagnostic systems rather than their appropriate use, especially when it comes to the diagnostic acceleration evident in relation to several specific conditions over recent decades.

There are many examples of this, including rising rates of diagnosis of juvenile bipolar disorder (Scull, 2019) and, perhaps most commonly, increased diagnosis of autism spectrum disorder (ASD) in recent times. ASD arguably provides the clearest demonstration of this complex trend which finds its roots in a combination of a legacy of under-diagnosis, recent changes in diagnostic criteria, and likely use of diagnosis for ancillary purposes, such as admittance to treatment, access to education, or entitlement to social supports. This is a nuanced picture that is partly attributable to the absence of biological tests for many disorders, but also an increased desire for diagnosis of all kinds of conditions, psychiatric and non-psychiatric, across society.

These complexities are especially clear in the context of ASD. Many factors appear relevant to the distribution of ASD diagnoses across communities. One recent study examined the prevalence of ASD among eight-year-olds in New York and New Jersey from 2000 to 2016 (Shenouda et al., 2023). This research found that 81% of eight-year-olds with ASD in this area were male, 20% were non-Hispanic Black, 26% were Hispanic, and 45% were non-Hispanic White. While some of the study's findings relating to gender might reflect the biology of the condition and its epidemiology, some findings might reflect other factors linked to availability of services or socio-economic issues that influence access to diagnosis.

This study also identified a two-fold increase in the prevalence of diagnoses of ASD with intellectual disability over the period studied (i.e., between 2000 and 2016) and a five-fold increase in diagnoses of ASD without intellectual disability. Children who lived in affluent areas were 80% more likely to be identified as having ASD without intellectual disability compared to children in underserved areas. A greater proportion of children identified as having ASD with intellectual disability lived in vulnerable areas compared to children who had ASD without intellectual disability.

The increase in ASD diagnoses and the patterns identified across this population were widely discussed in the media at the time (e.g., Mac Ghlionn, 2023). What led to this dramatic rise? Is the increase real or apparent? If it is real, why did it happen? There are many possible explanations, some potentially linked to genuine increases in rates, some linked with a correction of past under-diagnosis, and some potentially associated with access to diagnosis or other services. It is worth considering some of these in detail.

First, it is likely that ASD was significantly under-recognised and under-diagnosed in the past, so there might be a correction occurring as children who had undiagnosed ASD are finally assessed and can now access the supports they need. If so, this is a positive development for these children and for adults in a similar position who require assistance and support. This would hopefully correct a legacy of neglect, help some people to achieve greater understanding and self-acceptance, and facilitate access to appropriate treatment and support.

Even taking this into account, however, a five-fold increase in diagnoses over 16 years seems excessive and suggests that other factors are relevant. The variations in diagnoses across socio-economic groups indicate possible biases in terms of access to diagnostic services, the making of diagnoses, and/or the provision of support. It is entirely possible that ASD is truly distributed differently across various socio-economic groups, although this would require more study to establish definitively. Either way, the uneven distribution of diagnoses is cause for concern, especially the socio-economic gradients.

A further factor in this equation is the possibility that diagnostic thresholds for ASD are being driven downwards as a means to access services (Fombonne, 2023). In other words, a child with specific needs in terms of reading, writing, or some other developmental area might gain access to, and benefit from, greater educational supports if they have a diagnosis of ASD, even if this diagnosis is not fully justified in strict clinical terms. While providing a diagnosis in this situation is understandable at the individual level, it changes the purpose of diagnosis significantly by influencing the interpretation of criteria outlined in international classification systems.

This kind of diagnostic expansion is neither biologically based nor necessarily helpful in the long term. For some people with ASD, such a diagnosis brings relief, acceptance, access to services, and improved quality of life. For others, however, especially people with mild features of ASD, diagnosis can be an unhelpful, disempowering event that radically alters their self-view and leads to expectations of 'treatment' that might not be met. The moment of diagnosis is always a powerful one in terms of self-image and future expectations, so it needs to be considered with care in the particular context of each individual concerned.

Either way, the trend towards increased diagnosis of ASD appears to be gathering pace. This echoes developments across the rest of medicine beyond psychiatry, as diagnostic thresholds fall rapidly everywhere (Burns, 2013). Increasingly, doctors treat symptomless people for problems that might increase risk of future illness (e.g., impaired glucose tolerance, hypertension, etc.), in addition to people who present with active symptoms. Even among those with symptoms, diagnostic cut-offs for many medical conditions change over time, generally moving downwards in recent years, just like in psychiatry. This hunger for diagnosis is not limited to mental health: we live in an era of medicalisation of everyday life. For better or worse, psychiatry is part of that *Zeitgeist*.

Diagnosis as a Tool for Shared Understanding

This chapter has focused on 'Diagnosing Mental Illness', looking at the purpose of diagnosis in psychiatry, the merits and demerits of specific diagnostic approaches, and the appropriate use of diagnostic systems in research and mental health care. Inevitably, any such discussion encompasses the DSM and ICD, as well as general approaches to diagnosis in clinical practice. The emphasis in this chapter has been on thoughtful use of diagnosis as a tool for shared understanding and research, rather than rigid approaches to symptom-based syndromes in individual people.

It is essential that the core tasks of psychiatry and mental health care do not become obscured by diagnosis or the many controversies surrounding it. The key goals remain providing care and treatment to people in states of psychiatric and psychological distress, developing health and social care systems that promote wellness, enhancing human rights in the provision of services, deepening social inclusion, and enhancing autonomy at all times. Careful, thoughtful use of the DSM and ICD can assist with these tasks provided their use is accompanied by an awareness of the limitations of diagnostic systems and underpinned by a commitment to genuine therapeutic engagement with individuals and their families. Diagnosis is useful and sometimes essential, but nothing can replace compassionate, ethical clinical care.

With all of this in mind, and despite the limited role of biological tests in psychiatry, diagnosis remains necessary in order to create a common language about psychiatric conditions and human suffering, perform research into new treatments, identify the causes of mental illness, and protect human rights, especially in the setting of admission and treatment without consent. The history of psychiatry suggests that the latter task is especially important and deserves particular attention. Used wisely, diagnosis helps with all of these matters, and can also reduce stigma and advance self-understanding, provided the diagnostic process is approached honestly, openly, and with humility. These qualities are essential in all aspects of psychiatry and they create the context for clear, collaborative diagnosis.

Against this background, it has always intrigued me that the DSM is sometimes described as the 'psychiatrist's bible'. I think that those who say this mean to suggest that psychiatrists regard every word of the DSM as sacred and inviolable, and do not deviate from it in theory or in practice. Although rhetorically catchy and very common, the 'psychiatrist's bible' epithet is something of a strawman. In fact, diagnostic systems such as the DSM and ICD are rarely used in this rigid, inflexible way. No clinician who truly listens to a patient can fail to notice that nobody fits any category perfectly. Life is vastly more complicated than the DSM or ICD could possibly reflect. Human suffering is infinitely variable. As a result, diagnostic criteria need to be held lightly, if at all.

On the other hand, describing the DSM as a 'bible' is not entirely wrong, given the way that most people use their 'bible' or other sacred text in their lives. The vast majority of people who have a 'bible' or bible-equivalent do not take every word literally. Most people ignore vast tracts of their chosen religious text, interpret some parts as metaphors rather than literal truths, and adhere to other parts some of the time, but rarely always. In other words, sacred texts, although held in high esteem, are inevitably interpreted with nuance and awareness, and are sometimes ignored completely, even by self-professed believers.

It is necessary, useful, and wise to treat the DSM and ICD in a similar way. Certain parts of these systems will prove useful in individual cases, other parts might need interpretation, and some sections can be safely ignored. As with religious texts, many of the problems with the DSM and ICD stem from over-literal approaches that try to adhere to every word, but fail to apply the overall messages in a flexible, realistic, compassionate way. Fundamentalism helps nobody: it misses the big picture, ignores the human dimension, and leads to absurdity at best and harm at worst.

In other words, diagnostic systems are helpful guides in uncertain landscapes, but the person always comes first. Human existence is vastly more variegated than the DSM or ICD can ever fully describe, and so is human suffering. For practitioners, recognition of this complexity is deepened by engaging with diagnostic systems in a constructive but critical way, and by listening carefully to what patients and their families tell us. They often have both the problems and the solutions, if we listen with humility and hear what is said.

It is useful to complement awareness of psychiatric classification systems with engagement with accounts of mental illness from different perspectives, not just psychiatric viewpoints. Rachel Aviv's book *Strangers to Ourselves: Stories of Unsettled Minds* is an especially valuable contribution to the literature on this theme (Aviv, 2022). Aviv's fascinating volume examines the lived experience of mental illness from a variety of angles in a range of settings with insight, awareness, and restraint. Understanding takes time, but it is time well spent.

The overall message from this chapter is that the DSM, ICD, and other classification systems have important uses and essential roles, but there is no single interpretative framework that makes sense for everyone all the time. While we have much in common when we suffer, each person is different in many ways. So is their mental illness, and so is their pathway to recovery.

Kate, the 16-year-old school girl whom we met at the start of this chapter, decided to cut her wrists in an effort to 'fill the emptiness, and take the tension away'. Kate was alone in the house at the time, and nobody was expected home for a few hours. Kate inflicted superficial cuts on both her wrists. Afterwards, she felt that the tension was 'partly relieved for a few minutes', but then she felt ashamed. What if her parents found out? What if her brother or sister saw her? Soon, Kate felt 'empty' again, as well as ashamed. She wondered if she should cut herself some more, but resisted.

Kate covered her wrists and told nobody what she had done. She didn't even write it in her journal. Kate continued to attend school and meet her friends, but she also slipped into the habit of harming herself repeatedly, cutting different parts of her body. Soon, this became a regular habit. Kate felt worse on each occasion, but also found it hard to stop. Soon, Kate felt ashamed all the time. She still told no one, but wrote in her journal: 'Still empty. Always empty. What's happening?'

Kate continued to see the school counsellor. Kate spoke to the counsellor about feeling 'empty' and 'ashamed', but did not tell her about the self-harm. The counsellor was nevertheless concerned. She arranged for Kate to see a psychiatrist. The psychiatrist spoke with Kate at length. The psychiatrist recognised that Kate was distressed and experiencing upsetting emotions, but did not appear to be 'mentally ill'. Kate told the psychiatrist about the self-harm, but Kate was clear that she was trying to 'relieve tension', not to end her life. The psychiatrist recognised that Kate had a good relationship with the counsellor and recommended that Kate continue to see her. The psychiatrist did not feel that any particular diagnosis would be either accurate or helpful in Kate's case.

Kate was relieved by the discussion with the psychiatrist and continued to attend the counsellor, although she did not initially share the extent of her self-harm. The counsellor, however, was very experienced and suspected that Kate was harming herself quite frequently. When Kate downplayed this, the counsellor did not press the point. The counsellor felt that maintaining her relationship with Kate was the most important thing, and that Kate would confide more in time.

The counsellor was right. Kate told her more over the following weeks and months. Eventually, Kate showed her wrists to the counsellor, who – to Kate's astonishment – was not shocked by Kate's behaviour. The counsellor said that while she was concerned about Kate, she had seen similar behaviour many times. In other words, the counsellor both demonstrated and told Kate that Kate was not alone in this distress. The feelings and behaviours that overwhelmed Kate did not overwhelm her counsellor when Kate told her about them. Together, they read through the criteria for depression in the ICD. Both Kate and the counsellor felt that Kate did not meet all of these criteria, but Kate recognised some of the symptoms in her own life. Also, she saw that other people were familiar with this general situation, these problems, this behaviour. Kate was not alone.

This was a turning point for Kate. It was not necessary for Kate to be formally diagnosed with a mental illness or to receive formal psychiatric treatment. Kate just needed to know that she was not alone, and that the emotions and actions that seemed to overpower Kate, did not overpower her counsellor, who could listen calmly, nod, and absorb whatever Kate said. The counsellor allowed this to happen by remaining calm but deeply interested in Kate's experiences. The counsellor offered a safe, reliable space. Her demeanor, behaviour and discussion about the ICD let Kate know that other people felt the same 'emptiness' that Kate felt, other people behaved in similar ways, other people felt ashamed, and – with support – other people found a way through this.

Kate found a way to cope, too. With the help of her counsellor, Kate explored her feelings and behaviours, developed new coping mechanisms, invited her parents to two of the counselling sessions, and managed to reduce her self-harming behaviour over time, and eventually stop. With the support of her counsellor and family, Kate moved on with her life, leaving this period in her past, without any need for a psychiatric diagnosis or formal psychiatric care.

Diagnosis is essential and even lifesaving for some people with specific sets of symptoms and problems in their lives. But Kate's story shows that, sometimes, no diagnosis is the best diagnosis of all, especially if the person is already engaging with care and support on their own terms. And, as the psychiatrist in this story demonstrates, sometimes no psychiatry is the best psychiatry of all.

Key Messages

- How to diagnose specific mental illnesses, and to what extent it is useful to do so, have been topics of discussion and debate in psychiatry throughout its history and remain controversial today.
- The symptom-based diagnostic systems most commonly used are the American Psychiatric Association's *Diagnostic and Statistical Manual of Mental Disorders (Fifth Edition) (Text Revision)* (DSM) and the World Health Organization's *ICD-11: International Classification of Diseases (Eleventh Revision)* (ICD).
- Diagnoses based on these classification systems do not necessarily map onto biological conditions; these diagnoses are links between symptoms

and clinical signs on the one hand, and understanding and treatment on the other. They are tools and guides, rather than ends in themselves, and they can always change.

- Used wisely, diagnostic systems create a common language for sharing experiences of mental illness, psychiatric symptoms, and psychological suffering. They also facilitate the study of the causes of, and treatments for, specific collections of symptoms or mental illnesses.
- Clear, published diagnostic systems can bring clarity and accountability to the diagnosis of mental illness and provision of treatment. In this way, they can help prevent the politicisation and misuse of psychiatry and protect human rights, especially in the context of admission and treatment without consent under mental health legislation.
- Risks of diagnostic systems include over-literal interpretation of criteria in individual cases, diagnostic acceleration and diagnostic expansion in order to access services, and general lack of flexibility; the DSM warns explicitly against the latter risk.
- Other potential benefits of the DSM and ICD, once they are used thoughtfully, include reducing stigma, alleviating disproportionate guilt or blame that individuals or families might feel, helping create networks of people affected by similar symptoms, and assisting people in choosing the best treatments.
- Ultimately, the DSM, ICD, and other classification systems have important uses and essential roles, but there is no single interpretative framework that makes sense for everyone all the time. Diagnoses need to be applied and considered in the context of each individual's life, and used as tools for building a shared understanding, rather than rigid categorisation.

References

American Psychiatric Association. *Diagnostic and Statistical Manual of Mental Disorders* (Fifth Edn, Text Revision). Washington, DC: American Psychiatric Association Publishing, 2022.

Aviv R. *Strangers to Ourselves: Stories of Unsettled Minds.* London: Harvill Secker, 2022.

Bhugra D, Popelyuk D, McMullen I. Paraphilias across cultures: contexts and controversies. *Journal of Sex Research* 2010; 47: 242–56 (https://doi.org/10.1080/00224491003699833).

Blazer DG. *The Age of Melancholy: 'Major Depression' and its Social Origins.* New York and Hove: Routledge, 2005.

Bloch S, Reddaway P. *Russia's Political Hospitals: The Abuse of Psychiatry in the Soviet Union.* London: Victor Gollancz, 1977.

Bloch S, Reddaway P. *Soviet Psychiatric Abuse: The Shadow Over World Psychiatry.* Boulder, CO: Westview Press, 1985.

Brown GW, Harris T. *Social Origins of Depression: A Study of Psychiatric Disorder in Women.* London: Tavistock Publications, 1978.

Burns T. *Our Necessary Shadow: The Nature and Meaning of Psychiatry.* London: Allen Lane, 2013.

Clare AW. *Psychiatry in Dissent: Controversial Issues in Thought and Practice.* London: Tavistock Publications Limited, 1976.

Fombonne E. Editorial: is autism overdiagnosed? *Journal of Child Psychology and Psychiatry* 2023; 64: 711–14 (https://doi.org/10.1111/jcpp.13806).

Garfinkel P. *A Life in Psychiatry: Looking Out, Looking In.* Toronto, ON: Barlow, 2014.

Horowitz AV. *Creating Mental Illness.* Chicago and London: The University of Chicago Press, 2002.

Jauhar S, Johnstone M, McKenna PJ. Schizophrenia. *Lancet* 2022; 399: 473–86 (https://doi.org/10.1016/S0140-6736(21)01730-X).

Kelly BD. Compassion, cognition and the illusion of self: Buddhist notes towards more skillful engagement with diagnostic classification systems in psychiatry. In: Shonin E, Van Gordon W, Griffiths MD (eds), *Mindfulness and Buddhist-Derived Approaches in Mental Health and Addiction* (pp. 9–28). Cham: Springer, 2016 (https://doi.org/10.1007/978-3-319-22255-4_2).

Kelly BD. *Mental Health in Ireland: The Complete Guide for Patients, Families,* Health Care Professionals and Everyone Who Wants to Be Well. Dublin: The Liffey Press, 2017.

Kelly BD. *In Search of Madness: A Psychiatrist's Travels Through the History of Mental Illness.* Dublin: Gill Books, 2022.

Kelly BD. *Psychiatry in Dissent*: Anthony Clare's critique, defence and reinvigoration of psychiatry. *BJPsych Advances* 2023; 29: 426–7 (https://doi.org/10.1192/bja.2023.29). (Link to licence: https://creativecommons.org/licenses/by/4.0/) (accessed 7 November 2023).

Mac Ghlionn J. Doctor who helped broaden autism spectrum 'very sorry' for over-diagnosis. *New York Post*, 24 April 2023 (https://nypost.com/2023/04/24/doctor-who-broadened-autism-spectrum-sorry-for-over-diagnosis/) (accessed 23 July 2023).

Munro R. *China's Psychiatric Inquisition: Dissent, Psychiatry and the Law in Post-1949 China.* London: Wildy, Simmonds and Hill Publishing Ltd., 2006.

Pietikainen P. *Madness*: A History. London and New York: Routledge, 2015.

Scull A. *Psychiatry and its Discontents.* Oakland, CA: University of California Press, 2019.

Shenouda J, Barrett E, Davidow AL, Sidwell K, Lescott C, Halperin W, Silenzio VMB, Zahorodny W. Prevalence and disparities in the detection of autism without intellectual disability. *Pediatrics* 2023; 151: e2022056594 (https://doi.org/10.1542/peds.2022-056594).

Shorter E. *What Psychiatry Left Out of the DSM-5: Historical Mental Disorders Today.* New York and London: Routledge, 2015.

Vrigkou E, Stamatakis R, Umla-Runge K. Frequency of diagnostic classification systems' usage by mental health professionals in day-to-day clinical practice. *BJPsych Open* 2022; *8*: S77–8 (https://doi.org/10.1192/bjo.2022.257). (Link to licence: https://creativecommons.org/licenses/by/4.0/) (accessed 23 July 2023).

Watters E. *Crazy Like Us: The Globalization of the American Psyche.* New York: Free Press, 2010.

World Health Organization. *ICD-11: International Classification of Diseases (Eleventh Revision)*. Geneva: World Health Organization, 2019.

World Health Organization. *Basic Documents: Forty-Ninth Edition (Including Amendments Adopted up to 31 May 2019)*. Geneva: World Health Organization, 2020 (https://apps.who.int/gb/bd/) (accessed 23 July 2023).

4   Treating Symptoms and Disorders

Harper was 50 years of age and lived with their partner, CJ. Harper worked as an accountant and usually enjoyed their work. Harper liked to go hiking at the weekend and take long walks with their dog. From earliest childhood, Harper loved being outdoors: working in the garden, hiking, or swimming in the sea.

In the months following their fiftieth birthday, Harper began to feel depressed. Their mood was low, especially in the morning, and they had very little energy. Harper's sleep was also disturbed. They had problems getting to sleep, and, when they eventually fell asleep, they woke many times during the night with strange, disturbing dreams. Harper began to wake early in the morning, at around 4 am, and could not get back to sleep. They felt tired all the time, lost their appetite, and had no desire to spend time in the garden. They rarely went hiking or swimming anymore. CJ almost always walked the dog.

CJ was concerned. Harper was clearly unhappy and possibly depressed. Some days, Harper seemed to despair completely and said they felt hopeless about the future. CJ urged Harper to see their general practitioner (family doctor) to seek treatment and support. Harper was reluctant, saying: 'I don't think anyone can help me'. But, just to keep CJ happy, Harper went to the doctor and told the doctor what was happening.

The doctor suggested that Harper should see a clinical psychologist for treatment for depression. Harper told the doctor that they did not believe in 'talking therapies' and would prefer medication. The doctor felt that Harper had moderate depression which was affecting their life, and which would benefit from a psychological approach or medication. In the end, the doctor arranged for Harper to see the clinical psychologist and also prescribed antidepressant medication. The doctor and Harper had a long discussion about the advantages and disadvantages of psychological therapy and medication, and eventually agreed on this dual treatment plan. The doctor also advised Harper to do their best to walk the dog or at least accompany CJ and the dog because physical activity is helpful, even if it sometimes feels hard. Harper agreed to try.

Over the following three months, Harper's mood and other symptoms improved. They attended appointments with the clinical psychologist and used the insights and techniques that the psychologist identified. Harper also took the antidepressant medication, and experienced no side-effects from it. Harper tried

DOI: 10.4324/9781003378495-5

to walk the dog as much as possible, even though this was hard at first. It took time, but as the months passed, Harper felt better, resumed many of their old activities, and managed to sleep through most nights. CJ was pleased with the improvement. Soon, Harper was fully well again.

A year later, after discussing this episode with their doctor, Harper gradually stopped taking their antidepressant medication. This did not cause any problems. Harper remained well and still used the coping skills and techniques that the clinical psychologist recommended.

Two years later, Harper became depressed again, for no apparent reason. This time, their doctor re-started the antidepressant medication that had helped last time and re-referred Harper to the clinical psychologist. Unfortunately, Harper remained depressed two months later, so the doctor referred Harper to see a psychiatrist. The psychiatrist listened to Harper's concerns and reviewed the treatment options with them. After a detailed discussion, the psychiatrist recommended a different antidepressant medication. Harper tried this for eight weeks, along with attending the clinical psychologist, but still felt deeply depressed. Their mood was low, their appetite was poor, and they had virtually no energy or enthusiasm for anything. 'It's much worse this time', Harper said. CJ agreed.

Soon, Harper began to lose hope and experience suicidal thoughts. Harper did not tell CJ, for fear of upsetting them, but there were days when Harper wondered if life was worth living. One day, Harper even considered ending their own life. Harper had never felt this bad before. At their next appointment with the psychiatrist, Harper asked, in despair: 'Can anything be done?'

Introduction

Treatment can be challenging in psychiatry, just as it often is in other areas of medicine and clinical care. Deciding which treatment to offer depends on a range of factors including a person's presenting symptoms, other conditions or illnesses they might have, their past history of psychiatric treatment (if any), and their personal preferences for one form of treatment over another. While some people prefer psychological approaches to mental health problems, others specifically request medication to help alleviate their symptoms. These preferences need to be taken into account to optimise the likelihood of reaching agreement on a sustainable therapeutic plan and producing the best outcome in the end.

In addition, mental health needs change over time, so treatments and supports that are offered at one point might not prove equally effective at another time. In Harper's case, the treatments that helped Harper initially did not help sufficiently when their problems recurred some years later. This is not uncommon: treatments that helped in the past are usually the best first choice if similar problems recur at a later point, but sometimes a different solution is needed in a new situation. Change is constant.

Against this background, this chapter looks at how treatments are chosen in psychiatry in the first place. Once a problem is described or a diagnosis is made (see Chapter 3: 'Diagnosing Mental Illness'), what is the next step? What is the evidence to support commonly used interventions, such as cognitive-behaviour therapy (CBT), other psychological therapies, mindfulness, antidepressant medication, and antipsychotics? What about other treatments, such as electroconvulsive therapy (ECT), or newer approaches, such as ketamine or psilocybin combined with psychotherapy? How can we choose between these treatments in individual cases? Do they work? Should they be used? If so, when? And for whom?

These issues are central to the practice of psychiatry and lie at the heart of this chapter, which focusses on 'Treating Symptoms and Disorders'. To begin, the chapter outlines the over-arching bio-psycho-social approach to mental health care, and then looks at the evidence-bases for key treatments such as CBT, interpersonal psychotherapy, certain mindfulness-based approaches, antidepressants, ECT, antipsychotics, and some other approaches (e.g., involving ketamine or psilocybin combined with psychotherapy). These discussions are based on systematic reviews, meta-analyses, and guidelines for each treatment, where available. The aim is to describe the benefits of certain treatments, point to evidence to support their use, and note the importance of weighing up adverse effects against benefits. While therapeutic decisions are always specific to the individual involved and their life situation, it is important to understand the underpinning evidence in order to offer the interventions which are most likely to help.

Certain topics require and receive particular attention throughout the chapter. These include suicide and antidepressants, the metabolic side-effects of antipsychotics, and controversies surrounding ECT. Topics such as these form an important part of discussions about psychiatric care, so it is essential that they are weighed against the demonstrated benefits of treatments, and that balanced conclusions are reached.

Bio-Psycho-Social Psychiatry

The bio-psycho-social model of health, illness, and health care was described by George L. Engel, a professor of psychiatry and medicine, in *Science* in 1977 (Engel, 1977). The essence of this framework lies in its acknowledgement of biological, psychological, and social dimensions to health, illness, and health care. In other words, while each illness might have a physical cause (known or unknown), there are also psychological and social aspects to risk, causation, symptoms, treatments, and outcomes. As humans, we are complex actors in complicated environments, subject to a range of different forces and influences which shape our experiences in profound ways over time. All these factors – biological, psychological, and social – must be considered for a full understanding of the causes of illness, its manifestations, preventive paradigms, treatment approaches, and therapeutic outcomes.

In terms of psychology, for example, human behaviour clearly affects the distribution of illnesses which are caused by smoking, alcohol, drug misuse, and other risk-related activities. Analyses of causation, prevention initiatives, or programmes of treatment that ignore the psychological dimensions of these behaviours will have very limited impact. Similarly, the experience of physical symptoms is shaped by the psychology of individuals and groups, as is willingness to seek and accept treatment, along with long-term therapeutic outcomes.

From a social perspective, the distribution of symptoms and illnesses across populations is far from random, as multiple factors determine who gets which illness, how it manifests, when it is treated (if at all), and what the likely outcome will be. These social factors include poverty, inequality, living arrangements, socio-economic circumstances, access to preventive programmes, political stability (or lack thereof), and a range of other matters. Access to care is similarly patterned by social forces, economic conditions, and political contexts, as are the efficacy of interventions which are offered, and outcomes. In short, we are social creatures living in societies, and, as such, the social landscape inevitably has a determinative effect on health, illness, and health care.

This combination of biological, psychological, and social considerations is especially clear in psychiatry, where conditions such as depression and anxiety not only find some of their roots in psychological experiences and social circumstances, but also manifest with a combination of psychological and biological symptoms (see Chapter 3: 'Diagnosing Mental Illness'). In consequence, treatment of depression is based on a bio-psycho-social approach, at least in theory. Treatment can include physical or 'biological' treatments (such as antidepressant medication, antipsychotics, or ECT, reflecting the 'physical' elements of the disorder), psychological therapies (such as CBT, interpersonal psychotherapy, or mindfulness-based approaches, reflecting the 'psychological' or 'mental' dimensions), and social interventions (reflecting the personal, social, and economic contexts in which depression develops) (Kelly, 2017).

Often, specific treatments reflect two or three of the dimensions of this bio-psycho-social model, such as antidepressants that improve sleep, boost mood, and help to re-build social function. The biological, the psychological, and the social are not separate categories: they reflect the same underlying processes. In an ideal world, biological, psychological, and social approaches to any given condition are combined to meet the needs and reflect the circumstances of each individual concerned.

This bio-psycho-social approach can be usefully applied not only to conditions in psychiatry (e.g., depression, schizophrenia, bipolar affective disorder, etc.), but also to illnesses in other areas of medicine (e.g., cardiovascular disease, diabetes mellitus, stroke). All of these conditions, and their treatments, are affected by biological, psychological, and social forces which act (both together and separately) to influence risk, genesis, diagnosis, management, and outcomes. While the relative salience of each of these dimensions varies between illnesses, between people, and over time, all are relevant to varying degrees for most people most of the time. We are complex, multi-dimensional beings who suffer, heal, and help each other in complex, multi-faceted ways.

This bio-psycho-social model is often articulated in contradistinction to what is described as a 'biomedical model', a term which suggests an approach that is based solely on biology and does not take account of psychological or social determinants of health, illness, and health care. The term 'biomedical model' is often used as a strawman in discussions about models of care, especially in psychiatry. It is, at best, an over-simplification or exaggeration, and, at worst, an unjust mischaracterisation of medical approaches to illness and treatment, which have always recognised psychological and social dimensions. It is simply impossible for any practitioner to be unaware of the psychological and social aspects of human suffering and of clinical care, or to have a purely 'biomedical' approach in practice.

Writing about the bio-psycho-social model, Bolton suggested, in 2022, that 'an alternative way of looking at this kind of terminology is that the terms serve as shorthand for methodological assumptions or hypotheses as to where causes and cures will be found, along with whatever evidence supports them':

> In this spirit, I suggest that we can make use of the term 'biopsychosocial model' as a shorthand for methodological assumptions that causes and/or cures of specific conditions at specific stages, including matters of adjustment and quality of life, will generally – across a wide range of conditions – include biological, psychological and social factors, and interactions between them. The contrast is then with the 'biomedical model', which deals with biological factors only.
>
> (Bolton, 2022; p. 229)

There are many challenges to the full and systematic use of a bio-psycho-social approach to mental illness. These challenges relate to both resource limitations in mental health services and changing views about various forms of treatment. The role of psychopharmacology, for example, continues to evolve as the benefits and limitations of different medications are better described and understood over time (Shorter, 2021). While there is strong evidence that psychiatric medications are no less effective than medications in other areas of medicine and are sometimes more efficacious (Leucht et al., 2012), the precise role of various psychotropics remains the subject of discussion in the literature (Dean, 2021). This is precisely as it should be. Debate is essential.

This continued robust discussion also presents an opportunity to better articulate the importance of *non-pharmaceutical* approaches to mental illness, including psychological therapies and social interventions. Many forms of psychotherapy have developed especially strong evidence bases which support their use across multiple conditions (see the discussion of CBT below, for example). Combinations of medication, psychological care, and social support are often the most effective ways to relieve symptoms and improve outcomes. One size does not fit all, and the bio-psycho-social framework has sufficient flexibility to reflect this in practice.

In terms of psychiatry, the bio-psycho-social paradigm raises an interesting issue about 'integrated treatment' by psychiatrists; i.e., the extent to which an individual psychiatrist should both prescribe medication and provide psychotherapy themselves, as opposed to attending only to the pharmaceutical element of care and referring the patient to a separate psychotherapist for psychological treatment. Gabbard and Kay argued, in 2001, that combining medication with psychological care appeared effective (consistent with the bio-psycho-social model), but added that one-person treatment, in which the psychiatrist both prescribes medication and provides psychotherapy, offers specific advantages (Gabbard & Kay, 2001).

In modern, multi-disciplinary mental health teams, it is common that different roles are dispersed across multiple mental health professionals, with psychiatrists looking after the medication element of care and often providing team leadership; trained therapists delivering psychotherapy (e.g., clinical psychologists, nurse specialists, counsellors, or psychiatrists with psychotherapy training); and social workers or others providing social support, employment assistance, and other social interventions. Other team members can include speech and language therapists, dieticians, addiction counsellors, and others.

While this multi-disciplinary structure can optimise the use of different skill sets and provide important diversity in care, it relies on effective teamwork to prevent fragmentation. Used wisely, however, the multi-disciplinary approach is more than the sum of its parts, and strongly supports an assertive renewal of the bio-psycho-social approach in contemporary mental health care. In 2022, Williamson argued that the bio-psycho-social model is 'not dead, but in need of revival':

> There is a disconnect between the education we receive, the competencies we are trained in and the psychiatry that we practice. The biopsychosocial model is valid and useful, but it can be of no use to our patients if we fail to implement it. As such, a concerted effort is required to revive it in practice. Senior psychiatrists should lead by example and formulate, with the appreciation that individuals are more than their diagnoses.
>
> (Williamson, 2022; p. 234)

Against this background, and bearing in mind the overarching bio-psycho-social approach, it is essential that all individual treatments provided within that framework are based on clear evidence of effectiveness. A complete summary of research supporting every treatment in psychiatry is beyond the scope of this (or any) book. Useful summaries of evidence-based interventions in certain areas are provided elsewhere. *The Maudsley Prescribing Guidelines in Psychiatry (14th Edition)*, for example, summarise pharmaceutical approaches to many conditions (Taylor et al., 2021).

Instead of attempting to replicate this and other comprehensive summaries of this nature, the remainder of this chapter examines selected examples of common interventions to illustrate the nature and strength of evidence that is available. It is useful to start with CBT, a psychological therapy that has grown enormously over recent decades, along with interpersonal psychotherapy and mindfulness-based interventions for various conditions.

Cognitive-Behaviour Therapy and Other Psychological and Social Therapies

CBT is a psychological therapy that focusses on the use of cognitive strategies (i.e., techniques related to thinking patterns and habits) and behavioural strategies (i.e., techniques related to actions and behavioural habits), in an effort to re-frame distressing thoughts, enhance coping strategies, reduce symptoms, and promote recovery. The patient will usually meet the psychotherapist over a number of therapeutic sessions and, together, identify errors or unhelpful thinking patterns which may deepen or prolong psychological symptoms. The patient and psychotherapist develop ways to address these errors and habits, and improve symptoms and outcomes.

CBT can be delivered as individual sessions, in group format, online, or though manuals and self-help materials. The ideas that underpin this therapeutic approach can be traced to several ancient philosophies and traditions, including stoicism and Buddhist psychology. CBT as it is currently understood emerged in the mid-twentieth century, as Sigmund Freud's psychoanalysis went into decline and a new cognitive and behavioural paradigm started to emerge. Thought leaders included Albert Ellis and Aaron Beck who developed what became known as the 'cognitive revolution'. In essence, attention shifted from the unconscious mind, which lay at the heart of psychoanalysis, to the conscious mind, which forms the focus of attention in CBT (Rothman, 2023).

Today, there is strong evidence that CBT is highly effective in the management of a range of conditions, including depression, generalised anxiety disorder, panic disorder, social phobia, and post-traumatic stress disorder (Kelly, 2017). For some people with mild or moderate depression, the benefits of CBT can exceed those of antidepressant medication, although both treatments are often used simultaneously.

The dominance of CBT today is both merited and interesting. In 2018, David and colleagues argued that CBT has become 'the *gold-standard* psychological treatment – as the best standard we have in the field currently available – for the following reasons':

(1) CBT is the most researched form of psychotherapy. (2) No other form of psychotherapy has been shown to be systematically superior to CBT; if there are systematic differences between psychotherapies, they typically favor CBT. (3) Moreover, the CBT theoretical models/mechanisms of change have been the most researched and are in line with the current mainstream paradigms of human mind and behavior (e.g., information processing). At the same time, there is clearly room for further improvement, both in terms of CBT's efficacy/effectiveness and its underlying theories/mechanisms of change. We further argue for an integrated scientific psychotherapy, with CBT serving as the foundational platform for integration.

(David et al., 2018; p. 1)

Looking at specific mental illnesses, the published evidence in favour of CBT is consistently clear and reliable. One systematic review of randomised controlled trials in adults with a primary diagnosis of depression which included a CBT intervention identified 91 studies and reported strong evidence that CBT interventions delivered a larger short-term decrease in depression scores compared to treatment-as-usual (López-López et al., 2019). If possible, further research is needed into the use of technology in delivering CBT (e.g., hybrid or multi-media approaches), but the overall message is clear: CBT works for many people with depression.

The evidence is similarly compelling for anxiety disorders. In 2023, a systematic review and network meta-analysis of CBT treatment delivery formats for panic disorder identified 74 trials with 6,699 participants and found clear evidence to support various formats of CBT:

group, guided self-help and individual CBT delivery formats are all superior to treatment as usual having similar effect sizes, and no relevant differences emerged when they were compared head-to-head. On the other hand, CBT delivered as unguided self-help was not superior to treatment as usual. CBT delivered in any format was consistently as accepted as treatment as usual in terms of overall trial dropout rates.

(Papola et al., 2023; p. 621)

Similarly for eating disorders, another systematic review and meta-analysis found that therapist-led CBT was more effective than inactive (waiting lists) and active (any psychotherapy) comparisons in people with bulimia nervosa and binge eating disorder (Linardon et al., 2017). The authors concluded that CBT is effective for eating disorders, although they, too, noted that higher quality clinical trials are needed.

The dominance of CBT should not detract from the benefits of other forms of psychotherapy, which are sometimes overshadowed by CBT. Interpersonal psychotherapy, for example, is a time-limited, manual-based, pragmatic, focused therapy which, like CBT, usually lasts for a few months and is undertaken with a trained psychotherapist (Kelly, 2017). In the context of depression, this approach emphasises that the occurrence of depression is not the patient's fault, and that the disorder has developed in the patient's specific psycho-social context, which is significant in terms of recovery. One meta-analysis of interpersonal psychotherapy for depression identified 38 relevant studies including 4,356 patients and concluded that interpersonal psychotherapy is effective in depression, both as an independent treatment and in combination with pharmacotherapy (Cuijpers et al., 2011). Like CBT, therefore, interpersonal psychotherapy works well for many people with depression.

Other psychotherapies tend to have less clear evidence to support them but still find a place in the infinitely variegated world of psychological approaches to human distress. Psychoanalysis, for example, is still practised, although systematic evidence of its effectiveness is not as clear as the evidence supporting CBT or interpersonal psychotherapy (De Maat et al., 2013). There is, however, considerable variability in how people respond to different therapeutic approaches, so the persistence of psychoanalysis is welcome, even if more evidence is needed before it can be systematically recommended for specific conditions.

Social interventions also commonly function on both social and psychological levels. This reflects the bio-psycho-social origins and effects of many conditions. In the context of depression, for example, there are established relationships between depressive symptoms, traumatic life-events, stressful circumstances, and deficits in social support. Social interventions include provision of social support, measures to increase social engagement, and befriending services for people who are lonely, isolated, or otherwise unsupported. Many of these interventions have both social and psychological dimensions, reflecting the integrated, multi-dimensional nature of mental illness and (ideally) its management. Complex, multi-layered states of mind require complex, multi-layered responses, rooted in the bio-psycho-social framework.

Mindfulness-Based Interventions

Perhaps the most interesting development in recent decades has been the emergence of psychotherapeutic approaches that find some of their roots in Buddhist tradition. Many of these initiatives centre on the practice of 'mindfulness' which became a buzzword in psychotherapy and popular culture in many countries towards the end of the twentieth century.

Mindfulness means paying attention to the present moment, as simply and directly as possible (Kelly, 2019). It involves developing a careful, curious awareness of the sensations, thoughts, and emotions that are present, but not changing or judging them. It involves staying focussed on the present moment as much as possible, and when the mind wanders, gently re-directing it back to direct sensations: the feeling of your feet on the floor, the texture of this book in your hands. The idea of mindfulness is rooted in Buddhist and early Hindu psychology and forms a key part of meditative practices in both traditions. It is an ancient art which also echoes through other psychological and spiritual traditions, many of which incorporate some form of contemplative practice or prayer.

Over recent decades, mindfulness has become part of psychotherapeutic approaches to a range of mental illnesses and psychological symptoms. More specifically, there is now compelling evidence that particular courses of mindfulness-based therapies, provided over an eight-week period, help to prevent relapse of depression (Segal et al., 2018). Data to support this approach have accumulated rapidly but steadily in recent times and merit close attention.

In 2021, one 'systematic review and network meta-analysis' of 'mindfulness-based cognitive therapy [MBCT] for prevention and time to depressive relapse' identified 23 relevant publications of which 17 were randomised controlled trials (McCartney et al., 2021). The results strongly supported the effectiveness of MBCT compared to treatment as usual (TAU):

> MBCT is more effective than TAU in the long-term in preventing relapse of depression and has statistically significant advantages over TAU and placebo for time to relapse of depression. No statistically significant differences were observed between MBCT and active treatment strategies for rate of relapse or time to relapse of depression.
>
> (McCartney et al., 2021; p. 6)

Learning the skills of mindfulness and how to apply them is clearly a powerful technique for preventing relapse in depression, albeit that this practice does not appeal to everyone. Some people prefer approaches that are based primarily on other forms of psychotherapy or medication, so it is vital to understand the patient's views about mindfulness before, during, and after treatment. Seeking to 'systematically review and synthesise the experiences of participants with depression taking part in MBCT', one 'systematic review and meta-ethnographic synthesis' of MBCT in major depression identified 21 qualitative studies of fair quality on this theme:

> Across 21 studies of participants with current or previous depression who had participated in MBCT, three overarching themes were developed: 'Becoming skilled and taking action', 'Acceptance' and 'Ambivalence and Variability'. Participants became skilled through engagement in mindfulness practices, reporting increased awareness, perspective and agency over their experiences. Participants developed acceptance towards their experiences, self and others. There was variability and ambivalence regarding participants' expectations and difficulties within mindfulness practices.
>
> (Williams et al., 2022; p. 1494)

The authors noted that 'many studies were conducted in MBCT-research centres that may hold conflicts of interest' and 'did not address the impact of the participant–researcher relationship thus potentially affecting their interpretations'. Even so, these 'findings help to enhance participant confidence in MBCT, alongside understanding the processes of change and the potential for difficulties. MBCT is beneficial and provides meaningful change for many but remains challenging for some' (pp. 1494–5). Other approaches which involve mindfulness include ACT (acceptance and commitment therapy) which is beyond the scope of the present chapter but is beneficial for many people (Sun et al., 2022).

Despite compelling evidence to support various mindfulness-based interventions, mindfulness has become a victim of its own popularity. Too often, caricatured versions of mindfulness are presented as simple solutions to complex problems, or as easy ways to side-step challenging inter-personal issues that need to be addressed (Purser, 2019). These misrepresentations are regrettable. Mindfulness is a very useful tool but is not the answer to everything. While more research is needed in certain areas, various levels of evidence now support mindfulness-based psychological therapies for some people with mild and moderate depression, anxiety disorders, self-harming behaviour, substance misuse, obsessive-compulsive disorder, and eating disorders (Kelly, 2017). These conditions can be difficult to treat in practice, so any new therapies which are supported by evidence are welcome.

Mindfulness can also help to promote holistic health in chronic medical illness, deepen psychological care during cancer treatment, and assist in terminal care settings. There is particular evidence of benefit in depression, pain conditions, smoking, and addictive disorders (Goldberg et al., 2018). Finally, for some people without psychological problems or mental illness, mindfulness can offer a powerful way to improve general psychological wellbeing. The benefits can be subtle but profound, once mindfulness is practised with diligence, care, and commitment (Segal et al., 2018).

Antidepressant Medication and Electro-Convulsive Therapy

Harper, whom we met in the case history at the start of this chapter, was prescribed an antidepressant medication as part of their treatment for depression. Whenever any medication is considered, it is important that such a prescription forms part of a comprehensive bio-psycho-social treatment plan. Some people are very keen on medication, while others prefer an emphasis on psychological therapies, such as CBT, interpersonal psychotherapy, or mindfulness-based approaches. Working with these preferences can help to strengthen the therapeutic relationship, generate a collaborative management plan, and optimise therapeutic understanding during treatment and recovery.

If an antidepressant medication is to be commenced, clinical guidelines recommend newer agents (e.g., selective-serotonin re-uptake inhibitors) as first-line medications for depression, rather than older agents (e.g., tricyclic anti-depressants or monoamine oxidase inhibitors) (Taylor et al., 2021). Newer antidepressants have fewer side-effects than older ones and are safer, so they are the logical choice if medication is being considered for depression.

But do antidepressants work? This question continually arises during public discussions about depression and merits attention here. The simple answer is that antidepressants are very helpful tools for alleviating depression in many people if they are prescribed with care, used appropriately, monitored sensibly, and form part of a broader treatment plan. Not everyone with depression requires an antidepressant, especially if they have mild or moderate depression which responds to psychological therapy such as CBT. But for some people with moderate or severe depression, antidepressants can help to alleviate a great deal of suffering and can even prove to be lifesaving.

In terms of evidence, one 'systematic review and network meta-analysis' of the 'comparative efficacy and acceptability of 21 antidepressant drugs for the acute treatment of adults with major depressive disorder' published in *The Lancet* in 2018 'identified 28,552 citations and of these included 522 trials comprising 116,477 participants' (Cipriani et al., 2018; p. 1357). The results were unambiguous:

> All antidepressants were more efficacious than placebo in adults with major depressive disorder. Smaller differences between active drugs were found when placebo-controlled trials were included in the analysis, whereas there was more variability in efficacy and acceptability in head-to-head trials.
>
> (Cipriani et al., 2018; p. 1357)

In terms of efficacy, 'in head-to-head studies, agomelatine, amitriptyline, escitalopram, mirtazapine, paroxetine, venlafaxine, and vortioxetine were more effective than other antidepressants'. In terms of 'acceptability, agomelatine, citalopram, escitalopram, fluoxetine, sertraline, and vortioxetine were more tolerable than other antidepressants'. Overall, the authors 'found few differences between antidepressants when all data were considered' (p. 1363). In short, antidepressants work for many people, and the variations between specific antidepressants are small.

In clinical practice, the choice of antidepressant (if medication is to be used) will depend on the severity of the depression, the patient's treatment history, and the patient's preference. It is important that the decision to start an antidepressant is made jointly between the patient and the doctor or mental health team, and is carefully reviewed after approximately six weeks to see if progress is occurring (Kelly, 2017). If progress is not satisfactory, treatment can be adjusted or reconsidered, and other therapeutic modalities considered (e.g., CBT). Treatment is a dynamic process that often requires flexibility over time. Teamwork and good communication are essential.

In terms of side-effects, many people experience no adverse effects whatsoever from antidepressants. Others describe mild side-effects (e.g., transient nausea), but opt to stay on the medication on the basis that the positive effects (e.g., improved mood, better sleep) exceed any adverse effects. Other side-effects can include headache, drowsiness, weight change, and various other effects depending on the specific medication. In all cases, possible adverse effects should be discussed prior to prescription and reconsidered during treatment.

There has been particular discussion regarding antidepressants and suicidality. In 2003, widely publicised warnings from the US Food and Drug Administration about a possible increase in risk of suicidality with antidepressant use in young people were linked with decreased antidepressant use (Lu et al., 2014). Unfortunately, there were simultaneous increases in suicide attempts among young people. This highlights the importance of monitoring and reducing possible unintended consequences of such warnings and media reporting, even when such warnings have a basis in fact. Today, *The Maudsley Prescribing Guidelines in Psychiatry (14th Edition)* note that, in general, suicidality is reduced by antidepressants, but also that antidepressant treatment has been associated with an increased risk of suicidal thoughts and acts in some people, especially adolescents and young adults (Taylor et al., 2021; p. 309). As a result, it is recommended that patients are warned of this potential adverse effect during the early weeks of treatment and are told how to seek help if needed.

If antidepressant medication, CBT, and various other elements of bio-psycho-social treatment do not prove sufficient, and if a person's depression intensifies beyond a certain point, the option of electro-convulsive therapy (ECT) can be considered. ECT can be a controversial treatment, owing not least to its complicated, conflicted history (see Chapter 2: 'The History of Psychiatry'). Accumulated evidence, however, supports its use in specific circumstances. In 2003, the UK ECT Review Group published a systematic review and meta-analysis of the efficacy and safety of ECT in depressive disorders, and concluded that ECT is an effective short-term treatment for depression, and is likely more effective than drug therapy (UK ECT Review Group, 2003).

In 2010, the UK's National Institute for Clinical Excellence published a definitive assessment, recommending ECT for rapid, short-term improvement of severe symptoms after a trial of other treatments had been ineffective and/ or when the condition was potentially life-threatening, in people with severe depressive illness, catatonia, or severe or prolonged mania, following risk-benefit analysis (National Institute for Clinical Excellence, 2010). In 2018, a systematic review further confirmed ECT's role in catatonia (Pelzer et al., 2018) and recent guidelines affirm its role in treatment-resistant depression (Taylor et al., 2021; p. 321).

A full consideration of ECT, including its detailed indications, benefits, and potential adverse effects (which include memory problems), is beyond the scope of the present chapter, as is an account of the development, uses, and misuses of the treatment in the past (for further context, see: Shorter and Healy, 2007). It is, however, important to emphasise that the usual considerations regarding communication, teamwork, and monitoring can go a great distance towards rational, evidence-based use of ECT, optimising efficacy, minimising adverse effects, and strengthening the therapeutic bond. Communication is especially important in the context of ECT owing to widespread stigma and misunderstandings about this useful if controversial treatment.

Antipsychotic Medication

Similar considerations apply to antipsychotic medication. Good communication lies at the heart of rational prescribing and obtaining the best outcomes from antipsychotic medication, which is used in schizophrenia, severe depression with psychosis, mania (in bipolar affective disorder), other conditions involving psychosis, and certain other settings. These medications offer many benefits once they are used with care and consideration, and treatment is reconsidered at regular intervals.

The first effective antipsychotic, chlorpromazine, was developed in the 1950s and was followed by a number of related medications in tablet and injected forms (Kelly, 2017). These agents alleviated psychotic symptoms (e.g., delusions and hallucinations) and made it possible for some long-term patients to leave large psychiatric institutions and live with greater independence in the community. These 'first-generation' or 'typical' antipsychotics included fluphenazine, trifluoperazine, flupentixol, haloperidol, zuclopenthixol, sulpiride, and pimozide.

It was soon apparent that these medications, despite their benefits, can have significant adverse effects, including movement disorders (such as restlessness or Parkinsonism), dry mouth, constipation, sedation, effects on the heart (increasing the risk of sudden cardiac death), and various other effects (e.g., dizziness, sexual dysfunction). A number of strategies were introduced to manage these issues, and research focused on developing new treatments that would combine good clinical effects with fewer side effects. A series of 'second-generation' or 'atypical' antipsychotics was duly developed and introduced to clinical practice.

As a result, there is now a broad range of antipsychotic medications available, with different combinations of benefits and potential adverse effects. 'Atypical' antipsychotics include risperidone, olanzapine, quetiapine, aripiprazole, amisulpride, ziprasidone, and paliperidone. Some of these agents combine therapeutic efficacy with concerning side-effects, such as weight gain and other impacts on metabolism. Clozapine, another antipsychotic, is generally reserved for treatment-resistant schizophrenia. A more detailed consideration of individual medications, their profiles, and their individual roles is beyond the scope of the present chapter and is provided elsewhere (e.g., Taylor et al., 2021). For now, it is sufficient to say that each antipsychotic has its own combination of benefits and side-effects, and each has a different role in the treatment of various forms of psychosis and severe mental illness.

But, given that some of the antipsychotics can have significant adverse effects, what is the evidence that they work? Are the potential negative effects justified by the positive ones?

In 2013, Leucht and colleagues published a meta-analysis of the comparative efficacy and tolerability of 15 antipsychotics for the treatment of schizophrenia in *The Lancet* (Leucht et al., 2013). This research group identified 212 trials suitable for inclusion in the study, with data for 43,049 participants. All 15 antipsychotics were significantly more effective than placebo. The medications differed substantially in side-effects, and there were small but robust differences in efficacy. In addition, the data challenged a simple classification into 'first-generation' and 'second-generation' agents. Instead, the authors found that hierarchies in different domains could help clinicians to match antipsychotic drug choice to the needs of individual patients, rather than simply categorising these medications into two 'generations'.

But what about side-effects? In particular, some 'second-generation' antipsychotics are associated with weight gain. Might this lead to poor physical health, cardiovascular illness, and increased mortality? Many people with schizophrenia are on antipsychotic medication for years or even decades, so might certain long-term adverse effects have a cumulative impact over time? Are these medications worth it?

In 2020, Taipale and colleagues published a follow-up study of physical morbidity and mortality in the context of antipsychotic treatment among 62,250 patients with schizophrenia in Finland (Taipale et al., 2020). After following up these patients for a median of 14 years, this research group found no increase in the risk of hospitalisation for physical illness, including cardiovascular disease, among people with schizophrenia while on antipsychotics. This provides strong evidence that, despite metabolic and other side effects, antipsychotics do not increase the risk of serious physical illness requiring hospitalisation among those taking them. But what about the risk of death?

Taipale and colleagues found that the adjusted hazard ratio for all-cause mortality was 0.48 (95% confidence interval: 0.46–0.51) among people with schizophrenia while on antipsychotics (compared with not being on antipsychotics). There were similar reductions in cardiovascular mortality (0.62; 95% confidence interval: 0.57–0.67) and mortality from suicide (0.52; 95% confidence interval: 0.43–0.62). To put these findings another way, mortality rates during 14 years of follow-up were 46.2% for people with schizophrenia who were not on an antipsychotic, 25.7% for those taking any antipsychotic, and 15.6% for those taking clozapine. These mortality benefits persisted even after adjustment for gender, age, time since diagnosis, previous psychiatric hospitalisations, other medication use, non-adherence, previous suicide attempt, substance abuse, physical comorbidities, and various other factors.

Overall, these results indicate that long-term antipsychotic use does *not* increase the risk of serious physical illness requiring hospitalisation. In fact, antipsychotics are associated with a substantially *decreased* mortality rate among people with schizophrenia, especially those on clozapine. Again, the adverse effects of these medications must be considered in each individual case, not least because some people find the metabolic effects of certain medications so disturbing that they would prefer a different treatment, despite any benefits. Communication and flexibility are vital in this process, including communicating the substantial benefits of antipsychotics in the long term.

New Treatments for Mental Illness

So far in this chapter, we have considered the evidence to support certain treatments for specific mental illnesses: CBT, interpersonal psychotherapy, mindfulness-based approaches, antidepressants, ECT, and antipsychotics. New treatments are also emerging and there has been particular interest in substances such as ketamine and psilocybin recently. While these avenues of research attract a great deal of media attention, this should not distract from the requirement for sound scientific evidence before such substances come into widespread use as treatments for mental illness (if they ever do).

Ketamine, for example, is a dissociative anaesthetic that is also used for pain management and is misused outside medical settings despite considerable risk of adverse effects. In 2023, a systematic review of oral ketamine for depression identified 22 relevant studies, including 4 randomised clinical trials, 1 case series, 6 case-reports, 5 open-label trials, and 6 retrospective chart review studies involving 2,336 people (Meshkat et al., 2023). All the studies included in this review recorded significant improvement following ketamine administration, and good tolerance, but the trials had a high risk of bias owing to analysis methods and adverse events monitoring. More work is needed before ketamine can be systematically used for depression, but these findings are promising.

Notwithstanding the need for further research, one 2023 'systematic review of the print media representation of ketamine treatments for psychiatric disorders' identified 119 print and online news articles, 'peaking in March 2019 when the United States Food and Drug Administration approved esketamine':

Ketamine treatment was portrayed in an extremely positive light (n = 82, 68.9%), with significant contributions of positive testimony from key opinion leaders (e.g. clinicians). Positive research results and ketamine's rapid antidepressant effect (n = 87, 73.1%) were frequently emphasised, with little reference to longer-term safety and efficacy. Side-effects were frequently reported (n = 96, 80.7%), predominantly ketamine's acute psychotomimetic effects and the potential for addiction and misuse, and rarely cardiovascular and bladder effects. Not infrequently, key opinion leaders were quoted as being overly optimistic compared with the existing evidence base.

(Thornton et al., 2023; p. 1)

Over-enthusiastic media coverage such as this can instil false hope and generate expectations that might not be met. As *The Guardian* newspaper noted in response to this study:

Clinical studies show a dose of ketamine treatment does help people with serious clinical depression to rapidly feel better, but this effect usually lasts just a few days [...] The effects of the long-term, repeated use of ketamine treatments need to be more comprehensively studied, and researchers have called for better monitoring and reporting of ketamine-related side effects.

(Davey, 2023)

Similar concerns surround other substances, such as psilocybin (a naturally occurring psychedelic). In 2022, a randomised trial studied the effect of single doses of 25 milligrams, 10 milligrams, and 1 milligram of psilocybin, along with psychological support, for a treatment-resistant episode of major depression (Goodwin et al., 2022); three weeks after administration, 37% of the 25-milligram group had responded, 19% of the 10-milligram group, and 18% of the 1-milligram group. At week 12, the incidence of sustained response was 20% in the 25-milligram group, 5% in the 10-milligram group, and 10% in the 1-milligram group. These are encouraging data in a difficult-to-treat population, but they are neither dramatic nor revolutionary.

Despite careful, credible studies such as this one, with modest, promising results, the world is awash with giddy excitement about psychedelics (Kelly, 2022). People are 'micro-dosing', taking 'facilitated' drug trips, and reporting dramatic breakthroughs after using hallucinogens that have been used to alter minds since ancient times. Research is accumulating, pharmaceutical companies are gearing up, and venture capitalists hover with barely concealed delight at an emerging market.

Before getting carried away, though, it is useful to take a breath and figure out what is going on. Psychedelics are hallucinogenic drugs such as mescaline (derived from cacti), LSD (lysergic acid diethylamide or 'acid'), psilocybin (found in 'magic mushrooms') and DMT (N,N-dimethyltryptamine, a rapid-acting, intense psychedelic). Many of these substances have been used for centuries as part of rituals and religious ceremonies.

Initial effects of some of these drugs can include relaxation and euphoria, accompanied by hallucinations. Negative effects can include confusion, dizziness, diminished concentration, clumsiness, blurred vision, sweating, vomiting, numbness, hyperventilation, and fast or irregular heartbeat. Bad trips can be terrifying and these agents can have long-term effects on mental health.

The idea that some of these substances might be useful for mental illness is not novel. Psilocybin was researched in the 1960s, but abandoned until recently. Today, media discussions often focus on individual stories of psychedelic experiences that were followed by emotional breakthroughs. While these personal stories can be compelling, people with bad experiences are less likely to speak out.

Before psychedelics can be recommended widely, there needs to be systematic evidence that their positive effects outweigh the negatives, especially among people in distress. The recent wave of research suggests that some of these substances might play useful roles in certain circumstances in the future. As we have seen, findings on ketamine and psilocybin give reason for hope, but are not definitive. In the end, these approaches are unlikely to be transformative or appropriate for everyone, but it is probable that some sort of psilocybin-assisted psychotherapy (or similar) will be introduced in the coming years.

Already, esketamine – a variant of ketamine, a sort of psychedelic – is licenced for some people with depression in certain places. In Ireland, for example, the drug can be given in combination with an antidepressant to certain adults with a major depressive disorder who have not responded to at least two different treatments to date. It can also be given for acute short-term treatment of some psychiatric emergencies in specific circumstances. Esketamine can have side effects, so it is highly regulated and carefully supervised, but it is a start.

There is less evidence to support 'micro-dosing'. In 2021, a study of almost 200 people found some improvements after four weeks of taking small amounts of psychedelics, but the benefits were no greater than those in the placebo group (Szigeti et al., 2021). Again, more study is needed (Polito and Liknaitzky, 2022).

From a pragmatic viewpoint, both sides of the psychedelics' discussion are apparent in day-to-day clinical practice. On the one hand, mental health professionals commonly see people who struggle deeply with treatment-resistant depression and post-traumatic stress disorder (PTSD), among other conditions. There are many treatments that help, but more options would be very useful. On the other hand, the negative effects of psychedelics are also apparent: hallucinations, mood problems, lives destroyed by drug misuse, and people who do not recover from bad trips, whose lives are changed forever by magic mushrooms or LSD.

In the end, we need more systematic, randomised clinical trials before psilocybin and similar substances can be safely recommended in clinical care. The most probable outcome is that a number of psychedelics will offer benefits to some people with specific conditions, in combination with psychotherapy. Psychedelics are not a game-changer for psychiatry or the definitive answer to mental illness. Rather less dramatically, they might prove to be one tool among many for some people. While they are likely to be useful, they are unlikely to be first-line treatments for anything any time soon.

The incorporation of psychedelics into mainstream medicine will also change how we see these substances. Anyone with romantic memories of ayahuasca ceremonies on backpacking trips in South America should banish those images immediately. Today, the world of psychedelics is peopled by pharmaceutical executives and venture capitalists, rather than mystics and shamans. The scene is more corporate than counterculture, more pinstripe than tie-dye. That is the price we pay for the evidence we need to use these substances wisely and well (if we use them at all). This psychedelic trip is not over yet.

Harper, the person with recurring depression whom we met at the start of this chapter, did not benefit sufficiently from two different antidepressant medications or psychological therapy. Despite everyone's best efforts, Harper still felt depressed, exhausted, and, at times, suicidal. Sometimes, Harper felt they were 'beyond help'. Their partner, CJ, was increasingly worried.

At Harper's next appointment, the psychiatrist considered all the options and decided to discuss the possibility of electro-convulsive therapy (ECT). Harper was shocked: 'Do they still do that?' Harper had only seen ECT in movies. 'Yes', said the psychiatrist, 'ECT is still used in certain, very limited circumstances. This is one of those times: treatment-resistant depression that has become life-threatening'. This rang true with Harper, who often felt that they should end their life. 'But I'm not coming into hospital', Harper said: 'I want to stay at home'.

Harper asked the psychiatrist if CJ could take part in the discussion. CJ attended another appointment with Harper the next day. The psychiatrist explained about ECT: the reasons for using it, the nature of the treatment, and its possible side-effects, especially its potential impact on memory. Harper and CJ were surprised to hear that ECT was still used, but they were also aware of the severity of the situation. As CJ said: 'I don't think Harper will make it to next week unless we do something.' Despite all the treatment, all the support, and all the love that CJ provided, Harper remained suicidal. Even though Harper was in a state of deep despair and barely ate or slept, CJ was happy for Harper to stay at home if it meant that Harper would get some treatment that might benefit them.

Harper received ECT treatment twice per week over the following four weeks. Harper attended the ECT clinic as an outpatient, arriving for the treatment in the morning, and waiting around for a few hours after each treatment to ensure that they recovered fully from the anaesthetic. CJ came to the clinic with Harper each time and remarked on the improvement that became apparent after the second week. Progress was slow but definite. At the end of eight weeks, Harper's mood was significantly brighter and their suicidal thoughts had gone. Harper's appetite and sleep also improved, and they even took the dog for walks. Harper experienced no side-effects from ECT, only benefit.

After the course of treatment was finished, Harper remained on an antidepressant medication and continued to see the clinical psychologist. They paid particular attention to their diet, lifestyle, and stress levels, in order to try to remain well. Most of all, they devoted time and attention to their partner, CJ, who had been a steadfast support through everything. Harper had no more episodes of depression, and later commented: 'ECT saved my life, but CJ makes life worth living'.

Key Messages

- Deciding which treatment to use in psychiatry depends on a range of factors including a person's presenting symptoms, other conditions or illnesses they have, their past history of treatment (if any), and their personal preferences for one form of treatment over another.
- Mental health needs change over time, so treatments and supports that are offered at one point might not prove equally effective at another time. Communication and flexibility are essential to optimise outcomes.
- The bio-psycho-social model of mental health care acknowledges biological, psychological, and social dimensions to health, illness, and treatment. While each condition might have a physical cause (known or unknown), there are also psychological and social aspects to risk, causation, symptoms, treatments, and outcomes.
- Cognitive-behaviour therapy (CBT) is highly effective in the management of a range of conditions, including depression, generalised anxiety disorder, panic disorder, social phobia, and post-traumatic stress disorder. It is the form of psychotherapy that is best supported by evidence at present.
- Other psychological therapies include interpersonal psychotherapy for depression, mindfulness-based approaches for a wide range of conditions, psychoanalysis, and various others.
- Evidence strongly supports the effectiveness of antidepressants for many people with depression. Variations between antidepressants are small, so choice of antidepressant (if medication is to be used) depends on the severity of the depression, the patient's treatment history, and the patient's preference.
- Electro-convulsive therapy is recommended for rapid, short-term improvement of severe symptoms after a trial of other treatments has been ineffective and/or when the condition is potentially life-threatening, in people with severe depressive illness, catatonia, or severe or prolonged mania, following risk-benefit analysis. Potential adverse effects include memory problems.
- Evidence strongly supports the effectiveness of antipsychotic medication for psychotic conditions such as schizophrenia. Long-term antipsychotic use

does *not* increase the risk of serious physical illness requiring hospitalisation and is associated with a substantially *decreased* mortality rate among people with schizophrenia.

- Potential new treatments, such as ketamine and psilocybin, often in combination with psychotherapy, attract a great deal of attention, but this should not distract from the requirement for a sound evidence base before such substances come into widespread use (if they ever do). Initial results are promising, but more data are needed before they can be recommended for systematic use in day-to-day clinical practice.

References

Bolton D. Looking forward to a decade of the biopsychosocial model. *BJPsych Bulletin* 2022; 46: 228–32 (https://doi.org/10.1192/bjb.2022.34). (Link to licence: https://creativecommons.org/licenses/by/4.0/) (accessed 15 August 2023).

Cipriani A, Furukawa TA, Salanti G, Chaimani A, Atkinson LZ, Ogawa Y, Leucht S, Ruhe HG, Turner EH, Higgins JPT, Egger M, Takeshima N, Hayasaka Y, Imai H, Shinohara K, Tajika A, Ioannidis JPA, Geddes JR. Comparative efficacy and acceptability of 21 antidepressant drugs for the acute treatment of adults with major depressive disorder: a systematic review and network meta-analysis. *Lancet* 2018; 391: 1357–66 (https://doi.org/10.1016/S0140-6736(17)32802-7). (Link to licence: https://creativecommons.org/licenses/by/4.0/) (accessed 15 August 2023).

Cuijpers P, Geraedts AS, van Oppen P, Andersson G, Markowitz JC, van Straten A. Interpersonal psychotherapy for depression: a meta-analysis. *American Journal of Psychiatry* 2011; 168: 581–92 (https://doi.org/10.1176/appi.ajp.2010.10101411).

Davey M. 'Beyond the evidence': media reports overhype ketamine's use as a depression treatment, review finds. *Guardian*, 8 June 2023 (https://www.theguardian.com/australia-news/2023/jun/08/beyond-the-evidence-media-reports-overhype-ketamines-use-as-a-depression-treatment-review-finds) (accessed 17 August 2023). (Courtesy of Guardian News & Media Ltd.).

David D, Cristea I, Hofmann SG. Why cognitive behavioral therapy is the current gold standard of psychotherapy. *Frontiers in Psychiatry* 2018; *9*: 4 (https://doi.org/10.3389/fpsyt.2018.00004). (Link to licence: https://creativecommons.org/licenses/by/4.0/) (accessed 15 August 2023).

Dean CE. *The Skeptical Professional's Guide to Psychiatry: On the Risks and Benefits of Antipsychotics, Antidepressants, Psychiatric Diagnoses, and Neuromania*. New York and London: Routledge, 2021.

De Maat S, de Jonghe F, de Kraker R, Leichsenring F, Abbass A, Luyten P, Barber JP, Van R, Dekker J. The current state of the empirical evidence for psychoanalysis: a meta-analytic approach. *Harvard Review of Psychiatry* 2013; 21: 107–37 (https://doi.org/10.1097/HRP.0b013e318294f5fd).

Engel GL. The need for a new medical model: a challenge for biomedicine. *Science* 1977; 196: 129–36 (https://doi.org/10.1126/science.847460).

Gabbard GO, Kay J. The fate of integrated treatment: whatever happened to the biopsychosocial psychiatrist? *American Journal of Psychiatry* 2001; 158: 1956–63 (https://doi.org/10.1176/appi.ajp.158.12.1956).

Goldberg SB, Tucker RP, Greene PA, Davidson RJ, Wampold BE, Kearney DJ, Simpson TL. Mindfulness-based interventions for psychiatric disorders: a systematic review and meta-analysis. *Clinical Psychology Review* 2018; 59: 52–60 (https://doi.org/10 .1016/j.cpr.2017.10.011).

Goodwin GM, Aaronson ST, Alvarez O, Arden PC, Baker A, Bennett JC, Bird C, Blom RE, Brennan C, Brusch D, Burke L, Campbell-Coker K, Carhart-Harris R, Cattell J, Daniel A, DeBattista C, Dunlop BW, Eisen K, Feifel D, Forbes MK, Haumann HM, Hellerstein DJ, Hoppe AI, Husain MI, Jelen LA, Kamphuis J, Kawasaki J, Kelly JR, Key RE, Kishon R, Knatz Peck S, Knight G, Koolen MHB, Lean M, Licht RW, Maples-Keller JL, Mars J, Marwood L, McElhiney MC, Miller TL, Mirow A, Mistry S, Mletzko-Crowe T, Modlin LN, Nielsen RE, Nielson EM, Offerhaus SR, O'Keane V, Páleníček T, Printz D, Rademaker MC, van Reemst A, Reinholdt F, Repantis D, Rucker J, Rudow S, Ruffell S, Rush AJ, Schoevers RA, Seynaeve M, Shao S, Soares JC, Somers M, Stansfield SC, Sterling D, Strockis A, Tsai J, Visser L, Wahba M, Williams S, Young AH, Ywema P, Zisook S, Malievskaia E. Single-dose psilocybin for a treatment-resistant episode of major depression. *New England Journal of Medicine* 2022; 387: 1637–48 (https://doi.org/10.1056/NEJMoa2206443).

Kelly BD. *Mental Health in Ireland: The Complete Guide for Patients, Families,* Health Care Professionals and Everyone Who Wants to Be Well. Dublin: The Liffey Press, 2017.

Kelly BD. *The Doctor Who Sat For A Year.* Dublin: Gill Books, 2019.

Kelly BD. Psychedelic drugs as healthcare? This trip has a long way to go. *Irish Independent,* 9 July 2022 (https://www.independent.ie/life/health-wellbeing/ psychedelic-drugs-and-how-to-change-your-mind-are-the-mental-health-benefits -real/41823268.html) (accessed 17 August 2023).

Leucht S, Cipriani A, Spineli L, Mavridis D, Örey D, Richter F, Samara M, Barbui C, Engel RR, Geddes JR, Kissling W, Stapf MP, Lässig B, Salanti G, Davis JM. Comparative efficacy and tolerability of 15 antipsychotic drugs in schizophrenia: a multiple-treatments meta-analysis. *Lancet* 2013; 382: 951–62 (https://doi.org/10.1016 /S0140-6736(13)60733-3).

Leucht S, Hierl S, Kissling W, Dold M, Davis JM. Putting the efficacy of psychiatric and general medicine medication into perspective: review of meta-analyses. *British Journal of Psychiatry* 2012; 200: 97–106 (https://doi.org/10.1192/bjp.bp.111.096594).

Linardon J, Wade TD, De la Piedad Garcia X, Brennan L. The efficacy of cognitive-behavioral therapy for eating disorders: a systematic review and meta-analysis. *Journal of Consulting and Clinical Psychology* 2017; 85: 1080–94 (https://doi.org/10 .1037/ccp0000245).

López-López JA, Davies SR, Caldwell DM, Churchill R, Peters TJ, Tallon D, Dawson S, Wu Q, Li J, Taylor A, Lewis G, Kessler DS, Wiles N, Welton NJ. The process and delivery of CBT for depression in adults: a systematic review and network meta-analysis. *Psychological Medicine* 2019; 49: 1937–47 (https://doi.org/10.1017 /S003329171900120X). (Link to licence: https://creativecommons.org/licenses/by/4 .0/) (accessed 15 August 2023).

Lu CY, Zhang F, Lakoma MD, Madden JM, Rusinak D, Penfold RB, Simon G, Ahmedani BK, Clarke G, Hunkeler EM, Waitzfelder B, Owen-Smith A, Raebel MA, Rossom R, Coleman KJ, Copeland LA, Soumerai SB. Changes in antidepressant use by young people and suicidal behavior after FDA warnings and media coverage: quasi-experimental study. *BMJ* 2014; 348: g3596 (https://doi.org/10.1136/bmj.g3596).

McCartney M, Nevitt S, Lloyd A, Hill R, White R, Duarte R. Mindfulness-based cognitive therapy for prevention and time to depressive relapse: systematic review and network meta-analysis. *Acta Psychiatrica Scandinavica* 2021; 143: 6–21 (https://doi.org/10.1111/acps.13242). (Link to licence: https://creativecommons.org/licenses/by/4.0/) (accessed 16 August 2023).

Meshkat S, Haikazian S, Di Vincenzo JD, Fancy F, Johnson D, Chen-Li D, McIntyre RS, Mansur R, Rosenblat JD. Oral ketamine for depression: an updated systematic review. *World Journal of Biological Psychiatry* 2023; 24: 545–57 (https://doi.org/10.1080/15622975.2023.2169349).

National Institute for Clinical Excellence. *The Use of Electroconvulsive Therapy* (Update: May 2010). London: National Institute for Clinical Excellence, 2010 (https://www.nice.org.uk/guidance/ta59/resources/the-use-of-electroconvulsive-therapy-pdf-371522989) (accessed 16 August 2023).

Papola D, Ostuzzi G, Tedeschi F, Gastaldon C, Purgato M, Del Giovane C, Pompoli A, Pauley D, Karyotaki E, Sijbrandij M, Furukawa TA, Cuijpers P, Barbui C. CBT treatment delivery formats for panic disorder: a systematic review and network meta-analysis of randomised controlled trials. *Psychological Medicine* 2023; 53: 614–24 (https://doi.org/10.1017/S0033291722003683). (Link to licence: https://creativecommons.org/licenses/by/4.0/) (accessed 15 August 2023).

Pelzer ACM, van der Heijden FMMA, den Boer E. Systematic review of catatonia treatment. *Neuropsychiatric Disease and Treatment* 2018; 14: 317–26 (https://doi.org/10.2147/NDT.S147897).

Polito V, Liknaitzky P. The emerging science of microdosing: a systematic review of research on low dose psychedelics (1955–2021) and recommendations for the field. *Neuroscience and Biobehavioral Reviews* 2022; 139: 104706 (https://doi.org/10.1016/j.neubiorev.2022.104706).

Purser RE. *McMindfulness*: How Mindfulness Became the New Capitalist Spirituality. London: Repeater Books, 2019.

Rothman J. Can cognitive behavioral therapy change our minds? *New Yorker*, 10 July 2023 (https://www.newyorker.com/culture/annals-of-inquiry/can-cognitive-behavioral-therapy-change-our-minds) (accessed 15 August 2023).

Segal Z, Williams M, Teasdale J. *Mindfulness-Based Cognitive Therapy for Depression* (Second Edn). New York and London: The Guilford Press, 2018.

Shorter E. *The Rise and Fall of the Age of Psychopharmacology*. New York: Oxford University Press, 2021.

Shorter E, Healy D. *Shock Therapy: A History of Electroconvulsive Treatment in Mental Illness*. New Brunswick, NJ and London: Rutgers University Press, 2007.

Sun Y, Ji M, Zhang X, Chen J, Wang Y, Wang Z. Comparative effectiveness and acceptability of different ACT delivery formats to treat depression: a systematic review and network meta-analysis of randomized controlled trials. *Journal of Affective Disorders* 2022; 313: 196–203 (https://doi.org/10.1016/j.jad.2022.06.017).

Szigeti B, Kartner L, Blemings A, Rosas F, Feilding A, Nutt DJ, Carhart-Harris RL, Erritzoe D. Self-blinding citizen science to explore psychedelic microdosing. *eLife* 2021; 10: e62878 (https://doi.org/10.7554/elife.62878).

Taipale H, Tanskanen A, Mehtälä J, Vattulainen P, Correll CU, Tiihonen J. 20-year follow-up study of physical morbidity and mortality in relationship to antipsychotic treatment in a nationwide cohort of 62,250 patients with schizophrenia (FIN20). *World Psychiatry* 2020; 19: 61–8 (https://doi.org/10.1002/wps.20699).

Taylor DM, Barnes TRE, Young AH. *The Maudsley Prescribing Guidelines in Psychiatry* (14th Edn). Hoboken, NJ and Chichester: Wiley Blackwell/John Wiley & Sons, Inc., 2021.

Thornton NLR, Kawalsky J, Milton A, Klinner C, Schokman A, Stratton E, Loo CK, Glozier N. A systematic review of the print media representation of ketamine treatments for psychiatric disorders. *BJPsych Open* 2023; 9: e104 (https://doi.org/10 .1192/bjo.2023.75). (Link to licence: https://creativecommons.org/licenses/by/4.0/) (accessed 17 August 2023).

UK ECT Review Group. Efficacy and safety of electroconvulsive therapy in depressive disorders: a systematic review and meta-analysis. *Lancet* 2003; 361: 799–808 (https:// doi.org/10.1016/S0140-6736(03)12705-5).

Williams K, Hartley S, Langer S, Manandhar-Richardson M, Sinha M, Taylor P. A systematic review and meta-ethnographic synthesis of mindfulness-based cognitive therapy for people with major depression. *Clinical Psychology and Psychotherapy* 2022; 29: 1494–514 (https://doi.org/10.1002/cpp.2773). (Link to licence: https:// creativecommons.org/licenses/by/4.0/) (accessed 15 August 2023).

Williamson S. The biopsychosocial model: not dead, but in need of revival. *BJPsych Bulletin* 2022; 46: 232–4 (https://doi.org/10.1192/bjb.2022.29). (Link to licence: https://creativecommons.org/licenses/by/4.0/) (accessed 15 August 2023).

5   Treatment Without Consent

Peter was seventeen when he first heard voices. He had a happy childhood to that point, although he struggled with school from a young age. Peter found it difficult to concentrate on learning, and his grades were often low. He had one or two friends but tended to isolate himself, especially in his early teenage years. Peter did not like sports and rarely spoke with his sister, who was five years younger. Nonetheless, he seemed content.

When Peter was seventeen, he became more distant from his family and friends. He was now silent most of the time and spent long periods in his bedroom on the Internet. His parents thought he seemed depressed but also wondered if this might be usual teenage behaviour. They sometimes heard Peter talking in his room at night but did not know if he was talking with someone on the Internet or talking to himself. After several months, Peter's parents asked Peter to see their family doctor. Peter was now 18.

Peter told the doctor that he felt lonely. He also said he heard two voices talking to him. He said the voices came from outside his head and were as loud and clear as the doctor's voice. One voice was a man who made comments about Peter: 'Peter is sitting in his room. Peter has no friends. Peter is thinking too much.' The other voice was a woman, telling Peter things about another planet: 'Everything is different there. But you already know this. It is a purple planet. But you already know this, Peter, don't you?'

Peter was afraid to tell anyone about his experiences, but they frightened him every day. Some nights, he could not sleep at all. He was relieved to tell the doctor about the voices, but also scared: 'Am I losing my mind?'

Peter's doctor told him that other people experienced these symptoms too, that these were signs of a mental illness, and treatment was available. The doctor prescribed an anti-psychotic medication for Peter and arranged for him to see a psychiatrist later that week. Peter was relieved but also anxious. 'Am I losing my mind?', he asked again, as he left the doctor's consultation room. 'No', repeated the doctor, 'but treatment and support will help'.

The psychiatrist provided Peter with further explanation, linked him with a community mental health nurse to visit Peter and his family at home, and continued the medication that Peter's family doctor had started. A month later, however, the situation had deteriorated.

DOI: 10.4324/9781003378495-6

Peter changed his mind about taking medication, having read that it can have side effects. Instead, someone Peter met on the Internet offered to sell him cannabis which, the person said, would 'change Peter's mind'. Peter started to smoke cannabis in the hope of relieving his symptoms. Cannabis had the opposite effect: it made the voices stronger and more negative, and made Peter more paranoid about the 'purple planet'. The voices now told Peter that he was already on the 'purple planet' and that people would soon come to 'take him to another area and kill him'.

Soon, Peter refused to leave his bedroom for any reason. He was constantly talking or shouting to himself and did not sleep at night. Peter's parents were very worried and phoned the family doctor. When the doctor visited the house, Peter refused to talk with her, remaining entirely silent in his room until she left. Peter refused any treatment, saying: 'There's no point. You know what is happening. You all know. Stop pretending.'

Peter's parents spoke to the family doctor again, who advised that Peter might require involuntary admission and treatment in an inpatient psychiatric facility, like a psychiatric hospital or the psychiatric ward of a general hospital. Peter's parents had no idea how such treatment could be arranged. They asked the doctor: 'Is that even possible? Is it the right thing to do?'

Introduction

Involuntary admission and treatment for mental illness is, rightly, a controversial and contested topic. Any deprivation of liberty or treatment without consent represents a significant curtailment of a person's autonomy, an intrusion into their lives, and a limitation of the observance of fundamental human rights for a period of time. And yet, virtually every jurisdiction in the world has legislation that permits involuntary admission and treatment for serious mental illness provided certain conditions are met and specific safeguards are put in place to avoid injustice.

For Peter, involuntary admission and treatment would mean that his family or someone else starts a legal process that generally involves a number of assessments and ends with a decision by a psychiatrist or, in some jurisdictions, a judge about whether or not involuntary care is justified, and for how long. These assessments generally take account of the nature and severity of Peter's symptoms, the level of risk his illness seems to pose, Peter's decision-making capacity, and the likelihood of Peter benefiting from treatment.

This chapter explores various legal issues associated with this process, as well as its risks and benefits. The chapter starts by outlining, as an example, one legal model of involuntary care, in the Republic of Ireland. The chapter summarises relevant human rights standards developed by international bodies such as the World Health Organisation (WHO) and the United Nations (UN), especially the UN Convention on the Rights of Persons with Disabilities (CRPD;

United Nations, 2006) and the diametrically opposed views of various UN bodies. It then examines international variations in rates of involuntary admission and what these might indicate, and finally, asks whether involuntary treatment should ever occur.

Legal Models of Involuntary Care

Legislation governing involuntary psychiatric care varies across jurisdictions. For the purpose of illustration, the Republic of Ireland provides a good example of key issues raised by mental health legislation, most of which also arise in different ways across other jurisdictions. These issues centre on definitions of 'mental illness' or 'mental disorder' in law, the role of apparent dangerousness in involuntary admission, and the relevance of decision-making capacity in different jurisdictions.

Involuntary treatment in Ireland is governed by the Mental Health Act 2001. The 2001 Act states that 'a person may be involuntarily admitted to an approved centre pursuant to an application under section 9 or 12 and detained there on the grounds that he or she is suffering from a mental disorder' (Section 8(1)). The Act defines 'mental disorder':

> In this Act 'mental disorder' means mental illness, severe dementia or significant intellectual disability where –
>
> (a) because of the illness, disability or dementia, there is a serious likelihood of the person concerned causing immediate and serious harm to himself or herself or to other persons, or
>
> (b) (i) because of the severity of the illness, disability or dementia, the judgment of the person concerned is so impaired that failure to admit the person to an approved centre would be likely to lead to a serious deterioration in his or her condition or would prevent the administration of appropriate treatment that could be given only by such admission, and
>
> (ii) the reception, detention and treatment of the person concerned in an approved centre would be likely to benefit or alleviate the condition of that person to a material extent.
>
> (Section 3(1))

In relative terms, this is a quite specific definition of 'mental disorder'. It contrasts with the definition in the Mental Health Act 1983 in England and Wales (a neighbouring and broadly comparable jurisdiction), which defines 'mental disorder' very broadly, as 'any disorder or disability of the mind' (Section 1(2)). The Irish definition is more detailed because it also serves as the criteria for involuntary admission. Irish legislation goes on to define 'mental illness', 'severe dementia', and 'significant intellectual disability' in precise terms:

- 'Mental illness' means a state of mind of a person which affects the person's thinking, perceiving, emotion or judgment and which seriously impairs the mental function of the person to the extent that he or she requires care or medical treatment in his or her own interest or in the interest of other persons;
- 'Severe dementia' means a deterioration of the brain of a person which significantly impairs the intellectual function of the person thereby affecting thought, comprehension and memory and which includes severe psychiatric or behavioural symptoms such as physical aggression;
- 'Significant intellectual disability' means a state of arrested or incomplete development of mind of a person which includes significant impairment of intelligence and social functioning and abnormally aggressive or seriously irresponsible conduct on the part of the person (Section 3(2)).

Ireland's Mental Health Act 2001 specifies that a person shall not be involuntarily admitted 'by reason only of the fact that the person (a) is suffering from a personality disorder, (b) is socially deviant, or (c) is addicted to drugs or intoxicants' (Section 8(2)). There are similar (although not identical) exclusions in England and Wales in relation to 'learning disability' unless the 'disability is associated with abnormally aggressive or seriously irresponsible conduct' (Section 1(2A)); their 1983 Act also states that 'dependence on alcohol or drugs is not considered to be a disorder or disability of the mind' in this context (Section 1(3)).

While these provisions are similar to those in many other jurisdictions, there are variations on these themes around the world. In India, for example, the Mental Healthcare Act 2017 defines 'mental illness' more broadly than in Ireland, and specifically includes substance misuse but excludes learning disability:

'Mental illness' means a substantial disorder of thinking, mood, perception, orientation or memory that grossly impairs judgment, behaviour, capacity to recognise reality or ability to meet the ordinary demands of life, mental conditions associated with the abuse of alcohol and drugs, but does not include mental retardation which is a condition of arrested or incomplete development of mind of a person, specially characterised by subnormality of intelligence.

(Section 2(1)(s))

The Indian legislation specifies that 'mental illness shall be determined in accordance with such nationally or internationally accepted medical standards (including the latest edition of the International Classification of Disease of the World Health Organisation) as may be notified by the Central Government' (Section 3(1)). In addition:

(3) Mental illness of a person shall not be determined on the basis of (a) political, economic or social status or membership of a cultural, racial

or religious group, or for any other reason not directly relevant to mental health status of the person; (b) non-conformity with moral, social, cultural, work or political values or religious beliefs prevailing in a person's community.

(4) Past treatment or hospitalisation in a mental health establishment though relevant, shall not by itself justify any present or future determination of the person's mental illness (Section 3).

Returning to Ireland's criteria for 'mental disorder' and, thus, involuntary admission, there are two specific criteria, only one of which the person with 'mental illness, severe dementia or significant intellectual disability' must fulfil: (a) the 'risk' criterion, or (b) the 'treatment' criterion. A person can fulfil both criteria, but that is not necessary for involuntary admission to occur; only one is needed.

The 'risk' criterion requires that, 'because of the illness, disability or dementia, there is a serious likelihood of the person concerned causing immediate and serious harm to himself or herself or to other persons' (Section 3(1)(a). There are two problems with this criterion. First, this is an explicitly risk-based criterion, despite plentiful evidence that the accuracy of risk assessment in psychiatry is significantly limited (Connors and Large, 2023). Nobody can predict the future with sufficient reliability to justify deprivation of liberty, even in high-risk populations (Gulati et al., 2020). The second problem with Ireland's 'risk' criterion is that it does not include a requirement that the person will benefit from treatment. In theory, this permits involuntary admission of a person even if there is no prospect of them benefiting from that admission; were this to occur, it would be legal but, presumably, unethical.

The second criterion for involuntary admission in Ireland is the 'treatment' criterion, which requires that '(i) because of the severity of the illness, disability or dementia, the judgment of the person concerned is so impaired that failure to admit the person to an approved centre would be likely to lead to a serious deterioration in his or her condition or would prevent the administration of appropriate treatment that could be given only by such admission', and '(ii) the reception, detention and treatment of the person concerned in an approved centre would be likely to benefit or alleviate the condition of that person to a material extent' (Section 3(1)(b)).

While this criterion requires the 'judgment of the person' to be 'impaired' in a specific way, it is not an explicitly capacity-based criterion, with the result that a person who still possesses decision-making capacity could be admitted as an involuntary patient. This concern is mitigated in part, but not in full, by Section 57 of the 2001 Act (in which the word 'patient' means *involuntary* patient):

The consent of a patient shall be required for treatment except where, in the opinion of the consultant psychiatrist responsible for the care and treatment of the patient, the treatment is necessary to safeguard the life of the patient, to restore his or her health, to alleviate his or her condition, or to relieve his or her suffering, and by reason of his or her mental disorder the patient concerned is incapable of giving such consent.

(Section 57(1))

This creates the peculiar possibility that a person with decision-making capacity could be detained under the 'treatment' criterion, but then refuse all treatment. In this situation, it appears likely that the person would not meet the requirement of the 'treatment' criterion that 'the reception, detention and treatment of the person concerned in an approved centre would be likely to benefit or alleviate the condition of that person to a material extent' (Section 3(1)(b)(ii)). As a result, the patient would have to be discharged, but they could be detained under the 'risk' criterion (which has no 'treatment' requirement) if they are deemed to present sufficient risk.[1]

As a result, the Irish legislation's position on decision-making capacity is interesting and not entirely logical because it permits the involuntary admission of people who possess decision-making capacity, but not their involuntary treatment. Ireland is by no means alone in presenting rather convoluted criteria for involuntary admission and treatment, especially in relation to decision-making capacity. In India, the Mental Healthcare Act 2017 sets out criteria for 'supported admission' which include that 'the person is ineligible to receive care and treatment as an independent [voluntary] patient because the person is unable to make mental healthcare and treatment decisions independently and needs very high support from his nominated representative in making decisions' (Section 89(1)(c)). As a result, lack of decision-making capacity is part of the criteria for admission as this category of patient in India. In relation to treatment:

(7) If a person with the mental illness admitted under this section requires nearly hundred per cent. support from his nominated representative in making a decision in respect of his treatment, the nominated representative may temporarily consent to the treatment plan of such person on his behalf.

(8) In case where consent has been given under sub-section (7), the medical officer or mental health professional in charge of the mental health establishment shall record such consent in the medical records and review the capacity of the patient to give consent every seven days (Section 89).

While the Indian legislation differs significantly from the Irish legislation, both engage with the idea of decision-making capacity and regard it as relevant to varying degrees in relation to involuntary treatment. These issues are apparent in much mental health legislation around the world, although they are often managed in different ways.

In the case of Peter, the young man with psychosis whom we met at the start of this chapter, the Irish legislation outlines a three-step involuntary admission process. The first step involves a relative, member of the health service, police officer, or someone else completing an 'Application' form which requests that the person is involuntarily admitted to a specified inpatient psychiatry unit or hospital. The 'applicant' then arranges for examination by a medical doctor who is not linked with the named inpatient psychiatry unit or hospital, and this doctor can complete a 'Recommendation' that such admission is needed. Then, after the person arrives at the inpatient psychiatry unit or hospital, a consultant psychiatrist has 24 hours to complete the third step or 'Admission Order' if they conclude that the person meets criteria for 'mental disorder' in the legislation.[2]

This process is outlined in detail in Ireland's Mental Health Act 2001, which also provides for automatic reviews by mental health tribunals, appeals to courts, and mandatory, free legal representation for patients. All told, Ireland's legislation is relatively standard in international terms and highlights key issues that arise in many jurisdictions, including the complexities of legal definitions of 'mental illness' or 'mental disorder', the central role of risk in criteria for involuntary care (despite our very limited ability to assess risk), and the complex interaction between decision-making capacity and involuntary care in many countries. Like all mental health legislation, Ireland's 2001 Act also raises an overarching question which is addressed throughout this chapter and elsewhere in this book: should involuntary admission and treatment *ever* occur?

Human Rights Standards

In light of legislation which permits involuntary admission and treatment for mental illness, and given the complicated issues that arise in drafting and operating such laws, the issue of human rights is immediately and urgently engaged. The history of psychiatry supports the necessity to articulate, protect, and promote rights in the context of severe mental illness and, especially, involuntary care (see Chapter 2 of this book: 'The History of Psychiatry').

The evolution of explicit protections for the human rights of people with mental illness is a relatively recent development. Article 1 of the UN *Universal Declaration of Human Rights* states that 'all human beings are born free and equal in dignity and rights. They are endowed with reason and conscience and should act towards one another in a spirit of brotherhood' (United Nations, 1948). Article 2 emphasises the universal nature of rights:

> Everyone is entitled to all the rights and freedoms set forth in this *Declaration*, without distinction of any kind, such as race, colour, sex, language, religion,

political or other opinion, national or social origin, property, birth or other status.

This emphasis on universality is useful and necessary, not least because previous declarations of rights were commonly interpreted so as to exclude certain groups. While mental illness was not mentioned explicitly in the list of factors which were *not* to form the basis of discrimination, it could be included under 'other status'. In 1991, the UN made this explicit in its *Principles for the Protection of Persons with Mental Illness and the Improvement of Mental Health Care* which state that 'there shall be no discrimination on the grounds of mental illness' (United Nations, 1991; Paragraph 1(4)). In addition:

> Every person with a mental illness shall have the right to exercise all civil, political, economic, social and cultural rights as recognized in the *Universal Declaration of Human Rights,* the *International Covenant on Economic, Social and Cultural Rights,* the *International Covenant on Civil and Political Rights,* and in other relevant instruments, such as the *Declaration on the Rights of Disabled Persons* and the *Body of Principles for the Protection of All Persons under Any Form of Detention or Imprisonment.*
>
> (Paragraph 1(5))

In relation to admission without consent, the *Principles* stated that

> A person may (a) be admitted involuntarily to a mental health facility as a patient; or (b) having already been admitted voluntarily as a patient, be retained as an involuntary patient in the mental health facility if, and only if, a qualified mental health practitioner authorized by law for that purpose determines, in accordance with Principle 4 ['Determination of mental illness'], that person has a mental illness and considers:

> (a) That, because of that mental illness, there is a serious likelihood of immediate or imminent harm to that person or to other persons; or
> (b) That, in the case of a person whose mental illness is severe and whose judgement is impaired, failure to admit or retain that person is likely to lead to a serious deterioration in his or her condition or will prevent the giving of appropriate treatment that can only be given by admission to a mental health facility in accordance with the principle of the least restrictive alternative (Paragraph 16(1)).

In the case of (b), 'a second such mental health practitioner, independent of the first, should be consulted where possible. If such consultation takes place, the involuntary admission or retention may not take place unless the second mental health practitioner concurs'. This position and some of this wording are reflected in mental health legislation around the world (World Health Organization, 2005). The 1991 UN *Principles* also specified conditions under which 'a proposed plan of treatment may be given to a patient without a patient's informed consent' (Paragraph 11(6)) and a requirement for a review of involuntary admission 'as soon as possible' after it occurs (Paragraph 17(2)).

Five years after the UN *Principles*, the WHO Division of Mental Health and Prevention of Substance Abuse provided more detail in *Mental Health Care Law: Ten Basic Principles* (Division of Mental Health and Prevention of Substance Abuse, 1996a). These *Principles* include 'promotion of mental health and prevention of mental disorders'; 'access to basic mental health care'; 'mental health assessments in accordance with internationally accepted principles'; 'provision of the least restrictive type of mental health care'; 'self-determination'; 'right to be assisted in the exercise of self-determination'; 'availability of review procedure'; 'automatic periodical review mechanism'; 'qualified decision-maker' (i.e., official or surrogate decision-makers should be qualified for the role); and 'respect of the rule of law' (p. i).

There were more detailed recommendations regarding mental health legislation in this document and the WHO's *Guidelines for the Promotion of Human Rights of Persons with Mental Disorders* (Division of Mental Health and Prevention of Substance Abuse, 1996b). Many of these rights-based considerations were further underlined in the 2001 WHO World Health Report, devoted to *Mental Health: New Understanding, New Hope* (World Health Organization, 2001) and the 2005 *WHO Resource Book on Mental Health, Human Rights and Legislation* (World Health Organization, 2005).

A somewhat different emphasis became apparent in the 2004 WHO document on *The Role of International Human Rights in National Mental Health Legislation,* which stated that the UN *Principles* outlined 'a number of major exceptions' to Principle 11, that 'no treatment shall be given' without informed consent (Rosenthal and Sundram, 2004; p. 36). In 2000, 'a meeting of disability rights experts convened by UN Special Rapporteur Bengt Lindqvist at Almåsa, Sweden [...] adopted a resolution finding that any law is 'inherently suspect' as a form of discrimination if it permits coercive treatment for individuals with disabilities and not all other people' (pp. 36–7).

Two years later, the CRPD continued this incremental shift in tone, moving from acceptance of admission and treatment without consent (once certain conditions were met and safeguards provided) to the current, ambiguous position reflected in the CRPD and an associated commentary, which are explored next.

United Nations' Convention on the Rights of Persons with Disabilities

The UN CRPD is one of the most significant developments in the field of mental health and human rights over the past two decades (United Nations, 2006). The

CRPD entered into force on 3 May 2008 and now has 164 signatories, although fewer states have ratified it (i.e., consented to be bound by it).

The purpose of the CPRD 'is to promote, protect and ensure the full and equal enjoyment of all human rights and fundamental freedoms by all persons with disabilities, and to promote respect for their inherent dignity. Persons with disabilities include those who have long-term physical, mental, intellectual or sensory impairments which in interaction with various barriers may hinder their full and effective participation in society on an equal basis with others' (Article 1).

The 'general principles' of the CRPD are 'respect for inherent dignity, individual autonomy including the freedom to make one's own choices, and independence of persons; non-discrimination; full and effective participation and inclusion in society; respect for difference and acceptance of persons with disabilities as part of human diversity and humanity; equality of opportunity; accessibility; equality between men and women', and 'respect for the evolving capacities of children with disabilities and respect for the right of children with disabilities to preserve their identities' (Article 3).

The CRPD outlines extensive rights relating to 'equality and non-discrimination' (Article 5), 'equal recognition before the law' (Article 12), 'access to justice' (Article 13), 'liberty and security of person' (Article 14), 'freedom from torture or cruel, inhuman or degrading treatment or punishment' (Article 15), 'freedom from exploitation, violence and abuse' (Article 16), 'protecting the integrity of the person' (Article 17), and many other areas.

While several aspects of the CRPD have generated discussion, Articles 12 ('equal recognition before the law') and 14 ('liberty and security of person') arguably hold the greatest relevance to the issue of admission and treatment without consent. Among its provisions, Article 12 requires states to 'reaffirm that persons with disabilities have the right to recognition everywhere as persons before the law'; 'recognize that persons with disabilities enjoy legal capacity on an equal basis with others in all aspects of life', and 'take appropriate measures to provide access by persons with disabilities to the support they may require in exercising their legal capacity'.

Article 14, among its provisions, requires states to 'ensure that persons with disabilities, on an equal basis with others: (a) enjoy the right to liberty and security of person; (b) are not deprived of their liberty unlawfully or arbitrarily, and that any deprivation of liberty is in conformity with the law, and that the existence of a disability shall in no case justify a deprivation of liberty'.

In 2014, the UN Committee on the Rights of Persons with Disabilities, which monitors implementation of the CRPD, published a 'General Comment' on Article 12 (United Nations' Committee on the Rights of Persons with Disabilities, 2014). The Committee appeared to call for the abolition of the concept of mental capacity and the elimination of substitute decision-making, involuntary mental health care, and the insanity defence.

The Committee drew a distinction between 'legal capacity' and 'mental capacity':

Legal capacity and mental capacity are distinct concepts. Legal capacity is the ability to hold rights and duties (legal standing) and to exercise those rights and duties (legal agency). It is the key to accessing meaningful participation in society. Mental capacity refers to the decision-making skills of a person, which naturally vary from one person to another and may be different for a given person depending on many factors, including environmental and social factors.

(Paragraph 13)

The Committee wrote that

Mental capacity is not, as is commonly presented, an objective, scientific and naturally occurring phenomenon. Mental capacity is contingent on social and political contexts, as are the disciplines, professions and practices which play a dominant role in assessing mental capacity.

(Paragraph 14)

The Committee suggested that 'the provision of support to exercise legal capacity should not hinge on mental capacity assessments; new, non-discriminatory indicators of support needs are required in the provision of support to exercise legal capacity' (Paragraph 29(i)).

Regarding 'substitute decision-making', the Committee said that 'support in the exercise of legal capacity must respect the rights, will and preferences of persons with disabilities and should never amount to substitute decision-making' (Paragraph 17). Consequent to this, states' 'obligation to replace substitute decision-making regimes by supported decision-making requires both the abolition of substitute decision-making regimes and the development of supported decision-making alternatives' (Paragraph 28).

The Committee went on to dismiss the idea of involuntary mental health care:

States parties have an obligation to provide access to support for decisions regarding psychiatric and other medical treatment. Forced treatment is a particular problem for persons with psychosocial, intellectual and other cognitive disabilities. States parties must abolish policies and legislative provisions that allow or perpetrate forced treatment, as it is an ongoing violation found in mental health laws across the globe, despite empirical evidence indicating its lack of effectiveness and the views of people using mental health systems who have experienced deep pain and trauma as a result of forced treatment.

(Paragraph 42)

In addition, the Committee questioned the notion of the insanity defense:

States have the ability to restrict the legal capacity of a person based on certain circumstances, such as bankruptcy or criminal conviction. However, the right to equal recognition before the law and freedom from discrimination requires that when the State denies legal capacity, it must be on the same basis for all persons. Denial of legal capacity must not be based on a personal trait such as gender, race, or disability, or have the purpose or effect of treating the person differently.

(Paragraph 32)

There is little doubt that the CRPD offers a once-in-a-generation opportunity to advance the rights of people with mental illness and protect their legal capacity (Kelly, 2021). The interpretation of Article 12 by the UN Committee on the Rights of Persons with Disabilities has, however, been strongly contested. In 2014, the Essex Autonomy Project noted that the Committee 'is not correct in its claim that compliance with the CRPD requires the abolition of substitute decision making and the best-interests decision-making framework' (Martin et al., 2014; p. i):

it is important to be clear that the claims of the Committee's *General Comment* go beyond anything that is explicitly stated in the text of the CRPD. The CRPD itself does not actually say that substitute decision-making should be abolished. Indeed, the Convention itself makes no use of the term 'substitute decision-making' at all. Neither does the CRPD state that the best-interests paradigm must be replaced. Indeed the only thing that the Convention says about best interests is that the best interests of children must be a primary consideration.

(p. 13)

Since 2014, there has been broadening agreement among mental health service users and providers that, contrary to the Committee's view, the concept of 'capacity' is a valid one and is not inconsistent with the CRPD (Dawson, 2015; Freeman et al., 2015; Appelbaum, 2019). Gergel and colleagues reported the views of UK service users on these issues:

The endorsement by the majority of service user respondents of involuntary treatment on the basis of impaired decision-making abilities counters a widespread view, upheld by the UN Committee on the Rights of Persons with Disabilities, that psychiatric use of capacity assessment and involuntary treatment necessarily violate fundamental human rights. Researchers, clinicians, and policy makers should consider that some service users with severe mental health conditions wish to request their own future involuntary treatment, using self-binding directives as a way to self-manage their illness and increase autonomy. When assessing the ethical viability of self-binding directives, mental capacity, and involuntary treatment, human rights advocates need to take a broad range of service user views into account.

(Gergel et al., 2021; p. 600)[3]

Other United Nations' Views on Treatment Without Consent

The interpretation of the CRPD presented by the UN Committee on the Rights of Persons with Disabilities in 2014 is further undermined by the positions of other UN committees and bodies which often present radically different views (Doyle Guilloud, 2019) and generally support the retention of treatment without consent in certain circumstances, provided specific conditions are met and sufficient safeguards are in place. In 2014, the UN Human Rights Committee accepted deprivation of liberty under specific circumstances, once there is adequate oversight:

> The existence of a disability shall not in itself justify a deprivation of liberty but rather any deprivation of liberty must be necessary and proportionate, for the purpose of protecting the individual in question from serious harm or preventing injury to others. It must be applied only as a measure of last resort and for the shortest appropriate period of time, and must be accompanied by adequate procedural and substantive safeguards established by law. The procedures should ensure respect for the views of the individual and ensure that any representative genuinely represents and defends the wishes and interests of the individual.
>
> (United Nations Human Rights Committee,
> 2014; Paragraph 19)

Consistent with this, the UN Subcommittee on Prevention of Torture and Other Cruel, Inhuman or Degrading Treatment or Punishment in 2016 accepted that treatment without consent was both necessary and justified in specific circumstances:

> Exceptionally, it may be necessary to medically treat a person deprived of liberty without her or his consent if the person concerned is not able to: (a) Understand the information given concerning the characteristics of the threat to her or his life or personal integrity, or its consequences; (b) Understand the information about the medical treatment proposed, including its purpose, its means, its direct effects and its possible side effects; (c) Communicate effectively with others.
>
> (United Nations Subcommittee on Prevention of
> Torture and Other Cruel, Inhuman or Degrading
> Treatment or Punishment, 2016; Paragraph 14)

The Subcommittee added that, 'in such a situation, the withholding of medical treatment would constitute inappropriate practice and could amount to a form of cruel, inhuman or degrading treatment or punishment' (Paragraph 15). This statement presents deep challenges to the reductive position adapted by the UN Committee on the Rights of Persons with Disabilities in 2014, a position which mental health service users, researchers, and other UN bodies increasingly do not share.

The views of states parties to the CRPD also indicate clear divergence from the Committee's interpretation. Ireland, for example, ratified the CRPD in 2018 but declared 'its understanding that the Convention allows for compulsory care or treatment of persons, including measures to treat mental disorders, when circumstances render treatment of this kind necessary as a last resort, and the treatment is subject to legal safeguards'.[4] Ireland also declared

> its understanding that the Convention permits supported and substitute decision-making arrangements which provide for decisions to be made on behalf of a person, where such arrangements are necessary, in accordance with the law, and subject to appropriate and effective safeguards.

Both of these statements adhere to the majority interpretation of the CRPD, rather than the reductive interpretation presented by UN Committee on the Rights of Persons with Disabilities. Articulating these positions permitted Ireland to ratify the CRPD and proceed with implementing its provisions to better protect the rights and legal capacity of people with mental illness and disabilities. It is imperative that ideologically based interpretations of the CRPD, which are poorly supported by the text of the Convention, do not delay this urgent task and do not further impair the rights of people with mental illness.

With this in mind, it is puzzling that, notwithstanding the views of UN member states (including but not limited to Ireland), various other UN bodies, and mental health service users (Gergel et al., 2021), the position of the UN Committee on the Rights of Persons with Disabilities was evident in the draft *Guidance on Mental Health, Human Rights, and Legislation* published by the WHO and the Office of the United Nations High Commissioner for Human Rights (OHCHR) for consultation in 2022 (World Health Organization and Office of the United Nations High Commissioner for Human Rights, 2022). While this publication was a draft document and therefore did not necessarily represent the final position of the WHO or OHCHR, pre-consultation drafts often provide useful insights into the thinking that underlies the development of guidance.

This particular document appeared to support the UN Committee on the Rights of Persons with Disabilities' interpretation of the CRPD and was, in consequence, divorced from the lived experience of mental illness, disabilities, and treatment, and was also, at times, contradictory (Kelly, 2024). To take just one example, the draft guidance stated that

> if de-escalation fails and a situation of violence arises, crisis intervention teams could provide protection against interpersonal violence and support

law enforcement to ensure the person is safely taken into custody where the person could be offered appropriate accommodations and support.

(p. 62)

However, the draft also stated that 'police intervention' should be 'free from discrimination and any use of force or coercion' (p. 97). The draft guidance did not explore how 'law enforcement' could keep a person in 'custody' without 'any use of force or coercion'.

Overall, the WHO/OHCHR draft guidance tended to avoid addressing difficult situations adequately, ostensibly on the basis that 'hard cases make bad law' (p. 62). It also stated that 'sometimes there will be no optimal solution' (p. 65), which is a notably defeatist position in guidance which is supposed to address complex dilemmas that appear difficult to solve. When the draft guidance could not avoid the issue of violence, its suggestions were contradictory and deeply unsatisfactory. 'Hard cases' are precisely the times when advice is needed. Sadly, both the WHO/OHCHR draft guidance and the UN Committee on the Rights of Persons with Disabilities avoided addressing these situations and limited themselves to general advice about good practices which are already in place in many services around the world. Clinicians do not have the luxury of avoiding 'hard cases' and cannot suggest self-contradicting responses to challenging scenarios.

Overall, the potential of the CRPD to protect and promote the rights of people with mental illness has not been realised to date, owing largely to interpretations that go well beyond the text of the CRPD and are explicitly rejected by states parties who hold ultimate responsibility for national legislation. While this reflects a general democratic deficit in how the UN is operated, it is a particular tragedy for people with mental illness: the CRPD has potential to protect rights if it is interpreted as it is written, if ideology is set to one side, and if the views of mental health service users, states parties, and other UN bodies are taken into account. Unfortunately, there is scant evidence of this happening. While the Convention has generated a vast academic literature, it has conspicuously failed to impact substantially on national legislation in most jurisdictions or on clinical practice in most settings. An invaluable opportunity is being missed.

Variations in Rates of Involuntary Hospitalisation

The failure of the CRPD to impact substantially on legislation and clinical practice in most jurisdictions is especially troubling because of the gravity of the issues involved: deprivation of liberty and treatment without consent. While involuntary admission and treatment are governed by legislation, there are invariably concerns as well as benefits associated with such interventions.

Variations in rates of involuntary admission across jurisdictions, despite relatively consistent rates of mental illness, is one such concern (Conlan-Trant & Kelly, 2022). In 2019, Luke Sheridan Rains and colleagues published a valuable study of variations in patterns of involuntary hospitalisation and legal frameworks across jurisdictions in *Lancet Psychiatry* (Sheridan Rains et al., 2019). Sheridan Rains and colleagues noted that the incidence of involuntary hospitalisation was reportedly rising in England and certain other high-income countries, but there was no apparent reason for this. Against this background, they compared rates of involuntary hospitalisation between 2008 and 2017 (where possible) for 22 countries in Europe, Australia, and New Zealand.

Their study showed that the overall median rate of involuntary hospitalisation was 106·4 (inter-quartile range: 58·5 to 150·9) per 100,000 people, but this varied substantially across jurisdictions: Austria had the highest rate (282 per 100,000 people) and Italy the lowest (14·5). Interestingly, the study found no relationship between annual involuntary admission rates and characteristics of the legal framework, but higher involuntary admission rates were associated with a larger number of beds, higher gross domestic product per capita purchasing power parity, health care spending per capita, the proportion of foreign-born individuals, and lower absolute poverty.

The disparities across jurisdictions are both large and largely unexplained, although it is worth remembering that while these findings are convincing and consistent with previous literature, comparison across borders is always difficult. In Italy, for example, many people with mental illness are treated in residential facilities rather than hospital units, and these facilities are often excluded from bed counts; when they are included, the number of beds in Italy is similar to that in the UK and elsewhere (Kelly, 2019).

Even so, Sheridan Rains and colleagues focused on *involuntary* hospitalisation and they demonstrated substantial variations both between countries and over time, with annual rates increasing in certain jurisdictions (e.g., Spain) and decreasing in others (e.g., Italy). The authors' comparison of legislation across jurisdictions supports the idea that law as written cannot explain these differences, although it is, of course, the day-to-day operation of specific elements of law that has the greatest effect. For example, certain patients find statutory mental health review panels so unpleasant that they ask for their status to be changed from involuntary to voluntary just to avoid the reviews. Variations in clinical practice by doctors and other health professionals are also relevant to differences within and between countries, as well as over time.

Two key messages are apparent from these contrasting rates of involuntary hospitalisation across jurisdictions. First, the presence of such variations suggests that many involuntary admissions might be avoided, possibly if services such as community clinics, outreach teams, and peer-led support were more widely available. With this broader view, it is clear that the decisions of politicians and service managers are likely to have a greater impact on rights, especially the right to treatment and support, than the decisions of individual clinicians whose options are generally very limited at the level of individual care. As the Essex Autonomy Project suggests, responsibility should be distributed clearly and appropriately:

Statutory provisions regarding support in the exercise of legal capacity must be attributable. For example, statutes that state only that support *should be provided* must be supplemented with clear guidance about who bears the responsibility for providing that support.

(Martin et al., 2016; p. 53)

The second key message from contrasting rates of involuntary hospitalisation across jurisdictions is the need for greater understanding of the operation of law in clinical practice, rooted firmly in lived experience of mental illness, involuntary admission, and treatment without consent. Clearly, mental health legislation plays a critical role in this area, reflecting the fact that law and medicine are both fields that can deeply marginalise or greatly assist vulnerable members of society. As a result, the interaction between law and medicine in psychiatry presents both significant risks and valuable benefits that should not be missed.

The risks of mental health legislation include inappropriate or excessive limitation of the observance of specific rights in the name of treating mental disorder. This risk can be mitigated by better voluntary mental health services, clear distribution of responsibilities in health and social care, dedicated legislation that respects human rights, free legal representation for patients and families, and appropriate avenues for appeal.

The benefits of mental health legislation include treatment of mental illness at times when the condition is severe and impairs decision-making capacity, as well as providing a legal framework that facilitates accountability rather than informal restrictions that evolve without adequate safeguards. The history of psychiatry makes it clear that these are important tasks (see Chapter 2: 'The History of Psychiatry').

The other potential benefit of mental health legislation is the use of law to promote access to services, rather than focussing exclusively on involuntary admission and treatment. India's Mental Healthcare Act 2017, for example, states that 'every person shall have a right to access mental healthcare and treatment from mental health services run or funded by the appropriate Government' (Section 18(1)). As a result, the Indian legislation grants a legally binding right to mental health care to over 1.3 billion people, one sixth of the planet's population, rather than focussing exclusively (or even chiefly) on treatment without consent (Duffy and Kelly, 2019). Despite the clear resource challenges associated with such developments, using law in this positive way will hopefully increase access to care at an earlier stage and reduce the need for involuntary admission.

Should Admission and Treatment Without Consent Ever Occur?

So far in this chapter, we have examined one legal model of involuntary care (in Ireland), outlined relevant human rights standards developed by international bodies such as the WHO and UN, focused especially on the CRPD and the

diametrically opposed views of other UN bodies, and noted significant variations in rates of involuntary admission across jurisdictions. There are also other
international variations in practice: in some jurisdictions, judges play a greater
role in decision-making under mental health law, and, in certain countries, compulsory community treatment orders permit compulsory treatment outside hospital settings (Dawson, 2024).

In an ideal society with perfect systems of mental health and social care, there
might be a greatly diminished need for involuntary admission and treatment, or
maybe none at all. However, as the WHO/OHCHR draft *Guidance on Mental
Health, Human Rights, and Legislation* notes, 'no country has yet eliminated all
forms of coercion in mental health systems' (World Health Organization and
Office of the United Nations High Commissioner for Human Rights, 2022; p.
61). The issue of paternalism is clearly relevant here (Wilbush, 1990), along with
the idea of a right to mental health care, including a right to involuntary mental
health care if required (see Chapter 10 of this book: 'The Future of Psychiatry:
Person-Centred Care and System-Level Change').

Ultimately, though, until such time as systems of health and social care
greatly diminish or eliminate the need for admission and treatment without consent, such practices should be possible, rare, and codified in law. Much of the
recent published rhetoric on these topics, both from international bodies and
elsewhere, comprises lengthy idealistic musings by people with neither experience of mental illness nor responsibility for treating it. This has created a regrettable situation of parallel monologues on these themes, with one side arguing
that involuntary care must never occur, and the other side urging pragmatism
and incremental change (Kelly, 2024).

In 2023 in *BJPsych Open*, Bernadette McSherry, Piers Gooding, and Yvette
Maker explored the literature on this 'Geneva impasse' (Martin & Gurbai, 2019)
between 'those who argue that compulsory care and treatment can never comply
with human rights law and those who argue that they can if certain conditions
are met' (McSherry et al., 2023; p. 1):

Human rights debates about mental healthcare have traditionally focused on
the rights to liberty and autonomy in relation to the compulsory treatment
of persons with psychosocial disabilities. Commentaries on the CRPD have
largely focused on what the right to equal protection before the law means for
the existence of compulsory treatment schemes and whether such schemes
should be abolished or reformed. Breaking through the so-called 'Geneva
impasse' might seem difficult at first glance. However, although disagreements about the legitimacy of compulsory treatment and coercive practices
persist, there is optimism that these practices can be reduced and attention is
turning to how best to achieve this.

(p. 3)[5]

Clearly, the magnitude of these disagreements can be reduced, as can rates of involuntary care and coercive practices, through better preventive measures, more responsive mental health care, and improved social supports. Many countries with relatively low rates of coercive practices, such as Ireland, already have strategies in place for quite some time seeking to further reduce coercive practices (e.g., Mental Health Commission, 2014; see also: Sashidharan et al., 2019). Renewed emphasis on such reforms will likely help, but these must be accompanied by broader protection of all rights, especially those directly relevant to accessing care and support:

> An emphasis on all categories of human rights, be they civil, political, economic, social or cultural, would seem to provide a framework for how best to provide the mental healthcare and treatment that persons with mental health conditions and psychosocial disabilities need. That way, the 'Geneva impasse' may become the 'Geneva pathway' to promoting human rights and high-quality mental healthcare.
>
> (McSherry et al., 2023; p. 3)

Based on several decades of research in this field and experience with people with severe mental illness, I know that the vast majority seek, accept, and benefit from voluntary treatment. Hopefully, this proportion will increase over time owing to improvements in mental health and social services, buttressed by broader protections of civil, social, and economic rights that the CRPD can offer, if a wide-angle, cooperative approach is adopted.

Nonetheless, for the minority of people with severe or life-threatening mental illness whose understanding and decision-making capacity are substantially impaired, I agree with the UN Subcommittee on Prevention of Torture and Other Cruel, Inhuman or Degrading Treatment or Punishment that, 'exceptionally, it may be necessary to medically treat a person deprived of liberty without her or his consent', if certain conditions are met and safeguards provided (United Nations Subcommittee on Prevention of Torture and Other Cruel, Inhuman or Degrading Treatment or Punishment, 2016; Paragraph 14). I have seen this many times and the transformative benefit it can bring in people's lives.

I also agree with the UN Subcommittee that, 'in such a situation, the withholding of medical treatment would constitute inappropriate practice and could amount to a form of cruel, inhuman or degrading treatment or punishment' (Paragraph 15). We need to improve our models of voluntary care so as to decrease the need for involuntary care and ideally eliminate it. But in this process, we cannot neglect those who fall through the cracks, those who require involuntary care, those whose understanding is so impaired as to preventably but irreversibly damage their health and lives. To neglect these people, or pretend that they do not exist, is a profound denial of their rights.

Peter, the 18-year-old man with paranoid psychosis whom we met at the start of this chapter, refused to leave his room, declined all treatment, and heard voices continually. He was hugely distressed, constantly agitated, and in clear need of treatment and support.

Peter's parents discussed the situation with their family doctor who explained the process for involuntary admission under mental health legislation. This involved one of Peter's parents signing an 'Application' for involuntary admission, the family doctor assessing Peter and signing a 'Recommendation' if appropriate, and then staff from the psychiatric hospital bringing Peter to the inpatient facility for assessment by a psychiatrist. This process was not easy.

Peter's father completed the 'Application' form with the agreement and assistance of Peter's mother, but Peter refused to leave his bedroom to see his family doctor. The doctor came to the house and spoke with Peter as best she could through the closed bedroom door. She again offered Peter voluntary outpatient treatment and support at home, but Peter again declined. Peter confirmed that he was on the 'purple planet' and that two 'voices' were talking to him most of the time. Finally, he opened the bedroom door and shouted at the doctor: 'Go away. You know what is going on. You are part of it too. You know what I'm talking about. You all know. Why don't you stop pretending?' He then closed the bedroom door again.

At this point, the family doctor had the information she needed to sign the 'Recommendation' form, stating that Peter was severely mentally ill, and that involuntary admission was the only way he could receive treatment. Based on the 'Application' and 'Recommendation', staff from the hospital came to Peter's house and, after much explanation, persuaded Peter to open his bedroom door. When Peter saw the hospital staff, he asked: 'Why are you here? Where are you taking me?' Peter was upset and afraid: he thought they were taking him to 'another area' of the 'purple planet' to kill him.

The staff explained their role again and offered voluntary outpatient treatment and support at home again. Peter declined again. They then reassured Peter as best they could and took him to the psychiatric hospital for assessment.

At the hospital, Peter's psychiatrist examined him and, again, offered the option of voluntary outpatient treatment and support at home. Peter again declined, and the psychiatrist completed the 'Admission Order' which confirmed Peter as an involuntary patient. The psychiatrist explained the entire process to Peter, telling Peter that he was mentally ill to the point of failing to understand his situation and requiring treatment. Peter did not resist treatment but signalled his disagreement.

The psychiatrist informed Peter of his rights, told him that a legal representative would be appointed immediately, and said that Peter's involuntary status would be reviewed by an independent tribunal within two or three weeks if Peter was still an involuntary patient at that point. The psychiatrist also provided a written explanation and arranged for Peter to discuss this matter with a nurse again later in the day.

Peter cooperated with care in the hospital, albeit under protest. He received anti-psychotic medication and, after a few days, participated in the occupational therapy programme. Peter enjoyed the physical exercise classes, although not the yoga. After two weeks, Peter's symptoms were substantially improved, and his psychiatrist changed his status from 'involuntary' to 'voluntary'. Peter agreed to spend a further two weeks in the hospital, during which he met with other members of the multi-disciplinary team, including the community mental health nurse he had seen before and a clinical psychologist.

After four weeks in hospital, Peter was discharged home with a full outpatient treatment plan in place. He still heard voices from time to time, but they were less persistent and less negative, and Peter agreed that treatment helped. Overall, he was less preoccupied, less distressed, and more positive about the future.

Peter left the hospital with appointments to see the community mental health nurse and clinical psychologist, as well as an arrangement to talk with his psychiatrist some weeks later. Peter was also referred to a substance misuse counsellor, to discuss his cannabis use.

When asked about his experience of involuntary admission, Peter said: 'I guess I needed treatment, but I hope I never need to go through that again.' 'What was the worst part?', his father asked, worried that Peter was angry at him for arranging the admission or resentful that the clinical team treated him without consent initially. Peter responded without hesitation: 'I didn't like hospital, but the months I spent in my bedroom hearing voices, before I went to hospital, that was easily the worst part. Never again.'

Key Messages

- Involuntary admission and treatment for mental illness is, rightly, a controversial and contested topic. Deprivation of liberty or treatment without consent represents a significant limitation of the observance of fundamental human rights.
- Nevertheless, virtually every jurisdiction has legislation that permits involuntary treatment for serious mental illness if certain conditions are met and safeguards are provided.
- Key issues in mental health legislation centre on definitions of 'mental illness' or 'mental disorder', the role of apparent dangerousness, and the relevance of decision-making capacity.
- Interpretations of the United Nations' (UN) Convention on the Rights of Persons with Disabilities (CRPD) vary, but there is growing consensus among mental health service users, states parties, researchers, and UN bodies that the concepts of decision-making capacity and involuntary admission and treatment do not violate human rights standards and can protect rights.

- Benefits of mental health legislation include treatment of mental illness when the condition is severe and impairs decision-making capacity, as well as providing a legal framework that facilitates accountability.
- Risks of mental health legislation include inappropriate or excessive limitation of the observance of specific rights in the name of treating mental disorder. This risk can be mitigated by better voluntary services, clear distribution of responsibilities in health and social care, dedicated legislation that respects human rights, free legal representation, and appropriate avenues for appeal.
- Until such time as systems of health and social care greatly diminish or eliminate the need for admission and treatment without consent, such practices should be possible, rare, and codified in law.

Notes

1 Separate provisions apply to 'psycho-surgery' (Section 58), 'electro-convulsive therapy' (ECT; Section 59), 'administration of medicine' for over three months (Section 60), and 'treatment of children' (Section 61).
2 For someone who already is a voluntary inpatient, there is a different, two-step process to change from voluntary to involuntary status, involving assessments by two consultant psychiatrists (Sections 23 and 24). There is also a separate process for children (Section 25).
3 Licence: https://creativecommons.org/licenses/by/4.0/ (accessed 28 May 2023).
4 https://treaties.un.org/pages/ViewDetails.aspx?src=TREATY&mtdsg_no=IV-15 &chapter=4&clang=_en (accessed 28 May 2023).
5 Licence: https://creativecommons.org/licenses/by/4.0/ (accessed 29 May 2023).

References

Appelbaum PS. Saving the UN Convention on the Rights of Persons with Disabilities – from itself. *World Psychiatry* 2019; 18: 1–2 (https://doi.org/10.1002%2Fwps.20583).

Conlan-Trant R, Kelly BD. England's rate of involuntary psychiatric admission is double that of the Republic of Ireland: why? A consideration of some possible causes. *Medicine, Science and the Law* 2022; 62: 64–9 (https://doi.org/10.1177 /00258024211029071).

Connors MH, Large MM. Calibrating violence risk assessments for uncertainty. *General Psychiatry* 2023; 36: e100921 (https://doi.org/10.1136/gpsych-2022-100921).

Dawson J. A realistic approach to assessing mental health laws' compliance with the UNCRPD. *International Journal of Law and Psychiatry* 2015; 40: 70–9 (https://doi .org/10.1016/j.ijlp.2015.04.003).

Dawson J. Compulsory community treatment: is it the least restrictive alternative? In: Kelly BD, Donnelly M (eds), *Routledge Handbook of Mental Health Law* (pp. 356–70). London and New York: Routledge, 2024.

Division of Mental Health and Prevention of Substance Abuse. *Guidelines for the Promotion of Human Rights of Persons with Mental Disorders.* Geneva: World Health Organization, 1996b (https://apps.who.int/iris/handle/10665/41880) (accessed 27 May 2023).

Division of Mental Health and Prevention of Substance Abuse. *Mental Health Care Law: Ten Basic Principles*. Geneva: World Health Organization, 1996a (https://apps.who .int/iris/handle/10665/63624) (accessed 27 May 2023).

Doyle Guilloud S. The right to liberty of persons with psychosocial disabilities at the United Nations: a tale of two interpretations. *International Journal of Law and Psychiatry* 2019; 66: 101497 (https://doi.org/10.1016/j.ijlp.2019.101497).

Duffy RM, Kelly BD. India's Mental Healthcare Act, 2017: content, context, controversy. *International Journal of Law and Psychiatry* 2019; 62: 169–78 (https://doi.org/10 .1016/j.ijlp.2018.08.002).

Freeman MC, Kolappa K, de Almeida JMC, Kleinman A, Makhashvili N, Phakathi S, Saraceno B, Thornicroft G. Reversing hard won victories in the name of human rights: a critique of the General Comment on Article 12 of the UN Convention on the Rights of Persons with Disabilities. *Lancet Psychiatry* 2015; 2: 844–50 (https://doi.org/10 .1016/S2215-0366(15)00218-7).

Gergel T, Das P, Owen G, Stephenson L, Rifkin L, Hindley G, Dawson J, Ruck Keene A. Reasons for endorsing or rejecting self-binding directives in bipolar disorder: a qualitative study of survey responses from UK service users. *Lancet Psychiatry* 2021; 8: 599–609 (https://doi.org/10.1016/S2215-0366(21)00115-2). (Link to license: https://creativecommons.org/licenses/by/4.0/) (accessed 26 April 2024).

Gulati G, Dunne CP, Kelly BD. Violence risk assessment in psychiatry: nobody can predict the future. *BMJ Opinion*, 17 November 2020 (https://blogs.bmj.com/bmj /2020/11/17/violence-risk-assessment-in-psychiatry-nobody-can-predict-the-future/) (accessed 25 May 2023).

Kelly BD. Variations in involuntary hospitalisation across countries. *Lancet Psychiatry* 2019; 6: 361–2 (https://doi.org/10.1016/S2215-0366(19)30095-1).

Kelly BD. Mental capacity, human rights, and the UN's Convention on the Rights of Persons with Disabilities. *Journal of the American Academy of Psychiatry and the Law* 2021; 49: 152–6 (https://jaapl.org/content/49/2/152.long) (accessed 25 May 2023).

Kelly BD. The right to mental health care in mental health legislation. In: Kelly BD, Donnelly M (eds), *Routledge Handbook of Mental Health Law* (pp. 384–402). London and New York: Routledge, 2024.

Martin W, Gurbai S. Surveying the Geneva impasse: coercive care and human rights. *International Journal of Law and Psychiatry* 2019; 64: 117–28 (http://dx.doi.org/10 .1016/j.ijlp.2019.03.001). (Link to license: https://creativecommons.org/licenses/by/4 .0/) (accessed 26 December 2023).

Martin W, Michalowski S, Jütten T, Burch M. *Achieving CRPD compliance: is the Mental Capacity Act of England and Wales Compatible with the UN Convention on the Rights of Persons with Disabilities? If Not, What Next? An Essex Autonomy Project Position Paper*. Colchester: University of Essex, 2014 (https://autonomy.essex.ac.uk /resources/achieving-crpd-compliance-is-the-mental-capacity-act-of-england-and -wales-compatible-with-the-un-convention-on-the-rights-of-persons-with-disabilities -if-not-what-next/) (accessed 25 May 2023).

Martin W, Michalowski S, Stavert J, Ward A, Ruck Keene A, Caughey C, Hempsey A, McGregor R. *Three Jurisdictions Report: Towards Compliance with CRPD Art. 12 in Capacity/Incapacity Legislation Across the UK. An Essex Autonomy Project Position Paper*. Colchester: University of Essex, 2016 (https://autonomy.essex.ac.uk/resources /eap-three-jurisdictions-report/) (accessed 25 May 2023).

McSherry B, Gooding P, Maker Y. Human rights promotion and the 'Geneva impasse' in mental healthcare: scoping review. *BJPsych Open* 2023; 9: E58 (https://doi.org/10.1192/bjo.2023.50) (Link to license: https://creativecommons.org/licenses/by/4.0/) (accessed 26 April 2024).

Mental Health Commission. *Seclusion and Restraint Reduction Strategy.* Dublin: Mental Health Commission, 2014 (https://www.mhcirl.ie/sites/default/files/2022-09/Seclusion-and-Restraint-Reduction-Strategy.pdf) (accessed 26 May 2023).

Rosenthal E, Sundram CJ. *The Role of International Human Rights in National Mental Health Legislation.* Geneva: World Health Organization, 2004.

Sashidharan SP, Mezzina R, Puras D. Reducing coercion in mental healthcare. *Epidemiology and Psychiatric Sciences* 2019; 28: 605–12 (https://doi.org/10.1017/s2045796019000350).

Sheridan Rains L, Zenina T, Dias MC, Jones R, Jeffreys S, Branthonne-Foster S, Lloyd-Evans B, Johnson S. Variations in patterns of involuntary hospitalisation and in legal frameworks: an international comparative study. *Lancet Psychiatry* 2019; 6: 403–17 (https://doi.org/10.1016/S2215-0366(19)30090-2).

United Nations. *Universal Declaration of Human Rights.* New York: United Nations, 1948 (https://www.un.org/en/about-us/universal-declaration-of-human-rights) (accessed 28 May 2023).

United Nations. *Principles for the Protection of Persons with Mental Illness and the Improvement of Mental Health Care.* Geneva: Office of the United Nations High Commissioner for Human Rights, 1991 (https://www.ohchr.org/en/instruments-mechanisms/instruments/principles-protection-persons-mental-illness-and-improvement) (accessed 27 May 2023).

United Nations. *Convention on the Rights of Persons with Disabilities.* New York: United Nations, 2006 (https://social.desa.un.org/issues/disability/crpd/convention-on-the-rights-of-persons-with-disabilities-crpd) (accessed 25 May 2023).

United Nations' Committee on the Rights of Persons with Disabilities. *General Comment No. 1 (Article 12).* New York: United Nations, 2014 (https://www.ohchr.org/en/documents/general-comments-and-recommendations/general-comment-no-1-article-12-equal-recognition-1) (accessed 25 May 2023).

United Nations Human Rights Committee. *General Comment No. 35 (Article 9).* New York: United Nations, 2014 (https://www.ohchr.org/en/documents/general-comments-and-recommendations/general-comment-no-35-article-9-liberty-and-security) (accessed 25 May 2023).

United Nations Subcommittee on Prevention of Torture and Other Cruel, Inhuman or Degrading Treatment or Punishment. *Approach of the Subcommittee on Prevention of Torture and Other Cruel, Inhuman or Degrading Treatment or Punishment Regarding the Rights of Persons Institutionalized and Treated Medically Without Informed Consent.* New York: United Nations, 2016 (https://documents-dds-ny.un.org/doc/UNDOC/GEN/G16/011/96/PDF/G1601196.pdf?OpenElement) (accessed 25 May 2023).

Wilbush J. Patient care and paternalism: dilemmas of family practice. *Canadian Family Physician* 1990; 36: 703–8 (https://www.ncbi.nlm.nih.gov/pmc/articles/PMC2280587/).

World Health Organization. *Mental Health: New Understanding, New Hope.* Geneva: World Health Organization, 2001 (https://apps.who.int/iris/handle/10665/42390) (accessed 27 May 2023).

World Health Organization. *WHO Resource Book on Mental Health, Human Rights and Legislation.* Geneva: World Health Organization, 2005 (https://digitallibrary.un.org/record/565952?ln=en) (accessed 27 May 2023).

World Health Organization and Office of the United Nations High Commissioner for Human Rights. *Guidance on Mental Health, Human Rights, and Legislation (Draft).* Geneva: World Health Organization and Office of the United Nations High Commissioner for Human Rights, 2022 (https://www.ohchr.org/en/calls-for-input/calls-input/draft-guidance-mental-health-human-rights-legislation-who-ohchr) (accessed 25 May 2023).

6   Neuroscience and Psychiatry

Taraji was 20 years old when she had her first episode of mania. Taraji worked as a hairdresser. In her spare time, Taraji liked to run. She competed in local road races and, most years, she ran a marathon. At weekends, Taraji either worked extra shifts at the hairdressing salon or spent time with her friend, Mandisa. Taraji and Mandisa liked to take long walks, starting in the early morning, and ending late at night at one of their houses. Taraji and Mandisa could walk all day, talking together about everything under the sun.

One day, Taraji woke early and went for an extra-long morning run. She felt brilliant and bounced into work, full of enthusiasm. Taraji felt like this all week, the best she had ever been. At the weekend, Taraji suggested that she and Mandisa go for a hike. Taraji said they could camp overnight in the countryside. Mandisa did not enjoy camping, but Taraji was so enthusiastic that Mandisa agreed. The hike went well, but Mandisa noticed that Taraji barely slept at all. Taraji said she wanted to spend the night gazing at the stars.

Taraji became more and more energetic over the following weeks. She arrived in work early, but often left in the middle of the day. She could be gone for hours before returning to the hairdressing salon at closing time and offering to work into the night. Taraji's boss did not know what to do but said that if Taraji continued to behave like this, she would lose her job. Taraji didn't seem to mind. She just laughed and said she had to do a lot of shopping.

Taraji felt she needed very little sleep over this period, and sometimes did not go to bed at all. One night, Taraji phoned Mandisa at 3 am, asking her to come for a run 'under the glorious stars of heaven'. Mandisa switched off her phone and went back to sleep but was increasingly worried about Taraji.

Finally, early one Saturday morning, Taraji was arrested by the police. They found her standing on the roof of a building at 4 am singing at the top of her voice. When the police shouted up to her to come down, Taraji refused, telling them that she could fly. Taraji asked the police: 'Do you want me to fly down to you? I can fly like a bird. Will you watch me fly?'

Deeply alarmed, the police told Taraji to stay where she was and called the fire brigade. Three fire officers climbed onto the roof and encouraged Taraji to come down. Taraji still refused and continued to sing at the top of her voice. A police woman climbed up and tried to persuade Taraji to come down. Still,

DOI: 10.4324/9781003378495-7

Taraji refused, saying: 'I must be here. I must sing to save the world.' In the end, the police woman had to arrest Taraji to force her down from the roof to safety.

The police took Taraji to the police station, where they did a test for drugs and alcohol, and asked Taraji whom they could phone. Did she have a partner or family member they could contact? It was clear that Taraji needed help and support.

Taraji had lost her phone and the only number that she remembered was Mandisa's mobile phone number. The police phoned Mandisa who was horrified to hear that her friend had been arrested. Mandisa rushed to the police station and could scarcely believe what she saw: Taraji was sitting in a police cell, singing at the top of her voice, and either laughing or crying whenever she drew a breath.

'Is she on drugs?' Mandisa asked the police. 'Her tests showed no drugs or alcohol', the police woman said: 'But I think she is mentally ill.' 'I'm sure you're right', said Mandisa, bewildered by the situation.

Taraji had an episode of mania. She had increased energy, disinhibition, reduced need for sleep, grandiose ideation, and a delusion that she could fly. When the police called her friend Mandisa, it was clear to Mandisa that something needed to be done. At the suggestion of the police, Mandisa brought Taraji to the hospital. Taraji saw no reason for this but agreed to do what Mandisa suggested because she was her friend.

At the hospital, a psychiatrist spoke to Taraji, but she did not want to talk to him for very long. Taraji said that she had too much to do. The psychiatrist also spoke to Mandisa, who told him the full story.

The psychiatrist recommended that Taraji should be admitted to an inpatient psychiatry unit in a general hospital for treatment for mania. After some discussion, Taraji agreed: 'But only because I'm tired', she said. The psychiatrist told Taraji that she needed treatment. Taraji said: 'Let's talk about that tomorrow. Do you know that I can fly?'

The next morning, Taraji was full of energy when the doctor came to see her. After a great deal of negotiation, as well as encouragement from Mandisa, Taraji agreed to stay in the psychiatry unit, where she was treated with an antipsychotic medication and saw a clinical psychologist. At some level, Taraji was aware that something was wrong, even if she did not know exactly what.

Introduction

Taraji was mentally ill. She had lost touch with reality in a number of ways: she believed that she could fly and that her singing would save the world. Her behaviour was unusual and, eventually, she posed a serious risk to herself and possibly others. Taraji was not drinking alcohol or taking drugs (either illicit or prescribed) when she became unwell. After she went to the hospital, Taraji was examined by a psychiatrist who made a diagnosis of elation or mania, most likely in the context of undiagnosed bipolar affective disorder (previously known as manic depression).

Taraji's story is not uncommon. Bipolar affective disorder is frequently seen in mental health services and often presents substantial challenges to patients, families, and mental health professionals. The condition is associated with a substantial reduction in psychosocial functioning and the loss of approximately 10 to 20 potential years of life on average, owing chiefly to excess deaths from cardiovascular disease and suicide (McIntyre et al., 2020). Bipolar affective disorder can also be highly disruptive in a person's life and the lives of their family, often as a result of disinhibited behaviour and risk-taking, as demonstrated by Taraji's story. The condition is, however, treatable, so it is essential that interventions are provided in a timely, sustainable way.

Perhaps one of the most interesting parts of Taraji's case is the fact that biological tests, such as brain scans and blood tests, do not play a significant role in confirming a diagnosis of bipolar affective disorder. These tests can be used to rule out certain other conditions (e.g., brain tumours, hyperthyroidism, etc.), but there are no biological tests to confirm a diagnosis of bipolar affective disorder, depression, schizophrenia, anxiety disorder, or many other mental illnesses. Most psychiatric diagnoses are based on symptoms and signs, rather than biological tests, as discussed in Chapter 3 ('Diagnosing Mental Illness').

This chapter examines 'Neuroscience and Psychiatry'. While acknowledging the contributions that neuroscience has made to certain areas within this field, this chapter outlines the failure of neuroscience to substantially increase our understanding of the causes of common mental illnesses or to substantially inform new therapies. The chapter provides suggestions for a more focused, realistic, proportionate approach to neuroscience in psychiatry, optimising the promise of studies of imaging, genetics, inflammation, and new treatments, while remaining aware of the cost and opportunity cost of so much neuroscience over the past decades.

The chapter concludes by outlining the need for a plurality of research methodologies in psychiatry – a true synthesis of techniques and understandings across neuroscience, medicine, law, history, spirituality, and other fields. Neuroscience needs to be contextualised as part of this broader search for knowledge, meaning, and understanding. Genuine progress requires radical, interdisciplinary thought and practice. This matters deeply to everyone who develops mental illness, their families, their friends, and all who try to alleviate their suffering. That is to say: this matters to everyone.

Why are there no diagnostic tests for most mental illnesses? Despite certain technological advances and decades of costly neuroscience, why are there no biological markers for conditions such as bipolar affective disorder, depression, schizophrenia, and others? Their absence is remarkable, but explicable, not least because symptom-based syndromes are unlikely to map directly onto discrete biological entities.

Unravelling the Brain

Today, we know more about the human brain and nervous system than we have ever known. The brain contains approximately 86 billion neurons (nerve cells) and many billions of other types of cells that nourish and support the neurons (Kelly, 2022a). Each neuron communicates with thousands of other neurons using a range of different neurotransmitters (brain chemicals) which pass across synapses (gaps between cells). The resulting patterns of communication are infinitely variable, stretching across a network of between 100 trillion and 1,000 trillion connections, all discharging in different ways, at different times, in different combinations. The brain is an extraordinary creation, likely the most intricate in the world, and probably the most complicated object that has ever existed.

And that is just the brain, which is only one part of the even more complex nervous system which, in turn, forms just one element within the yet more complex human organism. The entire human body is infinitely connected, infinitely complicated, infinitely capable.

In view of this enormous complexity, it is little wonder that (a) detailed data about the brain is accumulating at pace, thanks to radical advances in neuroscience; but (b) even the masses of data that have been gathered to date do not come close to providing a complete picture of how the brain functions, let alone how the broader nervous system works, or how the human organism as a whole operates. Therefore, while the language of neuroscience is endlessly seductive, the therapeutic yield from recent neuroscience is bewilderingly low in practical terms in psychiatry (Legrenzi & Umiltà, 2011; Kelly, 2020). Given the resources devoted and effort applied to psychiatric neuroscience over recent decades, we might have expected greater advances by random chance alone. But, to date, the impact is very limited indeed.

Moreover, even if complete data about the brain were available (which they are not), the task of assembling such data into information and extracting understanding from it is still far distant from where we stand today. And even if we understood how the brain works when it is functioning well, that is quite different to understanding how it operates under conditions of illness, let alone when treatments are provided that further affect brain function.

Incredibly, the situation becomes even more complex when we consider that key brain functions which are disordered in mental illness, such as cognition, are not necessarily individual functions, but collective ones. Sloman and colleagues make this point with devastating clarity in *Frontiers in Systems Neuroscience*:

> Years of research in psychology, cognitive science, philosophy, and anthropology have shown that human cognition is a collective enterprise and is therefore not to be found within a single individual. Human cognition is an emergent property that reflects communal knowledge and representations that are distributed within a community [citations omitted]. By 'emergent'

property we mean nothing elusive or mysterious, but simply certain well-documented properties of groups that would not exist in the absence of relevant properties of individuals, but are not properties of any individual member of the group, or any aggregation of properties of some or all members of the group.

(Sloman et al., 2021; p. 2)

All told, we now have a great deal of scientific data about the biological nervous system, but, when it comes to something as complex as brain function, these scientific data amount to very little in terms of understanding mental illness and designing treatments. Our operational ignorance on this subject is vast, as is our lack of biological understanding of disordered mental function and its amelioration. The idea that certain brain activities which appear to be individual functions are, in fact, collective enterprises adds another dimension to our lack of knowledge, which is, as a result, vast, multi-dimensional, and essentially infinite.

Interestingly, despite this ocean of unknowing, and against all the scientific odds, there is strong evidence that many treatments for mental illness are highly effective (see Chapter 4: 'Treating Symptoms and Disorders'). Key psychiatric medications are just as useful as, or better than, treatments in other areas of medicine (Leucht et al., 2012). The fact that we do not know why many psychiatric treatments work is troubling, but that does not undermine evidence of their effectiveness. Antidepressants, for example, help to alleviate depression, so, even if we do not know why they work, they can still be usefully prescribed in accordance with treatment guidelines (Cipriani et al., 2018; Taylor et al., 2021).

All of this places psychiatry in a very unusual position: generally effective in treating symptom-based syndromes but lacking any compelling biological rationale to explain this. This situation is attributable, at least in part, to psychiatry's rather unlikely dual affiliations to (a) evidence-based treatment, and (b) diagnoses which are largely based on psychological symptoms rather than biological tests. As Pernu (2022) points out:

Two things make psychiatry unique among the sciences. First, psychiatry occupies an uneasy place between the physical and the mental ways of viewing the world. This is something that psychiatry has in common with psychology and the neurosciences, or 'the cognitive sciences' in general. Second, psychiatry is not simply disinterested, purely academic study of the body and the mind, but a discipline whose aim is distinctly pragmatic: to provide effective treatments to those who are suffering. This is something that psychiatry has in common with other essentially pragmatic disciplines, medicine in particular. What makes psychiatry unique is the way that its pragmatic goal lies at the intersection of two radically different ways of viewing the world; psychiatrists are, as it were, physicians operating in a non-physical realm.

(Pernu, 2022; p. 166)

The neuroscientific research of recent decades has sought to navigate these complex waters in a number of ways: investigating specific diagnoses, developing trans-diagnostic dimensional approaches, and going on broad-sweep fishing trips to identify patterns across vast datasets of genetic information or imaging data. The cost of this research has been enormous and the therapeutic yield remarkably low (Kelly, 2022a). While fields such as neuroimaging, genetics, inflammation studies, and various other areas are undoubtedly promising, they have been promising for several decades now and there comes a point when hope is no longer enough. It is time to think again.

The dispiriting truth is that, despite many decades of scientific research about the brain, there are still no biological tests to diagnose any common mental illness apart from some cases of dementia. Technologies such as brain scans and genetic sequencing have not significantly changed the diagnosis or treatment of common psychiatric disorders such as bipolar affective disorder, depression, schizophrenia, or anxiety disorder. Neuroscientific research in these areas might help with background understandings of possible origins for certain illnesses in specific people, and out-ruling 'non-psychiatric' diagnoses in particular cases, but they have not systematically altered diagnosis, treatment, or outcomes across psychiatry more broadly. This is a severe disappointment.

Neuroscience and Mental Illness

Overall, and while acknowledging the contributions that neuroscience has made to certain areas within psychiatry, it remains the case that recent brain science has not substantially increased our understanding of the causes of most common mental illnesses or provided new, science-driven treatment options. This situation merits closer thought and attention. Depression provides a good example of some of the issues involved.

As discussed in Chapter 4 ('Treating Symptoms and Disorders'), antidepressants help to alleviate a great deal of suffering for many people with moderate or severe depression (Cipriani et al., 2018), and can even prove lifesaving in some cases. These conclusions are based on the outcomes of clinical trials and, subsequently, the experience of prescribing antidepressants in day-to-day clinical practice. These conclusions are not based on any proposed neurochemical theories of depression (which would only be speculative) or on any proposed mechanism of action of the medications (which cannot be reliably stated, owing to limited neuroscientific understandings of the brain, mental illness, and its treatment).

Given that many effective antidepressants appear to affect serotonin, however, it was reasonable to wonder if a problem with serotonin might cause or increase the risk of depression in the first place, or if serotonin might be involved in some other way in the genesis of the condition. While such an explanation would likely only be part of a complicated, multi-factorial pathway to depression, it would nonetheless be useful to establish if serotonin dysfunction was somehow implicated along the way, even in some people. The apparent mechanism of action of certain antidepressants suggested that it might be. Could neuroscientific studies clarify this matter further? Might the largely serendipitous identification of effective antidepressants point towards one of the causes or neurochemical correlates of the condition? Such a finding would be enormously valuable and would hopefully increase understanding and help in the *systematic* search for better treatments.

In 2023, Moncrieff and colleagues published 'a systematic umbrella review of the evidence' relating to 'the serotonin theory of depression' (Moncrieff et al., 2023). This group 'aimed to synthesise and evaluate evidence on whether depression is associated with lowered serotonin concentration or activity':

> 17 studies were included: 12 systematic reviews and meta-analyses, 1 collaborative meta-analysis, 1 meta-analysis of large cohort studies, 1 systematic review and narrative synthesis, 1 genetic association study and 1 umbrella review [...] Our comprehensive review of the major strands of research on serotonin shows there is no convincing evidence that depression is associated with, or caused by, lower serotonin concentrations or activity. Most studies found no evidence of reduced serotonin activity in people with depression compared to people without, and methods to reduce serotonin availability using tryptophan depletion do not consistently lower mood in volunteers. High quality, well-powered genetic studies effectively exclude an association between genotypes related to the serotonin system and depression, including a proposed interaction with stress.
>
> (Moncrieff et al., 2023; pp. 3243, 3253)

In other words, according to the authors, 'the main areas of serotonin research provide no consistent evidence of there being an association between serotonin and depression, and no support for the hypothesis that depression is caused by lowered serotonin activity or concentrations' (Moncrieff et al., 2023; p. 3243). This comes as no surprise: it was long recognised that depression is a heterogeneous syndrome from genetic, clinical, biological, and pharmacotherapeutic viewpoints and does not map onto any single disorder of a single neurotransmitter (Rihmer et al., 2022). Depression is vastly more complex than that, and the idea that serotonin is involved in at least some people retains validity: after all, the medications work (see Chapter 4).

Where there is modest progress in certain areas of neuroscience, therefore, and while there are treatments that help substantially, scientific progress is incremental and does not yet provide clinically actionable information for the most part. Recent genetics research provides another example of the limitations of current knowledge and its reported potential. In 2023, a review of the last decade of research in psychiatric genetics found that psychiatric illnesses (as currently conceived) are influenced by thousands of genetic variants which act together, seem to be on genetic continua with each other, and share a large amount of genetic risk (Andreassen et al., 2023). This rather unsatisfying situation is likely to continue to be the case unless genetic or other research can meaningfully replace current symptom-based diagnostic categories with biologically defined categories which might not only elucidate causation but also point towards better treatments.

In the meantime, the contribution of much recent neuroscience to clinical care is extremely limited (Steele & Paulus, 2019). While its modest contribution and future potential need to be acknowledged, a sense of proportion is also needed, especially given a generally low baseline understanding of neuroscience, particularly in media (Washington et al., 2022). Brain images are especially seductive in press releases and news reports, and often fuel over-enthusiastic accounts of extremely modest findings from small neuroscientific studies (Satel and Lilienfeld, 2013). This is not helpful. As Raymond Tallis pointed out in *The Observer* in 2013:

> The greatest excitement, orchestrated by the most extravagant press releases, surrounds the discovery of correlations between the responsiveness of certain areas of the brain and particular aspects of our personality […] The idea that we are our brains, and that we are destined to act in certain ways prescribed by this biologically evolved organ, relieves us of some of the responsibility for our behaviour […] Neuroprattle that locates our experiences, propensities and character in the activity of parts of our brain […] gets in the way of the humanist project of truly understanding ourselves.
>
> (Tallis, 2013)

Despite such commentary, it remains a fact that overstatements and misunderstandings of neuroscience are long-standing (Tallis, 2011) and persistent, especially in psychiatry (Kelly, 2022a). This situation is somewhat perplexing, given the clearly limited impact of neuroscience on treatment for most mental illnesses. Considering this dearth of yield, why does such disproportionate fascination persist? The lure of technology, combined with hope for the future and modest progress, appear to underpin the excessive beguilement of current models of neuroscience, although the lack of therapeutic impact is a stubborn, unwelcome reminder of the limits of recent progress.

In 2020, David Kingdon addressed this issue in *BJPsych Bulletin*, asking: 'Why hasn't neuroscience delivered for psychiatry?':

> Neuroscience and genetic research findings have made major contributions to the understanding of a range of disorders. Substantial advances have been possible over the past two decades in the treatment of migraine (triptans), multiple sclerosis (beta interferon, copolymer, fingolimide and dimethyl fumarate), acute stroke (tissue plasminogen activator) and epilepsy (rapamycin). Genetic research is now delivering on its promise to transform therapeutics for blood disorders and 'gene silencing' for porphyria. Dementia research has developed an understanding of the neurological basis for these disorders. In contrast, the major mental illnesses psychosis, bipolar disorder, anxiety disorders, anorexia nervosa and depression have proved remarkably resistant to similar developments. Unfortunately, it is still not possible to cite a single neuroscience or genetic finding that has been of use to the practicing psychiatrist in managing these illnesses.
>
> (Kingdon, 2020; pp. 107–8)

As discussed in Chapter 4 ('Treating Symptoms and Disorders'), some of the most prominent new treatments in psychiatry such as ketamine or psilocybin combined with psychotherapy are not, in fact, new (they date from the 1960s or earlier) and are not based on recent neuroscientific advances (they derive from ancient traditions). While it is true that neuroscience has changed understandings of certain biological correlates of mental illness to a degree (Sinclair, 2020), the lack of therapeutic advances based in neuroscience remains a real concern.

The history of psychiatry suggests that, if biological research takes a step forward, it is likely to upturn current, symptom-based diagnostic categories, rather than simply providing new treatments for existing diagnoses. In other words, the questions currently being asked of neuroscience will likely turn out to be the wrong ones, and there will be a paradigm shift that changes the landscape rather than answers the questions we currently pose.

Recognition of anti-NMDA (N-methyl-D-aspartate) receptor encephalitis in the early 2000s is a good example of the kind of changes that likely lie ahead. Following the description of this autoimmune condition, certain patients with progressive psychiatric symptoms, cognitive impairment, seizures, abnormal movements, and various other complaints are now diagnosed with the biologically defined anti-NMDA receptor encephalitis, rather than a mental illness (Dalmau et al., 2019). Approximately 90% of people with anti-NMDA receptor encephalitis have prominent psychiatric or behavioural symptoms which make their condition difficult to differentiate from psychiatric disorders. Many would have been previously diagnosed with, and treated for, schizoaffective disorder, depression, mania, or other mental illnesses. Now, they are diagnosed with anti-NMDA receptor encephalitis and effectively treated with immunotherapy and other treatments, primarily by specialists other than psychiatrists.

A similar process of migration from psychiatry to another medical discipline occurred more than a century earlier when epilepsy was found to have a neurological basis, and shifted from being considered a fundamentally psychiatric condition to being treated primarily by general practitioners and neurologists, often in consultation with psychiatry (Kelly, 2022b). Future neuroscience is likely to produce similar paradigm changes, rather than neat answers to current questions based on the diagnostic categories of today. In other words, neuroscience, which has changed very little in psychiatry to date, might yet change everything. But when?

Bringing Realism, Pragmatism, and Context to Neuroscience

Taraji, whom we met in the case history at the start of this chapter, was examined by a psychiatrist who made a diagnosis of elation or mania, most likely in the context of bipolar affective disorder. This condition features strongly in the history of psychiatry and is now commonly treated with lithium, a mood-stabilising medication (Taylor et al., 2021). American poet Robert Lowell (1917–1977) suffered from bipolar affective disorder and underwent psychological therapy before being prescribed lithium. Once he received the medication, Lowell's condition improved dramatically. He commented: 'All the psychiatry and therapy I've had, almost 19 years, was as irrelevant as it would have been for a broken leg' (quoted in Jamison, 2017; p. 179).

The discovery of the therapeutic usefulness of lithium was largely empirical, rather than driven by neuroscience, but its impact demonstrates how a biological discovery can radically change psychiatry. Just as the recognition of anti-NMDA receptor encephalitis fundamentally shifted some patients from the ambit of psychiatry into another area of medicine, the discovery of the therapeutic value of lithium radically improved the treatment of bipolar affective disorder for many people. Can modern neuroscience systematically deliver similar improvements in understanding and treatment in the future? Is there a way to generate such insights routinely, rather than arbitrarily, using theory, logic, and science, instead of hunches and chance observations?

Despite the limited progress to date, a more focused, realistic, proportionate approach to neuroscience in psychiatry is entirely possible, optimising the promise of studies of imaging, genetics, inflammation, and new treatments while remaining aware of the cost and opportunity cost of much of the neuroscience of recent decades. In other words, we can do better, provided we are honest about the limited progress to date and provided we recognise the need to recalibrate, rebalance, and, to an extent, redirect research attention over the coming decades. Progress is possible but by no means inevitable.

Stein and colleagues, writing in *World Psychiatry*, argue that, while progress is undoubtedly gradual, there has been a steady accretion of knowledge and understanding in psychiatry, which bodes well for the future (Stein et al., 2022). In a similar vein, Misiak and colleagues, in *European Psychiatry*, note that 'ongoing progress in clinical neurosciences has provided new perspectives for a better understanding of processes underlying the pathophysiology of schizophrenia':

> Combining a variety of already proposed approaches to address clinical and etiological heterogeneity across the psychosis spectrum might help to dissect valid diagnostic constructs. Translation of approaches from other disciplines and medical specialties, including neurology, might further improve the diagnostic process in psychiatry. For clinical practice, the intersection between psychiatry and neurology indicates the necessity to follow routine collaboration of both disciplines in several clinical situations. This might be of particular importance in case of diagnosing psychotic disorders when organic causes need to be ruled out or in case of emergent psychotic symptoms in the course of diagnosed neurological disorders, including MS [multiple sclerosis].
>
> (Misiak et al., 2023; p. 8)

These authors add, however, that 'it is necessary to evoke the social context and indicate the importance of listening to patients and their relatives in shaping the ease and use of future diagnoses'. In *Frontiers in Neuroscience*, Gómez-Carrillo and colleagues, too, emphasise the need to locate neuroscientific approaches within their broader context, possibly through the prism of the bio-psycho-social model of mental health care:

> To be of maximum clinical utility and avoid over-generalization [...] the neuroscientifically based explanations and interventions sought by precision psychiatry must be situated in a larger ecosocial, systemic view of symptom networks, interpersonal interactions, and adaptations. More integrative multi-level system approaches can begin to realize the original promise of the biopsychosocial approach by showing how neurobiological models can be integrated with close attention to the social-cultural contexts that give rise to psychiatric disorders. This integrative approach can bridge the precision of mechanistic explanation with the person-centeredness of phenomenology in research and practice
>
> (Gómez-Carrillo et al., 2023a; p. 11)

An overreliance on decontextualised neuroscience presents many risks which can be mitigated by (a) being aware of the limits of current biological understandings of the human brain and nervous system more generally, and (b) remaining mindful of the broader context within which neuroscientific findings are discovered and are to be considered or applied. In a similar vein, Pernu and

Elzein, reflecting on the relationship between neuroscience and the law, note that, 'when deeming a biological basis of decisions and actions dysfunctional, we need to employ psychological and social considerations':

> The mind is dependent, in a crucial way, on its biological basis, the nervous system in particular. Information about this basis should, therefore, have a straightforward impact on our moral and legal reasoning, and, ultimately, on practical jurisprudence. However, despite advances of the neurosciences, neuroscientific evidence has not played a significant role in recent legal cases. Why is that?
>
> [...] Although we can often point to clear neural changes as being associated with the sort of a behavior, *actus reus*, that is under scrutiny in court proceedings, it is wrong to think that we should conclude that these neural changes are causally responsible for the behavior in question. All behavior has a neural basis, not only the sort that we find morally or legally concerning. We need, therefore, some independent, and ultimately psychologically and socially based, grounds for thinking that a particular neural change or feature is of such a sort that it should be designated as a cause of some behavior. When deeming a biological basis of decisions and actions dysfunctional, we need to employ psychological and social considerations.
>
> (Pernu & Elzein, 2020; p. 18)

More broadly, there is now growing awareness that findings from neuroscience not only need to be contextualised in this way, but are commonly overinterpreted and oversold, especially in the field of business, with specialist areas such as 'neuro-finance' and 'neuro-marketing' emerging in recent years (Horvath, 2023). Careful thought, humility, and expectation management are needed in order to avoid overinterpretating neuroscientific findings in these areas, in order to promote realistic evaluations of what has been achieved to date, and in order to understand what might follow in the future.

Searching for the 'Science' in Neuroscience in Psychiatry

So far in this chapter, we have discussed the limits of biological knowledge of the brain (and of mental illness), a tendency to overstate neuroscientific findings (especially in the media), and the idea that neuroscience needs to be contextualised as part of a broader search for knowledge and understanding (necessitating more radical, interdisciplinary approaches in the future). But if neuroscience really does hold substantial promise for the future (Cuttle & Burn, 2020), and if there really is poetry to be found in this science (Tracy, 2020), can more of this promise and poetry be harnessed *today*? What can we do now, for the patients of today, as opposed to the patients of some ever-receding future date when neuroscience has delivered its long-promised utopia?

The first point to note is that certain psychiatric treatments are advancing, albeit extremely slowly, based on biological knowledge of the body, including the brain. In 2023, the US Food and Drug Administration (FDA) approved zuranolone, a fast-acting, oral version of brexanolone, for treating postpartum depression (Rubin, 2023). Both zuranolone and brexanolone are neurosteroids and analogues of allopregnanolone, a derivative of progesterone, which rises in pregnancy, falls in the third trimester, and plummets after giving birth. While evidence of clinical effectiveness is compelling, zuranolone arrives with a 'black box' warning that it can impair a person's ability to drive and to perform other possibly hazardous activities. Notwithstanding this limitation, the advent of zuranolone is welcome and – at least in part – apparently biologically explicable. This will come as a huge relief both to those who will benefit from the treatment and to anyone who is concerned with the development of psychiatry; zuranolone seems to be an all-too-rare example of science and therapeutics finally connecting up in the field of mental health care. There is still some road to travel with this medication, but hopefully the promise of zuranolone will be borne out in practice.

In other areas of treatment, neuroscience is stimulating research into a variety of psychological processes which are relevant to psychiatric and psychotherapeutic practice to varying degrees (Mizen and Hook, 2020). While there is significant progress in these areas, however, there remain substantial gaps in understanding, and mental activity has properties which remain unexplained by knowledge of the biological brain (Paris, 2017). Similarly, in the field of addiction, functional neuroimaging is playing an important role in delineating the neurobiology of addictive behaviours, although future work could usefully focus more on replication, reliability, and the reproducibility of neuroscientific findings (Hayes et al., 2020). Studies of inflammation, too, show promise but have significant progress to make before direct clinical applicability (Kelly, 2022a; *Lancet Psychiatry,* 2023). There is lots of possibility, then, but limited delivery to date.

The difficulties with many of these areas of research lie not only with our limited biological knowledge of the brain and mental illness (which seriously hampers rational suggestions of novel treatments) but also the state of scientific research and publication in general. In 2022, Lee and colleagues, in the *British Journal of Psychiatry*, highlighted the problem of poor research integrity and noted that many research findings are incorrect, even when studies are performed correctly and published (Lee et al., 2022). Many registered clinical trials are never published, and questionable research practices are common, including outcome switching, selective reporting, and 'p-hacking'. While scientific publications can and should tighten their procedures for detecting poor practice and improving standards, those interventions are well down the road in the scientific process. There is also a need for educators to emphasise research integrity in order to improve standards of practice at all stages, not just at publication, along with funders insisting on greater clarity and accountability.

Perhaps the first step to improve integrity in psychiatric research is to adopt an attitude of humility towards what we already know about the brain in mental illness (remarkably little) and to value what we know from other fields about patterns of suffering and the occurrence of psychiatric disorders across populations (quite a lot). Charles E. Dean, in *The Skeptical Professional's Guide to Psychiatry: On the Risks and Benefits of Antipsychotics, Antidepressants, Psychiatric Diagnoses, and Neuromania*, sensibly points out that, even in an era of neuroscientific hubris, we already have reliable evidence that social stressors such as poverty and childhood abuse are associated with increased risks of depression and psychosis (Dean, 2021; p. 307). While these effects will likely prove to be biologically mediated, strategies for intervention need not await confirmation of the neuroscience of these associations. We can and should act now, in parallel with rational neuroscientific exploration.

This is central. We are currently failing to act sufficiently, even on the knowledge we have. These issues are explored further in Chapter 9 of this book, which is devoted to 'Global Injustice in Mental Health Care', and Chapter 10, which explores 'The Future of Psychiatry: Person-Centred Care and System-Level Change'. We already know a great deal about the risks of many mental illness and their distribution across populations, and we have treatments that work very well (Leucht et al., 2012). Even within a dense cloud of neuroscientific uncertainty and confusion, there is much that we can do better *today*. We should do it *now*.

Multidisciplinarity, Interdisciplinarity, Transdisciplinarity

So, where do we go from here, from a scientific perspective? If neuroscience has not delivered sufficiently to date, will it ever provide more answers? Or is the current model fundamentally broken, and in need of being replaced? Whither neuroscience in psychiatry?

First, it is important to acknowledge (yet again) that neuroscience already plays important, if limited, roles in day-to-day clinical psychiatry. Certain tests help to out-rule specific organic conditions during the diagnostic process (e.g., neuro-imaging for brain tumours); neuroscience contributes more in certain areas of psychiatry than others (e.g., dementia diagnosis, intellectual disability); and recent advances offer some specific treatments (e.g., in post-partum depression) and insights (e.g., in addiction) which will likely bear further fruit over future years (see above). The situation is far from perfect, but it is by no means hopeless. There is, however, a need to shift relative emphasis away from reifying current neuroscientific approaches which have delivered bewilderingly little in most areas of psychiatry to date, and towards other paradigms that can contribute more and differently, both now and in the future, in parallel with neuroscientific study (which should, of course, continue, despite its glacial progress).

Against this background, there is a need for a greater plurality of research methodologies in psychiatry, a true synthesis of techniques and understandings across neuroscience, medicine, law, history, spirituality, and other fields. Done well, this broad approach can amount to more than the sum of its parts, and can integrate research with understanding, understanding with treatment, and treatment with improved quality of life for patients and their families. The task is important, complex, and far from impossible – and it can proceed alongside a more chastened, humble, and evidence-based neuroscience.

The challenge is more acute in psychiatry than it is in other areas of medicine owing to psychiatry's continued reliance on symptom-based diagnostic categories. In 2023, George Ikkos argued, in *BJPsych Bulletin*, that 'psychiatry must forge its distinct identity':

> This will mean tolerating ignorance and uncertainty, sharing them intelligently with colleagues and the public and engaging creatively rather than concealing or denying them. At the same time continuing to chip away at ignorance and uncertainty where possible [...] For psychiatrists in Britain (and beyond), without losing passion for research, including in neuroscience (but also all other relevant areas), nor forsaking clinical and social commitment and hope, there is a need for ongoing recognition of affect as the object of psychiatric expertise, an attitude of humility about the state of advancement of our clinical science, attention to the sociology of ignorance, caution about adopting transatlantic healthcare policies and management techniques, and consistent commitment to intellectual and clinical pluralism.
>
> (Ikkos, 2023; p. 93)

Huxley and Poole, in response, note Ikkos's call 'for psychiatry to forge a new identity', implying 'that this should be more clearly social in nature', and they 'strongly support that proposition':

> Psychiatry and social science both work to understand and address the consequences of social adversity and injustice, even if psychiatry is sometimes reluctant to acknowledge this. Psychiatry has responsibilities at both population and individual levels. It is a fruitless enterprise to address the medical without attention to the social, but it is equally fruitless to suggest social solutions without attention to the actual illness experience and the relief of distress.
>
> (Huxley and Poole, 2023; p. 67)

Gómez-Carrillo and colleagues, writing in *Lancet Psychiatry* in 2023, agreed that any analysis of brain function which creates a separation between the brain and its social environment is too restrictive, will miss key determinants of mental health, and will hamper scientific advances in therapeutics (Gómez-Carrillo et al., 2023b). They note that while neuroscientific and sociocultural approaches remain largely separate in psychiatry, it is possible to bring them together in a multilevel explanatory framework that can advance psychiatric theory, research, and practice. The history of psychiatry strongly supports this conclusion.

In *Frontiers in Psychiatry,* Gómez-Carrillo and Kirmayer explore a 'cultural-ecosocial systems view for psychiatry' in some detail:

> While contemporary psychiatry seeks the mechanisms of mental disorders in neurobiology, mental health problems clearly depend on developmental processes of learning and adaptation through ongoing interactions with the social environment. Symptoms or disorders emerge in specific social contexts and involve predicaments that cannot be fully characterized in terms of brain function but require a larger social-ecological view. Causal processes that result in mental health problems can begin anywhere within the extended system of body-person-environment. In particular, individuals' narrative self-construal, culturally mediated interpretations of symptoms and coping strategies as well as the responses of others in the social world contribute to the mechanisms of mental disorders, illness experience, and recovery.
>
> (Gómez-Carrillo and Kirmayer, 2023; p. 1)

Against this background, Gómez-Carrillo and Kirmayer 'outline the conceptual basis and practical implications of a hierarchical ecosocial systems view for an integrative approach to psychiatric theory and practice' (p. 1). The 'cultural-ecosocial systems view' that they suggest 'understands mind, brain and person as situated in the social world and as constituted by cultural and self-reflexive processes'. It 'can be incorporated into a pragmatic approach to clinical assessment and case formulation that characterises mechanisms of pathology and identifies targets for intervention'.

Perhaps the most compelling aspect of this approach is not just its immediate clinical relevance to the lives of people with mental illness, but also the breadth of perspectives which are acknowledged as extant, relevant, and essential for understanding and progress. In order to realise the potential of this approach fully, there needs to be a significant move towards integrating research from diverse disciplines into psychiatric practice. This process can be multidisciplinary, interdisciplinary, transdisciplinary, or – ideally – all three at various times. Multidisciplinary approaches draw on knowledge from different disciplines but stay within their boundaries (Choi and Pak, 2006). Interdisciplinarity, by contrast, analyses, synthesises, and harmonises links between disciplines into a coherent and coordinated whole. Finally, transdisciplinarity integrates the natural, social, and health sciences in a humanities context, transcending their traditional boundaries in the process.

All three approaches are needed: multidisciplinarity, interdisciplinarity, and transdisciplinarity. The humanities are, perhaps, especially relevant in the context of psychiatry and conditions that affect the brain and human behaviour. Valtonen and Lewis make this point clearly in the *Journal of Medical Humanities*:

> The contemporary brain disorders debate echoes a century-long conflict between two different approaches to mental suffering: one that relies on natural sciences and another drawing from the arts and humanities. We review contemporary neuroimaging studies and find that neither side has won. The study of mental differences needs *both* the sciences and the arts and humanities.
>
> (Valtonen & Lewis, 2023; p. 291)

More specifically, Valtonen and Lewis conclude:

> It seemed, not so long ago, that empirical natural science and quantitative research were the only way forward for understanding mental health and that neuroscience would lead the way. But now, with a wealth of research on the limits of neuroscience for understanding mental health, it is time to reconsider how we research, teach, and practice mental health care [...] cognitive science, behavioral science, neuroscience, genetics, and medical science all have their place, and they all do what they can to help explain and predict aspects of mental difference. At the same time, the arts and humanities also provide us with a valuable understanding that cannot be achieved in any other way.
>
> (Valtonen and Lewis, 2023; p. 306)

Valtonen and Lewis are correct, and it is equally important that education in the humanities takes greater account of science in general and medical science in particular. A synthesis of understandings benefits all.

Moving Forward with Neuroscience

Developing a humbler, more evidence-based neuroscience that is integrated with approaches from other disciplines and more in tune with clinical realities is not an easy task, but it is an essential one. As discussed above, there is a serious problem with research integrity across much of science (Lee et al., 2022); research ethics boards face significant, complicated tasks assessing research, including risks to participants and researchers (Webber & Brunger, 2018); and the record of neuroscience in much of psychiatry is not especially inspiring to date (Kingdon, 2020). Even so, despite these challenges – or possibly because of them – something needs to change.

The copious resources devoted to current models of neuroscience have conspicuously failed to deliver sufficient progress in psychiatry to justify its domination over other areas of research (cultural, psychosocial, etc.) (Gardner and Kleinman, 2019). Promises of future benefit are justified to a degree, but are starting to wear thin. Surely, more could happen now? Given the prevalence and severity of mental illness around the world, the issue is a pressing one. Gardner and Kleinman argue convincingly that instead of contracting to focus solely on biological structure, research in psychiatry should expand if it is truly to meet the needs of people with mental illness who require care that is comprehensive and relational and that will alleviate their suffering effectively and humanely (Gardner & Kleinman, 2019). People with mental illness and their families have waited long enough. They deserve no less.

A humanistic commitment to understanding the lived experience of mental illness, its treatment, and its consequences is especially important. Anthropology has a particular role to play in this task. D'Arcy, for example, draws on ethnographic fieldwork in a community mental health system in Dublin, Ireland to explore the experiences of 'Sean', a man who was homeless and struggled with substance misuse, psychosis, and strong suicidal impulses:

> Though psychotic mental illness and substance use disorder are often identified as chronic illnesses that demand pharmacological management by biomedical institutions of care, cases of dual diagnosis like Sean's can easily be reframed as existential and ethical crises. Such a reframing can help to rethink the institutional politics inherent to treating such comorbidities, as well as the meaningful stakes of dual diagnosis for the people who engage with and sometimes withdraw from psychiatric care. Specifically, Sean's case has helped me to think through the doubling of these aforementioned experiences of rupture and marginality in the clinical, conceptual, and lived space of comorbidity; the concomitant doubling of the demands imposed by the psychiatric injunction to adhere to one category of medications and strenuously avoid another; and the degree to which my interlocutors' relationships to the nested assumptions *about* and clinical projections *regarding* the potential for transformations in my interlocutors' subjectivities were influenced by their respective proximities to an array of distinct but deeply interrelated substances. The ethical questions that remain – how to live in relation to these experiences and these substances – have given me further reason to return to considering the place of moral agency in the methadone clinic, the inpatient ward, and all of the spaces in between.
>
> (D'Arcy, 2023; pp. 7–8)

Reframing Sean's experiences and problems as 'existential and ethical crises', and considering them within an anthropological framework, opens a new window to connection, understanding, healing, and hope. Neuroscience will likely have much to offer in this process in the future, but neuroscience is not the only approach. Moreover, a decontextualised neuroscience, no matter how advanced it might be, would fail to address many of the human needs of people with mental illness, and fail to bring understanding to situations where it is desperately required.

Against this background, the current chapter acknowledges the contributions that neuroscience has made to certain, limited areas within psychiatry, but also recognises the failure of neuroscience to substantially increase our understanding of the causes of common mental illnesses or substantially inform new therapies for many conditions. We need a more focused, realistic, proportionate approach to neuroscience in psychiatry, optimising the promise of studies of imaging, genetics, inflammation, and new treatments, but remaining aware of the cost and opportunity cost of much neuroscience over the past decades. This involves a refreshed plurality of research methodologies and a true synthesis of techniques and understandings across neuroscience, medicine, law, history, spirituality, and other fields. Neuroscience needs to be contextualised as part of this broader search for knowledge and understanding, necessitating radical, interdisciplinary approaches that can truly elucidate the nature of mental illness and its treatment.

Taraji, the woman whom we met at the start of this chapter, had an episode of mania. She had increased energy, disinhibition, reduced need for sleep, grandiose ideation, and a delusion that she could fly. In the end, she agreed to inpatient psychiatric care.

After ten days of treatment, Taraji began to understand what had happened when she was arrested on the roof, singing songs, and believing she could fly. Taraji was enormously embarrassed. She had never been arrested before. Taraji asked the psychiatrist if she should contact the police and apologise, but the psychiatrist advised her to set that aside for the moment. Instead, Taraji went out for walks with Mandisa when she visited her in the hospital. Taraji confided to Mandisa that she had been depressed for several months in her late teens, but did not speak about it at the time. Together, they tried to make sense of what was happening. The psychiatrist told Taraji that she needed ongoing treatment for bipolar affective disorder to reduce the likelihood of further episodes of mania or depression. This made sense to Taraji: she never wanted anything like this to happen again.

Taraji was commenced on lithium, with appropriate monitoring and advice. Her antipsychotic medication was gradually stopped over a few weeks. Taraji spent three weeks in hospital and had follow-up appointments at the clinic with the psychiatrist and a clinical psychologist. She also saw a community mental health nurse who gave her his work phone number, to call him in any emergency. Taraji got back to work the following month and ran a marathon later that year. She even went camping again with Mandisa, who still disliked camping, but felt her friend deserved a break after this difficult period in her life.

Key Messages

- There is a great deal of scientific data about the human nervous system, but these data do not provide a complete picture of how the brain functions, let alone the biological basis of most mental illnesses or the biological correlates of treatment.
- Despite this lack of neuroscientific understanding, interventions such as anti-depressants help to alleviate a great deal of suffering, as evidenced by the outcomes of clinical trials and experience in day-to-day clinical practice – as opposed to proposed neurochemical theories of depression or proposed mechanisms of action, which remain unproven.
- Overreliance on decontextualised neuroscience presents many risks which can be mitigated by (a) being aware of the limits of current understandings of the human brain and nervous system, and (b) remaining mindful of the broader context within which neuroscientific findings are to be considered and applied; i.e., the personal, social, economic, and political landscapes in which mental illness develops (or does not develop), is diagnosed (or not diagnosed), and is treated (or not treated), as well as its long-term outcomes.
- While neuroscience continues to offer hope for the (perpetually distant) future, it is important that continued neuroscientific research is informed and accompanied by greater multidisciplinarity, interdisciplinarity, and transdisciplinarity in mental health research, services, education, and policy.
- Biological research should, of course, continue, but with enhanced aware-ness of the limited progress to date; renewed commitment to addressing the many problems across the scientific literature (e.g., outcome switching, selec-tive reporting, and 'p-hacking'); and greater integration with other areas of research and clinical practice.
- Neuroscience needs to be contextualised as part of this broader search for knowledge and understanding, embedded within a refreshed plurality of research methodologies and reflecting a more radical, fundamentally inter-disciplinary approach to psychiatric suffering and its alleviation.

References

Andreassen OA, Hindley GFL, Frei O, Smeland OB. New insights from the last decade of research in psychiatric genetics: discoveries, challenges and clinical implications. *World Psychiatry* 2023; 22: 4–24 (https://doi.org/10.1002/wps.21034).

Choi BCK, Pak AWP. Multidisciplinarity, interdisciplinarity and transdisciplinarity in health research, services, education and policy: 1. Definitions, objectives, and evidence of effectiveness. *Clinical and Investigative Medicine* 2006; 29: 351–64 (https://pubmed.ncbi.nlm.nih.gov/17330451/) (accessed 2 September 2023).

Cipriani A, Furukawa TA, Salanti G, Chaimani A, Atkinson LZ, Ogawa Y, Leucht S, Ruhe HG, Turner EH, Higgins JPT, Egger M, Takeshima N, Hayasaka Y, Imai H, Shinohara K, Tajika A, Ioannidis JPA, Geddes JR. Comparative efficacy and acceptability of 21 antidepressant drugs for the acute treatment of adults with major depressive disorder: a systematic review and network meta-analysis. *Lancet* 2018; 391: 1357–66 (https://doi.org/10.1016/S0140-6736(17)32802-7). (Link to licence: https://creativecommons.org/licenses/by/4.0/) (accessed 2 September 2023).

Cuttle G, Burn W. Neuroscience: the way forward. *BJPsych Advances* 2020; 26: 318–19 (https://doi.org/10.1192/bja.2020.72).

Dalmau J, Armangué T, Planagumà J, Radosevic M, Mannara F, Leypoldt F, Geis C, Lancaster E, Titulaer MJ, Rosenfeld MR, Graus F. An update on anti-NMDA receptor encephalitis for neurologists and psychiatrists: mechanisms and models. *Lancet Neurology* 2019; 18: 1045–57 (https://doi.org/10.1016/s1474-4422(19)30244-3).

D'Arcy M. 'Swallow them all, and it's just like smack': comorbidity, polypharmacy, and imagining moral agency alongside methadone and antipsychotics. *Medicine Anthropology Theory* 2023; 10: 1–25 (https://doi.org/10.17157/mat.10.1.6917). (Link to licence: https://creativecommons.org/licenses/by/4.0/) (accessed 2 September 2023).

Dean CE. *The Skeptical Professional's Guide to Psychiatry: On the Risks and Benefits of Antipsychotics, Antidepressants, Psychiatric Diagnoses, and Neuromania.* New York and London: Routledge, 2021.

Gardner C, Kleinman A. Medicine and the mind – the consequences of psychiatry's identity crisis. *New England Journal of Medicine* 2019; 381: 1697–9 (https://doi.org/10.1056/NEJMp1910603).

Gómez-Carrillo A, Kirmayer LJ. A cultural-ecosocial systems view for psychiatry. *Frontiers in Psychiatry* 2023; 14: 1031390 (https://doi.org/10.3389/fpsyt.2023.1031390). (Link to licence: https://creativecommons.org/licenses/by/4.0/) (accessed 2 September 2023).

Gómez-Carrillo A, Paquin V, Dumas G, Kirmayer LJ. Restoring the missing person to personalized medicine and precision psychiatry. *Frontiers in Neuroscience* 2023a; 17: 1041433 (https://doi.org/10.3389/fnins.2023.1041433). (Link to licence: https://creativecommons.org/licenses/by/4.0/) (accessed 2 September 2023).

Gómez-Carrillo A, Kirmayer LJ, Aggarwal NK, Bhui KS, Fung KP-L, Kohrt BA, Weiss MG, Lewis-Fernández R, Group for the Advancement of Psychiatry Committee on Cultural Psychiatry. Integrating neuroscience in psychiatry: a cultural-ecosocial systemic approach. *Lancet Psychiatry* 2023b; 10: 296–304 (https://doi.org/10.1016/s2215-0366(23)00006-8).

Hayes A, Herlinger K, Paterson L, Lingford-Hughes A. The neurobiology of substance use and addiction: evidence from neuroimaging and relevance to treatment. *BJPsych Advances* 2020; 26: 367–78 (https://doi.org/10.1192/bja.2020.68).

Horvath JC. The limits of neuroscience in business. *MIT Sloan Management Review* 2023; 64: 1–4 (https://sloanreview.mit.edu/article/the-limits-of-neuroscience-in-business/) (accessed 2 September 2023).

Huxley P, Poole R. Social psychiatry lives! *BJPsych Bulletin* 2023; 47: 65–7 (https://doi.org/10.1192/bjb.2022.77). (Link to licence: https://creativecommons.org/licenses/by/4.0/) (accessed 2 September 2023).

Ikkos G. Not doomed: sociology and psychiatry, and ignorance and expertise. *BJPsych Bulletin* 2023; 47: 90–4 (https://doi.org/10.1192/bjb.2022.60). (Link to licence: https://creativecommons.org/licenses/by/4.0/) (accessed 2 September 2023).

Jamison KR. *Robert Lowell, Setting the River on Fire: A Study of Genius, Mania, and Character.* New York: Alfred A. Knopf, 2017.

Kelly BD. Psychiatry's future: biology, psychology, legislation, and 'the fierce urgency of *now*'. *Indian Journal of Psychological Medicine* 2020; 42: 189–92 (https://doi.org /10.4103/IJPSYM.IJPSYM_492_19).

Kelly BD. *In Search of Madness: A Psychiatrist's Travels Through the History of Mental Illness*. Dublin: Gill Books, 2022a.

Kelly BD. Psychiatry is essential for now but might eventually disappear (although this is unlikely to happen any time soon). *Australasian Psychiatry* 2022b; 30: 171–3 (https:// doi.org/10.1177/10398562211048141). (Link to licence: https://creativecommons .org/licenses/by/4.0/) (accessed 2 September 2023).

Kingdon D. Why hasn't neuroscience delivered for psychiatry? *BJPsych Bulletin* 2020; 44: 107–9 (https://doi.org/10.1192/bjb.2019.87). (Link to licence: https:// creativecommons.org/licenses/by/4.0/) (accessed 2 September 2023).

Lancet Psychiatry. Integrating inflammation. *Lancet Psychiatry* 2023; 10: 235 (https:// doi.org/10.1016/s2215-0366(23)00064-0).

Lee W, Casey P, Poole N, Kaufman KR, Lawrie SM, Malhi G, Petkova E, Siddiqi N, Bhui K. The integrity of the research record: a mess so big and so deep and so tall. *British Journal of Psychiatry* 2022; 221: 580–1 (https://doi.org/10.1192/bjp.2022.74).

Legrenzi P, Umiltà C. *Neuromania: On the Limits of Brain Science*. Oxford: Oxford University Press, 2011.

Leucht S, Hierl S, Kissling W, Dold M, Davis JM. Putting the efficacy of psychiatric and general medicine medication into perspective: review of meta-analyses. *British Journal of Psychiatry* 2012; 200: 97–106 (https://doi.org/10.1192/bjp.bp.111.096594).

McIntyre RS, Berk M, Brietzke E, Goldstein BI, López-Jaramillo C, Kessing LV, Malhi GS, Nierenberg AA, Rosenblat JD, Majeed A, Vieta E, Vinberg M, Young AH, Mansur RB. Bipolar disorders. *Lancet* 2020; 396: 1841–56 (https://doi.org/10.1016 /S0140-6736(20)31544-0).

Misiak B, Samochowiec J, Kowalski K, Gaebel W, Bassetti CLA, Chan A, Gorwood P, Papiol S, Dom G, Volpe U, Szulc A, Kurimay T, Kärkkäinen H, Decraene A, Wisse J, Fiorillo A, Falkai P. The future of diagnosis in clinical neurosciences: comparing multiple sclerosis and schizophrenia. *European Psychiatry* 2023; 66: e58 (https:// doi.org/10.1192/j.eurpsy.2023.2432). (Link to licence: https://creativecommons.org/ licenses/by/4.0/) (accessed 2 September 2023).

Mizen CS, Hook J. Relational and affective neuroscience: a quiet revolution in psychiatric and psychotherapeutic practice. *BJPsych Advances* 2020; 26: 356–66 (https://doi.org /10.1192/bja.2020.63).

Moncrieff J, Cooper RE, Stockmann T, Amendola S, Hengartner MP, Horowitz MA. The serotonin theory of depression: a systematic umbrella review of the evidence. *Molecular Psychiatry* 2023; 28: 3243–56 (https://doi.org/10.1038/s41380-022 -01661-0). (Link to licence: https://creativecommons.org/licenses/by/4.0/) (accessed 26 January 2024).

Paris J. *Psychotherapy in An Age of Neuroscience*. New York: Oxford University Press, 2017 (https://doi.org/10.1093/med/9780190601010.001.0001).

Pernu TK. Methodological dualism considered as a heuristic paradigm for clinical psychiatry. *BJPsych Advances* 2022; 28: 166–9 (https://doi.org/10.1192/bja.2021 .56). (Link to licence: https://creativecommons.org/licenses/by/4.0/) (accessed 2 September 2023).

Pernu TK, Elzein N. From neuroscience to law: bridging the gap. *Frontiers in Psychology* 2020; 11: 1862 (https://doi.org/10.3389/fpsyg.2020.01862). (Link to licence: https://creativecommons.org/licenses/by/4.0/) (accessed 2 September 2023).

Rihmer Z, Dome P, Katona C. Serotonin and depression - a riposte to Moncrieff et al. (2022). *Neuropsychopharmacologia Hungarica* 2022; 24: 120–5 (https://mppt.hu/en/project/volume-24-issue-3-september-2022/) (accessed 2 September 2023).

Rubin R. A fast-acting pill received approval for postpartum depression – is it a game changer? *JAMA* 2023; 330: 902–4 (https://doi.org/10.1001/jama.2023.16499).

Satel S, Lilienfeld SO. *Brainwashed: The Seductive Appeal of Mindless Neuroscience.* New York: Basic Books, 2013.

Sinclair LI. What neuroscience has already done for us: commentary on… why hasn't neuroscience delivered for psychiatry? *BJPsych Bulletin* 2020; 44: 110–12 (https://doi.org/10.1192/bjb.2019.90).

Sloman SA, Patterson R, Barbey AK. Cognitive neuroscience meets the community of knowledge. *Frontiers in Systems Neuroscience* 2021; 15: 675127 (https://doi.org/10.3389/fnsys.2021.675127). (Link to licence: https://creativecommons.org/licenses/by/4.0/) (accessed 2 September 2023).

Steele JD, Paulus MP. Pragmatic neuroscience for clinical psychiatry. *British Journal of Psychiatry* 2019; 215: 404–8 (https://doi.org/10.1192/bjp.2019.88).

Stein DJ, Shoptaw SJ, Vigo DV, Lund C, Cuijpers P, Bantjes J, Sartorius N, Maj M. Psychiatric diagnosis and treatment in the 21st century: paradigm shifts versus incremental integration. *World Psychiatry* 2022; 21: 393–414 (https://doi.org/10.1002/wps.20998).

Tallis R. *Aping Mankind: Neuromania, Darwinitis and the Misrepresentation of Humanity.* Durham: Acumen Publishing, 2011.

Tallis R. Think brain scans can reveal our innermost thoughts? Think again. *Observer*, 2 June 2013 (https://www.theguardian.com/commentisfree/2013/jun/02/brain-scans-innermost-thoughts) (accessed 2 September 2023) (Courtesy of Guardian News & Media Ltd.).

Taylor DM, Barnes TRE, Young AH. *The Maudsley Prescribing Guidelines in Psychiatry* (14th Edn). Hoboken, NJ and Chichester: Wiley Blackwell/John Wiley & Sons, Inc., 2021.

Tracy DK. Keeping the brain in mind: why neuroscience matters to 21st-century psychiatrists. *BJPsych Advances* 2020; 26: 331–2 (https://doi.org/10.1192/bja.2020.13).

Valtonen J, Lewis B. The brain disorders debate, Chekhov, and mental health humanities. *Journal of Medical Humanities* 2023; 44: 291–309 (https://doi.org/10.1007/s10912-023-09786-1). (Link to licence: https://creativecommons.org/licenses/by/4.0/) (accessed 26 January 2024).

Washington N, Leone C, Niemi L. Neuroscience and mental illness. In: De Brigard F, Sinnott-Armstrong W (eds), *Neuroscience and Philosophy* (pp. 139–60). Cambridge, MA: MIT Press, 2022 (https://doi.org/10.7551/mitpress/12611.003.0009).

Webber V, Brunger F. Assessing risk to researchers: using the case of sexuality research to inform research ethics board guidelines. *Forum Qualitative Sozialforschung (Forum: Qualitative Social Research)* 2018; 19: 2 (https://doi.org/10.17169/fqs-19.3.3062).

7   Psychiatry, Culture, and Society

Miguel was 25 when he first heard the voices of two gods. The gods who spoke to him were not immediately familiar, although their message was one he knew well: that the world needs more love. This fitted with Miguel's religious beliefs and those of his community, who accepted multiple gods and believed that people needed to show more love towards each other.

Miguel first heard the gods when he was at home one afternoon, helping his children with their homework. Miguel lived with his wife and two children, aged eight years and six years. The children worked hard at school and did not cause their parents any trouble. Miguel helped with their homework every day. Soon, he was hearing the voices of the two gods every afternoon, as they repeated their message that the world needs more love.

At first, Miguel did not tell anyone about the voices. The gods, one female and one male, were kind and gentle. They told him things he already knew: that people do not love each other enough, that the modern world is too busy, and that most people ignore their spiritual side. The voices of the gods were very clear. The came from outside Miguel's head and were not the voice of his conscience. They were as loud and clear as the voices of Miguel's children, his wife, and his friends. The voices never said their names, but Miguel knew that they were gods.

One evening, Miguel told his wife what was happening. Miguel's wife, who shared his faith, wondered if Miguel had been selected for a special blessing. Together, they visited their priest, who listened carefully to Miguel's story. When Miguel finished talking, the priest sat in silence. After some time, he said: 'This is a very special experience. Treasure it'. Miguel was pleased to have shared his experiences with the priest, although the priest said that not everyone would understand, and some people might be jealous. The priest advised Miguel not to tell everyone about the two gods, but to be careful whom he spoke with. Miguel understood.

Over the following months, the gods talked to Miguel more and more. While Miguel initially welcomed their voices, he sometimes felt that he would like to have a break from them. Also, the tone of the voices changed. The gods now spoke less about love and began to criticise Miguel. They said that Miguel did not show enough love to the world. They said that Miguel was selfish because he

DOI: 10.4324/9781003378495-8

thought only about his children, his wife, and himself. The gods told Miguel that he must leave his home and bring a message of love to the wider world.

Miguel's priest told him to ignore these negative messages, but that was difficult for Miguel. The voices were persuasive. 'And maybe they are right', Miguel said. 'Maybe I need to go out into the world with a message of love?' The priest said that Miguel needed to decide this for himself, but he should think about his family and friends at home, who needed his love too.

One night, when the voices were especially strong, Miguel could no longer resist their urgings. He got out of bed, got dressed, and left his home alone at 3 am. He was going into the world to spread a message of love.

Introduction

Miguel's experience could be interpreted as a religious manifestation, a sign of mental illness (auditory hallucinations and possible delusions), or something else. Radically different interpretations can co-exist at the same time for some people, in which case attention focusses on whether or not the experience causes distress or problems in the person's life. In Miguel's case, the voices of the two gods were not immediately troublesome or disturbing: he welcomed their message of love, which fitted with his religious and spiritual positions, and made him feel that he had been chosen. The voices were also consistent with Miguel's cultural background and social setting, so there was no problem initially.

When the voices became more negative, however, and started to criticise Miguel, the situation changed considerably. Now, the voices were distressing Miguel and having a negative effect on his life. Finally, the two gods asked Miguel to leave his family and home, and set forth into the world on a mission to spread love. At this point, the voices were more persuasive and powerful. Miguel felt that he could no longer resist their commands. He acted on their advice and left his family behind to embark on an unplanned mission to an unknown location.

This case history highlights some of the tensions between specific mental experiences (in this case, hearing voices or auditory hallucinations) and the interpretative frameworks used to understand such phenomena (in this case, religious and cultural frameworks, rather than a psychiatric one). Against this background, this chapter explores the complicated relationship between psychiatry, culture, and society, reflecting the fact that psychiatry has always been a very social endeavour that is, for each individual, located in specific personal and social contexts. Psychological experiences or psychiatric symptoms inevitably emerge in particular social, cultural, and religious settings, with the result that the experience, interpretation, and treatment of psychiatric symptoms are inevitably shaped by society, culture, and other beliefs (such as religion and spirituality).

The chapter starts by outlining the relatively recent articulation of a clear relationship between psychiatry and culture, especially through the work of psychiatrist and anthropologist Arthur Kleinman in the 1980s. It then shifts focus to public expectations of psychiatry, particularly in terms of 'risk management', and how a 'culture of risk' can drive psychiatry in unhelpful directions. Linked with this, the chapter explores misuse of psychiatric diagnoses, practices, and institutions, both in history and today, and moves on to discuss professionalism in psychiatry and the current contract between psychiatry and society. This is followed by further discussion of 'cultural psychiatry' and what this means in theory and in practice. The chapter concludes by considering issues related to discrimination in psychiatry, including sexism, racism, and LGBTQIA+ (lesbian, gay, bisexual, transgender, queer, questioning, intersex, and asexual) issues, as well as ways to improve matters.

Throughout these discussions, there is emphasis on psychiatry as both a medical practice and a social endeavour, seeking to treat symptoms and alleviate distress, but doing so with an awareness of cultural and social context. Everyone's life is shaped by their personal beliefs, cultural milieu, and social surroundings, so their experience of psychological distress and psychiatric symptoms are inevitably influenced by similar considerations. Efforts at understanding, treating, and supporting recovery need to be informed by these realities and mindful of these powerful influences in everyone's lives. Psychiatry always has a social context. It ignores this at its peril.

Psychiatry and Culture

In 1980, Arthur Kleinman, a psychiatrist who also trained in anthropology, published a book titled *Patients and Healers in the Context of Culture: An Exploration of the Borderland between Anthropology, Medicine, and Psychiatry* (Kleinman, 1980). Kleinman argued in favour of an interdisciplinary approach to psychiatry, including ideas, methodologies, problem-frames, and solution-frames from both social science and clinical science. He argued that this was the best way to proceed in cross-cultural studies of health care. In this especially compelling volume, Kleinman recommended *mixing* disciplines alongside sharing ideas and approaches. In the book's epilogue, he noted the limited progress of medical anthropology in coming to terms with clinical reality and its different constructions in varied social structural and cultural settings.

Kleinman's observations were powerful and long overdue. Eight years later, in *Rethinking Psychiatry: From Cultural Category to Personal Experience*, he added that interdisciplinary relationships require work to flow in both directions (Kleinman, 1988), which is a point that is often missed in discussions of this topic: conversations work both ways. Kleinman further argued that psychiatry is a surprisingly good subject to re-examine from a cultural standpoint and offers particular opportunities to link anthropological theory to a much broader set of issues. This remains true today: bio-psycho-social psychiatry holds a very particular, multi-faceted mirror to society, exploring and illuminating areas of human culture and activity that other fields rarely approach. Often, mental health professionals work at the very edges of human experience.

The case of Miguel at the start of this chapter illustrates many of these points. Miguel's first framework for interpreting his experiences was a religious one, so he went to see a priest. The priest offered advice that was useful, sensible, and meaningful to Miguel and his family. In many cases, such advice might be all that is needed, not least because it accords with a pre-existing belief system (rather than introducing a new one) and fits into a familiar cultural framework (rather than imposing or constructing a different one). In Miguel's case, unfortunately, the advice from the priest did not prove sufficient over time, because the voices of the gods became more negative, persistent, and commanding. Even so, the initial impulse was clearly appropriate and wise: interpreting and responding to an unusual experience by using familiar concepts and coping strategies. That is how most people cope with most things, most of the time.

But the case of Miguel also illustrates the value of individual stories as a way of understanding the strengths *and* limitations of cultural interpretations of phenomena such as auditory hallucinations or paranoid delusions, which many cultures and societies ultimately associate with mental illness in one form or other. As a result, there is a specific role for ethnography within anthropology, and within the anthropologies of mental illness and psychiatry in particular, when individual case histories move beyond the bounds of the familiar and into the relative unknown, tugging at the edges of the knowable.

Ethnography, in this context, is the systematic description of peoples and cultures with their customs, habits, and differences. Ethnography forms a key part of social and cultural anthropology. Carefully conducted, this approach can not only deepen knowledge, but also advance engagement and understanding, with many consequent benefits. In fact, Lemelson and Tucker, in a detailed consideration of psychopathology and recovery in cultural context, argue that the issues, categories, factors, and domains which are identified in detailed, person-centred ethnography are directly related to *better health outcomes* (Lemelson and Tucker, 2015). This observation both reflects the value of experience-near ethnography and develops the idea that the understanding which results from it has identifiable therapeutic benefit.

This makes sense. As discussed in Chapter 3 ('Diagnosing Mental Illness'), most diagnoses in psychiatry are based on history, symptoms, and mental state examination, rather than biological tests. There are no blood tests or brain scans to confirm diagnoses such as schizophrenia, depression, bipolar affective disorder, or most other mental illnesses. As a result, it is virtually inevitable that cultural factors will play a role in expressions of distress, diagnostic practices, and provision of care. Bhugra and Gupta note a range of factors which are relevant, to varying degrees, in the relationship between culture and diagnosis and management in psychiatry, including ethnicity, race, racism, migration, life events, acculturation, and cultural identity (Bhugra & Gupta, 2010a). The culture of the individual is central, but also the cultures of organisations and clinicians, alongside cultural influences on treatments, ranging from psychotherapy to pharmacotherapy to social care. Understanding how these factors play out in practice requires near-person ethnography that illuminates lived experience rather than just theory.

In 1988, in *Rethinking Psychiatry: From Cultural Category to Personal Experience,* Kleinman argued that the decades at the end of the twentieth century and start of the twenty-first century would likely see the orientation of psychiatry swing from a western focus to encompass the broader world, including developing countries (Kleinman, 1988). This has occurred to a certain degree, as 'globalisation' (conceived as an intensifying of global interconnections) continues to change both perceptions of mental disorders and, possibly, some of their causes (Bhattacharya et al., 2010). Bhattacharya and colleagues point, in particular, to the potential effects of technology (such as television) on mental health, the cultural appropriateness of diagnostic practices, the consequences of economic disadvantage, risks of social fragmentation, and various other concerns and potential impacts of globalisation. Of course, these eventualities will not necessarily come to pass in all locations, and globalisation has many benefits, but these issues are worth considering from the perspective of cultural and social assimilation, and from the perspective of the evolving anthropology of psychiatry. The world changes, and how we suffer changes with it.

Integrating these perspectives into thought and practice is not always simple, especially in a rapidly shifting world. Writing in the context of anxiety disorders, Hinton and Simon propose a 'multiplex model' to describe the ways in which the biological mechanisms of anxiety and their psychological correlates are embedded in, shape, and are shaped by specific cultural contexts (Hinton & Simon, 2015). Composite, multi-level models are likely the best way to integrate these considerations in the future, and move towards a culturally informed neuroscience that truly mixes and assimilates knowledge from different sources, rather than maintaining contrasting kinds of knowing in separate conceptual boxes.

Incorporating culture into such models is important not only for improving understanding and treatment at the individual level, but also for shaping perceptions of psychiatry and mental health care at the level of societies and in the public arena. This topic is considered next.

Public Expectations of Psychiatry

Psychiatry has always been a social endeavour, as well as a medical one. From earliest times, societies routinely ostracised people with what would now be termed 'mental illness', treating them as different, dangerous, and 'other' (see Chapter 2: 'The History of Psychiatry'). While there were a small number of exceptions to this general rule, most societies expected that people with mental illness or other forms of unusual thought or behaviour would be either institutionalised or 'managed' in some way, often by psychiatry. Many times, the emergent profession of psychiatry colluded, implicitly or explicitly, in this task in an excessive or inappropriate way. This makes the relationship between psychiatry and society complicated, conflicted, and essential for understanding the history, present, and future of this discipline.

In 1977, Kathleen Jones, Professor of Social Administration at the University of York, delivered the 51st Maudsley Lecture before the Royal College of Psychiatrists, titled 'Society Looks at the Psychiatrist' (Jones, 1978). Jones proposed that, up until the early 1960s, psychiatrists had a key role as administrators, initially in asylum administration and then in the relatively more sophisticated administration of therapeutic communities and community psychiatry services, following the establishment of the National Health Service (NHS) in 1948. Since then, Jones argued, there was a growing tendency for psychiatrists to see themselves, and be seen, as doctors more than administrators, the emphasis shifting from their administrative roles to their medical ones.

Jones recommended that a balanced view should be taken of the anti-psychiatry movement of the 1960s and 1970s, which viewed psychiatrists as agents of social control. This critique was often taken to extremes but contained important lessons nonetheless, pointing to the potential for psychiatry to let itself become the vehicle for social vested interests or to serve the profession's own interests to an excessive degree. The history of psychiatry supports this concern (as outlined in Chapter 2).

Finally, Jones wrote that there was, in 1977, a new role for psychiatrists as innovators in an unstable situation of professional interaction, arguing that psychiatrists should always have one foot in medicine (which is psychiatrists' basic skill) and the other foot in the social sciences (because the practice of psychiatry moves well beyond medicine). There are philosophical issues, sociological factors, and inter-professional matters that inevitably shape psychiatry and its practices. Jones concluded that psychiatry had 'produced some great innovators in the past':

We need them now [...] if you take your professional title seriously, if you are prepared to work at the point where the *psyche* meets the *soma* and to accept the multiple roles which society thrusts upon you, you have a unique task.

(Jones, 1978; p. 332)

Jones's points remain fiercely relevant today, almost half a century later. Psychiatry should be cautious about accepting the roles that society seeks to assign it, and psychiatry should explicitly acknowledge the degree to which it is shaped by culture and society – and the ways in which a thoughtful psychiatry can interact with both, for the benefit of all. Two particular demands made of psychiatry require focused thought and attention today: society's demand that psychiatry become a repository of 'risk' (even when such risk is not linked with mental illness) and the demand for psychiatric medication even when it is not indicated ('a pill for every ill'). Both issues merit attention.

In many people's minds, mental illness is associated with a risk of harm to self or others. While there is a relationship between mental illness and various kinds of risk, there are significant limits to assessing the risk of violence at the individual level, even with the best tools available (Connors & Large, 2023). Notwithstanding clear evidence that such risk cannot be accurately assessed, society's demand for psychiatry to be a repository of risk of all descriptions is strong. In 1999, Holmes and Warelow argued that psychiatry had now become a system of risk management and that diagnostic classification facilitated and colluded in this process (Holmes and Warelow, 1999).

In 2019, Nikolas Rose, in *Our Psychiatric Future: The Politics of Mental Health*, wrote about this 'police' function of psychiatry and how it rests uneasily with efforts to destigmatise mental illness (Rose, 2019). This remains true today and is deeply regrettable. Mental health legislation in many jurisdictions has perpetuated the problem by incorporating 'risk' requirements into criteria for psychiatric admission and treatment without consent. For example, as discussed in Chapter 5 ('Treatment Without Consent'), Ireland's Mental Health Act, 2001 permits admission without consent if a person has 'mental disorder', which is defined as follows:

> In this Act 'mental disorder' means mental illness, severe dementia or significant intellectual disability where –
>
> (a) because of the illness, disability or dementia, there is a serious likelihood of the person concerned causing immediate and serious harm to himself or herself or to other persons, or
>
> (b) (i) because of the severity of the illness, disability or dementia, the judgment of the person concerned is so impaired that failure to admit the person to an approved centre would be likely to lead to a serious deterioration in his or her condition or would prevent the administration of appropriate treatment that could be given only by such admission, and
>
>   (ii) the reception, detention and treatment of the person concerned in an approved centre would be likely to benefit or alleviate the condition of that person to a material extent.
>
> (Section 3(1))

This emphasis on risk (especially in Section 3(1)(a)) is deeply regrettable and is not justified by the scientific evidence about risk assessment tools. Nobody can predict the future, so it is essential that psychiatry renegotiates its contract with society, so that deeply flawed risk assessments do not inadvertently lead to unjustified involuntary admissions (Gulati et al., 2020). This requires both legislative reform and addressing a culture of risk 'assessment' and risk aversion that is emerging in psychiatry and across society more broadly. This heavy emphasis on risk places psychiatry in a false position, likely results in significant injustice, and further stigmatises mental illness, psychiatry, and mental health care. It needs to stop.

The other key, disturbing societal demand of psychiatry, along with pressure for psychiatry to become a repository of ill-defined 'risk', is the demand for medication to treat both mental illness *and* the problems of day-to-day life: 'a pill for every ill'. This is considered next.

'A Pill for Every Ill'?

There is strong evidence to support the use of various medications for the treatment of mental illnesses such as depression, bipolar affective disorder, schizophrenia, and various other conditions (see Chapter 4: 'Treating Symptoms and Disorders'). This evidence, however, relates to diagnosed conditions only. Despite the many limitations of symptom-based diagnoses in psychiatry, they assist with identifying treatments that tend to help for specific sets of symptoms – but only for those particular conditions (see Chapter 3: 'Diagnosing Mental Illness'). That does not mean that such medications are necessarily useful for other conditions, for symptoms of lesser severity, or for general problems of living. These medications can, in fact, be actively unhelpful in such situations.

Despite these facts, there is a growing demand to medicalise many parts of everyday life, as diagnostic thresholds fall across all of medicine, including psychiatry (Burns, 2013). One of the consequences of this development is increased demand for diagnosis, treatment, and, in particular, psychiatric medication for reasons that are not necessarily related to diagnosed mental illness. This is a real concern which has grown in recent years and shows little sign of slowing down in the future.

In 2021, the Organisation for Economic Co-operation and Development (OECD), an intergovernmental organisation with 38 member countries, noted that consumption of pharmaceuticals has been rising for several decades, owing to increased need for medications to treat age-related and chronic diseases, and changes in clinical practice (Organisation for Economic Co-operation and Development, 2021). Use of antidepressant medications more than doubled in OECD member countries between 2000 and 2019. Why? What is driving this trend? What does it reflect?

In 2017, one study of rising rates of antidepressant use in the UK found that increased prescriptions between 1995 and 2011 appeared 'to be driven by an increase in long-term use of these medications' (Mars et al., 2017; p. 193), rather than new prescriptions:

> The prevalence of [antidepressant] prescribing doubled between 1995 and 2011, although levels remained relatively stable between 2002 and 2005, when there was a notable reduction in prescribing to those under 30 years. The overall rise in prescribing was largely driven by an increase in [selective serotonin reuptake inhibitors] and other [antidepressants]. Our findings suggest the observed rise in prescribing is not due to an increased number of people starting [medication], but rather appears to be explained by an increase in the duration of treatment.
>
> (Mars et al., 2017; pp. 197–8)

These authors recommended that, 'in the future, research, guidelines, and performance indicators should focus more on the appropriateness of long-term prescribing, and ensure regular review of patients who become established on long-term treatments' (Mars et al., 2017; p. 199). In addition to longer prescriptions, the overall increase in rates might also reflect better recognition of depression, expanded availability of treatment, evolving medical guidelines, or changes in the attitudes of patients and providers towards use of psychiatric medications in general. In other words, the trend is likely to be multi-factorial, with myriad different forces driving up prescription rates.

The role of non-medical factors in this phenomenon is suggested by the fact that there is significant variation in antidepressant use between countries (Organisation for Economic Co-operation and Development, 2023). Iceland, for example, reported the highest level of antidepressant consumption in the OECD in 2021, at a rate that was over seven times that of Latvia, which was the OECD's lowest. It is enormously unlikely that epidemiological differences in the occurrence of mental illness explain these variations fully, so social and cultural factors are undoubtedly relevant, including public and professional attitudes towards treatment and the structures of health and social care systems in different countries.

Overall, the general trend in psychiatric medication usage is upwards, and this shift appears primarily rooted in social factors rather than epidemiological ones. More broadly, the social contract between medicine and society is changing rapidly both in this way and in other ways, and merits close consideration and conscious renegotiation, rather than haphazard change that is poorly understood (Cruess & Cruess, 2011a). Ethics, too, are evolving in parallel with this in our increasingly globalised world, especially in the context of more informed service-users and stakeholders with expertise from both systematic study (across diverse fields) and personal experience (of illness and caring).

In relation to the ethics of psychiatry, Robertson and Walter argue that medical ethics have developed over recent decades in response to the scale of contemporary health care, the growth of interdisciplinary care and the bio-psycho-social approach, technical advancements, improved health care literacy, public policy, and the expectations of third parties (Robertson & Walter, 2011). Psychiatry has negotiated this change, they write, by adopting an ethical approach which can be seen as a social contract based on a three-way relationship with patients and other stakeholders in health care. Inevitably, ethical dilemmas emerge from tensions between responsibilities towards patients and responsibilities towards third parties.

These ethical tensions can be navigated in a number of ways, and Robertson and Walter suggest that social contract theory can help with deliberation on such matters. Consciously describing the social contract between psychiatry and society is an important first step, followed by examining psychiatry's relationship with society, and renegotiating this as needed. This process can usefully include honest acknowledgement of, and continued reflection on, the pressure for psychiatry to become a repository of ill-defined social 'risk' and the increased demand for psychiatric medications and other treatments to manage both diagnosed conditions *and* problems of everyday life which were not previously deemed to require interventions. These developments lie at the heart of key ethical tensions in psychiatry today. Articulating them clearly is an important first step towards understanding, learning, and resolution, including acknowledging psychiatry's own role in generating these trends.

Another area of concern regarding the contract between psychiatry and society is the continued risk of psychiatry being misused in ways that (explicitly or implicitly) seek to re-shape psychiatric thought, diagnoses, practices, or institutions in inappropriate ways or for inappropriate reasons. This is a long-standing issue in the history of psychiatry which persists today. It is considered next.

Misuse of Psychiatric Practices, Institutions, and Diagnoses

So far in this chapter, we have discussed the importance of culture in psychiatry (especially the work of Arthur Kleinman) and society's expectations of psychiatry, particularly its tendency to press certain roles upon psychiatry (and psychiatry's willingness to accept them), such as managing ill-defined 'risk' and providing medication for problems of living (in addition to evidence-based treatment of mental illness). Over-medicalisation is a broad problem across all areas of medicine, not just psychiatry, but it is especially concerning in psychiatry, not least because of the broader misuse of psychiatric diagnoses, practices, treatments, and institutions in the past and today.

This is a long-standing problem, dating from the earliest origins of the discipline of psychiatry. Chapter 2 examined 'The History of Psychiatry' in some detail and noted not only accounts of apparent mental illness in religious texts and ancient literature, and the emergence of psychiatry as a medical discipline, but also the history of psychiatric institutionalisation, deeply questionable treatments in the past (e.g., experimental surgical bacteriology, malaria therapy, insulin treatment, and lobotomy), and the many historical critics of psychiatry (especially, but not exclusively, during the 1960s and 1970s). Case histories from Richmond District Lunatic Asylum at Grangegorman in Dublin, Ireland were interspersed throughout that chapter to illustrate relevant points (Kelly, 2023), showing that, while the history of psychiatry certainly presents evidence of caring and progress, there was also excessive institutionalisation, harmful treatments, disproportionate deprivation of liberty, neglect of basic care, and violations of human rights.

Over the past century, the misuse of psychiatry for political reasons has been especially apparent and has proven difficult to eliminate completely. The most egregious example of this was the persecution of people with mental illness and intellectual disability in Nazi Germany where, in 1939, Adolf Hitler authorised a programme of systematic killing of people 'deemed incurably sick, after most critical medical examination' (Kelly, 2022). At least 275,000 people, generally with disability, mental disorder, or neurological illness, or elderly people, were killed at extermination centres located at psychiatric hospitals in Germany, Austria, occupied Poland, and what is now the Czech Republic. This killing programme ran from 1939 to 1945 and was known as 'Aktion T4', after Tiergartenstraße 4, the street address of the department set up in Berlin to administer the programme. Regrettably and shamefully, psychiatrists and other health professionals collaborated with this process in various ways.

While Aktion T4 was, perhaps, the most extreme persecution ever experienced by the mentally ill, there is also more recent evidence of the misuse of psychiatric diagnoses, treatments, and institutions in other countries. Robert van Voren notes that this matter gained attention during the 1970s and 1980s owing to evidence of systematic political abuse of psychiatry in the Soviet Union during this period, when around one third of political prisoners were incarcerated in psychiatric hospitals (Van Voren, 2010). Van Voren notes that this triggered a major division in the World Psychiatric Association, from which the Soviets were compelled to withdraw in 1983, although they returned conditionally in 1989. There is also evidence that political abuse of psychiatry occurred in other socialist countries, and on a systematic scale in Romania. In addition, van Voren points out, it became apparent during the first ten years of the current century that systematic political abuse of psychiatry was taking place in the People's Republic of China.

These misuses and abuses of psychiatry require investigation, remediation, and prevention for the future, wherever they are found. In addition, however, psychiatry can be misused or re-shaped in more subtle ways in many countries with apparently better records on human rights. In the UK, for example, Ikkos and colleagues write about the impact of sensational tabloid publicity on mental health policy, service provision, and even diagnosis:

To stem tabloid headlines, Tony Blair's Labour government practically invented a mental disorder which had no basis in science and the aim of which was not the treatment of mental ill health but the imagined protection of the public. Despite the opposition of all mental health professions, government, led by the Home Office rather than the Department of Health, spent £480 million on a 'treatment programme' for people with the invented disorder of 'DSPD' (dangerous and severe personality disorder). Results were predictably negative.

(Ikkos et al., 2023; p. 154)

This episode demonstrates what is, perhaps, psychiatry's most concerning Achilles heel: the diagnostic process. In the absence of definitive biological tests to positively diagnose mental illness, diagnosis can be subject to myriad influences, ranging from legitimate medical findings and genuine public interest to sensational media coverage and unhelpful political pressures. The potentially distorting role of powerful pharmaceutical corporations also merits attention, given that current medications are often effective but not curative and are therefore commonly prescribed for long periods.

Balancing these kinds of pressures and concerns with the social distribution of mental illness and the need for bio-psycho-social care is a challenging task. Poole and Robinson explore related themes in a 2023 paper in *BJPsych Bulletin*, titled 'Breaking out of the citadel: social theory and psychiatry':

Looking back at the impact of the 'Decade of the Brain' in the 1990s through the lens of what is now known about Big Pharma on the one hand and the role of urban deprivation in psychosis on the other, open-minded empiricists must acknowledge that some postmodern critiques have some scientific validity. An overemphasis on biological causes and treatments does tend to serve the interests of large corporations and tends to be associated with neglect of service users' social needs, irrespective of the effectiveness of biological treatment in relieving their symptoms. This acknowledgement does not imply acceptance that mental illness is a myth or that empirical psychiatry should be abolished. If we enter into a dialogue with those social theorists who respect empiricism, it is possible to see that psychiatrists relieve the suffering of many service users while also being part of a discourse that has some adverse sociocultural effects. To take an example, we should be able to acknowledge that while we fight stigma, psychiatry is part of the larger system that generates it.

(Poole and Robinson, 2023; p. 147)

Professionalism in Psychiatry

Psychiatry is a complicated endeavour, to state the matter at its mildest. In addition to its empirical basis in medicine and science, psychiatry is subject to myriad other influences including cultural factors (which can shape everything from expressions of distress to the acceptability of particular forms of treatment), social expectations (especially in terms of risk management and treating problems of everyday life), political pressures (from governments and others, sometimes leading to abuses of psychiatry), and the positives and negatives of big pharmaceutical corporations (which have both treatments that work and shareholders to satisfy, thus creating complex incentives). In short, the practice of psychiatry is convoluted, knotty, and possibly impossible to get fully right. Even so, we try.

Against this background, it is clear that a strong sense of professionalism is especially important if the discipline of psychiatry is to maintain its focus on treating mental illness, protecting rights, and continuing to develop as a part of medicine that is firmly rooted in evidence. The fact that most jurisdictions have mental health legislation which permits admission and treatment without consent in certain circumstances adds to the need for strong professionalism in this field, underpinned by clear responsibility, continual accountability, and transparent decision-making. These are challenging tasks, but essential ones for psychiatry.

In 2010, Bhugra and Gupta explored the issue of medical professionalism in psychiatry in particular depth in the journal *Advances in Psychiatric Treatment* (Bhugra & Gupta, 2010b). They wrote that the key principles of the primacy of patient welfare, patient autonomy, and social justice lie at the heart of medical and psychiatric professionalism, which also embraces the idea of fostering and celebrating good practice. They argued that the unwritten contract between psychiatry and society should be renegotiated regularly, as both a set of values and behaviours on the one hand, and relationships with patients, carers, and other stakeholders on the other. They identified various threats to medical professionalism over previous decades, linked with demoralisation among professionals. A perceived loss of autonomy and even learned helplessness appear to be significant factors in the 'loss' of professionalism, and they argued that part of the solution lies in psychiatry identifying its core attributes as a profession, as well as its competencies and skills.

These tasks are not easy but they are progressive, iterative, and essential. The core skills of a psychiatrist today are both similar to and different from those of a psychiatrist 50 or a 100 years ago. Key values persist, including, most notably, the centrality of patient care, supporting autonomy, maintaining compassion, adhering to evidence-based treatments, and certain other tenets of good practice which endure over time. But some essential skills change, such as learning how to practise new psychotherapies (e.g., mindfulness-based interventions) or staying abreast of advances in epidemiology or (to a lesser extent) neuroscience (see Chapter 6: 'Neuroscience and Psychiatry'). In addition, the balance between values shifts as society changes, with, for example, a more explicit emphasis on individual autonomy today, compared to a century ago. Many of these developments are deeply positive and long overdue, but all require recognition, attention, reflection, and, if needed, renegotiation.

George Ikkos, in a valuable contribution to a 2011 book, *Psychiatry's Contract with Society: Concepts, Controversies, and Consequences*, titled 'Psychiatry, professionalism, and society: a note on past and present', argues that the history of psychiatry suggests that psychiatrists should devote increasing attention to understanding values, working as part of teams, and managing systems, in addition to being proficient in both the art and the science of direct clinical assessment and treatment (Ikkos, 2011). Ikkos points to the 'integrative' nature of psychiatry, noting the role of 'culture' in the mix:

> Narrative, values, culture as well as science (social, psychological, and biological), and clinical skills are crucial to the practice of the speciality. It is a broadly integrative discipline.
>
> (Ikkos, 2011; p. 19)

In the same volume, Bhugra and colleagues explore 'Stakeholders' expectations of psychiatric professionalism' and note that diagnosis and managing medication are just one part of the professional role of psychiatrists (Bhugra et al., 2011). It is also necessary for psychiatry to speak to broader society and deliver services that are holistic, appropriate, and inspire confidence. They conclude that there is 'little doubt that professionalism in psychiatry is extremely important and it is up to the profession to explore this with stakeholders' (Bhugra et al., 2011; p. 69). Indeed it is.

Again, the 'integrative' nature of the psychiatric enterprise is evident here, necessitating a combination of medical practice and social engagement. In the end, all psychiatry is social, all psychiatry is personal, and all psychiatry should be evidence-based and accountable. It is a complex mix in practice and even more so in training, as the next generations of psychiatrists inculcate the knowledge, attitudes, and values that will shape their practice and careers.

Teaching professionalism is challenging and important, but modelling professionalism is even more impactful. Often, the structure of mental health services and the myriad pressures placed on psychiatry do not assist in either teaching or modelling professionalism to younger doctors. Impractical cost-saving in services and a growing culture of risk management can subtly undermine the education and training of a new generation of psychiatrists (Lydall & Malik, 2011). These factors can also imperil doctor wellbeing and even lead some trainees to leave psychiatry, given the impossible and often contradictory demands placed upon the discipline. Psychiatrists are routinely criticised for both admission and treatment without consent on the one hand, and adverse events such as patient suicide when admission does not occur on the other hand. The correct balance is difficult or even impossible to achieve. Either way, psychiatrists are blamed, mostly unjustly, for adverse outcomes that are largely beyond our control.

Teaching professionalism is a key part of addressing this issue, recognising the reasonable extent and limits of responsibility at the level of the individual psychiatrist in clinical practice. More broadly, teaching and modelling professionalism need to address issues such as leadership, allocation of responsibility, institutional culture, and experiential learning and reflection, among other matters (Cruess & Cruess, 2011b). Understanding the extent and limits of professional responsibility is central, along with developing a practice of personal reflection, providing collegial support, and actively cultivating compassion for all stakeholders in this complex arena: patients, families, colleagues, and ourselves.

Cultural Psychiatry

This chapter in the book focusses on 'Psychiatry, Culture and Society', looking at the socially and culturally embedded nature of mental illness (in the case history of Miguel at the start), the relationship between psychiatry and society (including public expectations of psychiatry, especially in terms of risk management), misuse of psychiatric diagnoses, practices, and institutions (in history and today), and the importance of professionalism in psychiatric training and practice. To complete the chapter's focus on culture, this section looks at the relevance of culture in clinical practice in relation to diagnosis and treatment. The final section explores issues related to discrimination in psychiatry, including sexism, racism, and LGBTQIA+ issues, as well as ways to improve matters in the future.

Practising psychiatry with an awareness of culture is a complex but essential task. It is helpful to consider this issue in relation to both the diagnosis of mental illness and its treatment. It makes sense to start with diagnosis.

In Chapter 3 of this book ('Diagnosing Mental Illness'), we noted increasing rates of diagnosis of various conditions, including rising rates of diagnosis of juvenile bipolar disorder and, perhaps most commonly, increased diagnosis of autism spectrum disorder (ASD) in recent times. While these rising rates might reflect a correction of previous under-diagnosis, it is also likely that culture plays a number of roles, ranging from shaping expressions of distress to influencing thresholds for help-seeking, and determining the acceptability of specific diagnoses and treatments.

The role of culture was apparent in the case history at the start of this chapter. Miguel heard the voices of two gods which were not immediately troublesome or disturbing, chiefly because they fitted with Miguel's religious beliefs and cultural background. He shared these experiences with his family and his priest, all of whom, like Miguel, interpreted them within a spiritual framework, rather than a medical or psychiatric one. This makes perfect sense and is sometimes all that is needed (although not in Miguel's case).

The role of culture in shaping expressions of mental distress and how such distress is understood has been explored in particular detail in the context of depression. Thinking in this area expanded notably in the 1980s and, in 1985, Marsella and colleagues contributed a compelling overview of 'cross-cultural studies of depressive disorders' to a book titled *Culture and Depression: Studies in the Anthropology and Cross-Cultural Psychiatry of Affect and Disorder*, edited by Arthur Kleinman and Byron Good (Marsella et al., 1985). Marsella and colleagues wrote that concepts equivalent to 'depression', as it is defined in North American and European contexts, were not found among certain non-European groups:

> That no conceptually equivalent terms for depression exist in many non-European cultures does not mean depressive disorders do not exist. Rather, it is possible that the subjective experience of depression, its behavioral manifestations, and the social responses to it may vary across cultures.
>
> (Marsella et al., 1985; p. 301)

They argued that, in order to understand depression, we needed to acknowledge the 'interdependency of culture, psychology, and biology' (p. 314). In the four decades since these comments, anthropological research and cross-cultural studies of depression and other conditions have confirmed this position: psychology, biology, and sociocultural factors strongly influence how we interpret psychological distress in ourselves, how we respond to it in others, the thresholds for help-seeking, and the kind of help we seek. Humans are social creatures, living in families, communities, and societies, so our sociocultural environment shapes a great deal of what we feel, think, and do. We influence each other.

Against this background, changes in the sociocultural environment will inevitably result in changes in diagnostic practices and treatment. Other factors are also relevant, including scientific advances and medical discoveries, but it seems that, in psychiatry at least, sociocultural factors are closely linked with shifts in terminology and understanding. Edward Shorter, in *How Everyone Became Depressed: The Rise and Fall of the Nervous Breakdown,* explores how the terminology for 'depression' changed over time and will likely change again, based on a broad range of influences (Shorter, 2013).

Culture is also relevant to treatment, as well as diagnosis, although the precise effects of culture on treatment are likely to vary between cultures, across conditions, and over time. Given the sheer breadth of this field, the number of treatments involved, and the diversity of cultures around the world, recent years have seen research start to look at specific treatments in particular sociocultural settings, so as to bring focus and therapeutic pragmatism to this vast thematic area.

A good example of this kind of work is provided by Li and colleagues, who conducted 'a systematic review and meta-analysis' of the 'efficacy of culturally adapted interventions for common mental disorders in people of Chinese descent', which was published in *Lancet Psychiatry* in 2023 (Li et al., 2023).

These authors noted that 'evidence suggests that culturally adapted psychological interventions have some benefits in treating diverse ethnic groups', so, they 'aimed to systematically assess the evidence for the efficacy of different cultural adaptations in treating common mental disorders in people of Chinese descent (i.e., ethnic Chinese populations)' (Li et al., 2023; p. 426). Following an extensive literature search, they included 67 records in their meta-analysis, encompassing 6,199 participants. They concluded that:

> Psychological interventions can be transported across cultures with appropriate modifications. Adaptations to interventions can be made by modifying evidence-based interventions, or in culturally specific ways that are rooted in the sociocultural context. However, findings are limited by the insufficient reporting of interventions and cultural adaptations.
>
> (Li et al., 2023; p. 426)

While further work is needed, these results suggest that, once psychological interventions are modified appropriately to a given culture, they can prove helpful even in different sociocultural contexts. This finding is important because over-attributing to culture might be just as harmful as under-attributing. Often, we have more in common than we think, even across cultures, provided we take the time to explore each other's perspectives. In psychiatry, pragmatic studies and reviews such as this are required to ensure that psychiatric treatments are culturally appropriate (with modifications, if needed), and then see if they retain effectiveness in diverse sociocultural settings. There is much to gain in this process. Sometimes, factors which are linked with culture, such as religion, can form part of important cross-cultural dialogues with psychiatry, and can be mediating factors in culture change (Bhugra, 1996). We ignore culture at our peril, and we explore it to the benefit of all.

Discrimination and Psychiatry

Finally, in any consideration of culture, it is necessary to consider the culture of psychiatry itself and, in particular, issues of sexism, racism, and discrimination. As a counterpoint, it is useful to articulate psychiatry's potential to overcome these issues and act as a vehicle for empowerment, especially for people who experience several kinds of discrimination and marginalisation at the same time.

In 1989, Joan Busfield, a senior lecturer in sociology, explored 'sexism and psychiatry' in the journal *Sociology* and concluded that psychiatry supported sexism by both 'contributing to the processes whereby social conformity is achieved' and helping with the construction and popularisation of 'conceptions of psychological normality which are gender-based' (Busfield, 1989; p. 360). Busfield argued that this conclusion did not mean that 'psychiatry is necessarily oppressive', but rather it necessitated examining 'the complex ways in which sexism may affect constructs and judgements', and 'the complex ways in which social relations generate mental sickness'. The former task lies firmly within psychiatry's remit, while the second lies not only within the ambit of psychiatry but also in the realms of social studies, politics, and economics.

The issue of sexism was evident in psychiatry not only at these conceptual levels, but also in the details of day-to-day clinical practice. In 1995, Hall and Deahl published a paper in the *Psychiatric Bulletin*, asking: 'Are psychiatrists sexist? A study of bias in the assessment of psychiatric emergencies' (Hall & Deahl, 1995). These authors examined 227 consecutive new patient assessments by psychiatry trainees and found that 'trainees were more likely to take alcohol, substance use and forensic histories from men, and more likely to take substance use histories from younger patients' (Hall and Deahl, 1995; p. 538). They 'concluded that trainees make sexist and ageist assumptions when they assess patients'. As a result:

> Sustained educational efforts are still required to increase the awareness of medical staff to the importance of substance use and alcohol histories in all patient groups, in order to overcome sexist and ageist clinical assumptions as demonstrated in our study.
>
> (Hall and Deahl, 1995; p. 540)

Psychiatric practice has changed in many ways in the three decades since Hall and Deahl's study, but addressing issues such as sexism, ageism, and racism is a continuous, iterative process. In 2021, for example, Joseph and Bhui noted that one 'concern for Black youth is that they are pathologised' through psychiatric diagnosis and 'sectioned' (under mental health legislation), and that some of this is linked with 'unconscious biases' or 'institutional racism' (Joseph and Bhui, 2021; p. 353). This is most apparent 'in detentions under the powers of the mental health act and in the forensic and criminal justice systems' (p. 358). How can this be addressed?

Appropriate use of diagnostic systems, maintenance of professional standards, and other quality assurance mechanisms can help identify and reduce such problems, but structural discrimination often requires structural solutions. These approaches must be rooted in psychiatric training, continuing professional development, and openness to cross-disciplinary work that identifies and addresses issues which might not be apparent to psychiatrists working within mental health systems, but might be readily identified from other perspectives. We need to be open and to learn.

Another area of concern for psychiatry is the position and treatment of members of LGBTQIA+ (lesbian, gay, bisexual, transgender, queer, questioning, intersex, and asexual) communities by and in psychiatry. Homosexuality was classified as a mental illness by the American Psychiatric Association until 1973 and by the World Health Organisation until 1990 (Kelly, 2017). Bartlett notes that the 'sickness model of LGBT people was dominant' in UK psychiatry (as it was elsewhere) for many years, and while more gay-affirming and positive therapies have been developed, 'many LGBT people report concerns' regarding their mental health care (Bartlett, 2021; pp. 343–4).

These issues require urgent, ongoing attention in the delivery of mental health care, but also in psychiatry more broadly, given the contingent nature of current conceptions of 'mental illness'. In other words, for as long as psychiatry relies on symptom-based diagnoses rather than diagnoses based on biological tests, psychiatry will remain uniquely susceptible to unconscious bias, discrimination, and the influence of various other inappropriate factors on diagnosis and treatment. These factors must be identified in the history of psychiatry (and apologies made), addressed today (in partnership with patients and families), and avoided in the future (through continued awareness, training, and education).

There is still much work to be done on these issues, but awareness is growing in psychiatry, as it is across broader society, especially during the last ten years. Poole and Robinson point out that 'organised psychiatry has become substantially more reflective over the past decade or so':

> The Royal College of Psychiatrists has apologised for previous abusive practices, such as aversion therapy to change sexual orientation. It has acknowledged the impact of structural racism in mental health services and as a cause of mental disorders. It has been respectful of sincere but flawed attempts to reinvent psychiatry.
>
> (Poole and Robinson, 2023; p. 148)

Today, the Royal College of Psychiatrists 'recognises and values the diversity amongst its members, associates, affiliates and staff', and 'is committed to eliminating discrimination on the grounds of gender, race, ethnic origin, sexual orientation, religion, belief, disabled status or any other unjustified condition' (Royal College of Psychiatrists, 2023). This value system is important, not least because psychiatry often has contact with people who already experience multiple kinds of discrimination in their lives and in the lives of their families. Psychiatry is, therefore, in a unique position to address, rather than amplify, disadvantage, and should make sure it does so.

This is a key mission for psychiatry today: eliminating the injustices experienced by people with mental illness and their families. Joseph and Bhui point out that mental health services are well positioned to act in response 'to societal harms to the marginalised' (Joseph & Bhui, 2021; p. 358). For the future, this will likely involve psychiatrists developing a new kind of professionalism that shifts further towards a partnership with patients and their families, rather than the models of medical professionalism that prevailed in the past (Borman, 2011). The need for this shift has never been greater. Some of these themes are revisited in Chapters 9 ('Global Injustice in Mental Health Care') and 10 ('The Future of Psychiatry: Person-Centred Care and System-Level Change') in this book, but they infiltrate most of the other chapters too: justice can only be achieved together.

Miguel, the 25-year-old man whom we met at the start of this chapter, heard the voices of 2 gods who told him to leave his home and spread a message of love in the world. Miguel duly departed in the middle of the night and got a train to a nearby city. There, he found a large monastery and spoke with a monk. Miguel told the monk that he wanted to spread a message of love. The monk sat down with Miguel, gave him some food, and asked where he was from. Miguel told the monk that he had two children at home, but the voices of two gods had told him to leave them behind and spread love in the world.

After listening to Miguel's story, the monk said that Miguel could stay the night at the monastery on one condition: Miguel had to telephone home to tell his family that he was safe. Miguel agreed to this and phoned his wife, who was very worried about him. She was relieved to hear that he was safe and offered to come to the city to collect him, but Miguel said he wanted to stay at the monastery for the night. Later, however, the voices told Miguel to leave the monastery. He slipped out the back door and walked along the motorway out of the city.

Some days later, Miguel's wife received a phone call from another monastery, telling her that Miguel was there, and appeared to be mentally ill. She collected him, but Miguel was not very happy to go home. As soon as they arrived back, Miguel walked away again, this time to the bus station. Miguel's wife collected him there and they spoke to their family doctor who arranged psychiatric assessment for Miguel in the local hospital. Miguel agreed to this only because his wife asked him to do it. The psychiatrist felt that Miguel was mentally ill, but his condition was not severe enough to meet the strict legal criteria for treatment against his wishes. Miguel refused voluntary treatment, declined all forms of support, went to the bus station, and travelled to another monastery in a distant city. His wife was distraught.

At that monastery, Miguel was given a room to sleep in, even though he was not a monk. He stayed for almost two months, before the monks asked him to move to a smaller room at the side of the nearby church. There, Miguel worked as a cleaner and caretaker in the church. He continued to hear the voices of the two gods, but they settled into a steady pattern. They were persistent but quieter. The priest was happy to let Miguel stay at the church in return for cleaning and minding the building. Over the following years, regular churchgoers became familiar with Miguel, as he swept and tidied the church, and opened and closed the building. All the time, Miguel muttered quietly to himself and to the gods, although nobody understood what he said.

Eventually, Miguel lost touch with his family, because he did not return their phone calls or talk to them when they tried to visit. Miguel lived the rest of his life as a church caretaker. When he died, some decades later, the new priest had no contact details for his family and he could not trace them, because he did not know Miguel's surname. Miguel was buried beside the church. His gravestone simply reads: 'Miguel'.

Key Messages

- Psychological experiences and psychiatric symptoms emerge in particular social, cultural, and religious settings, with the result that the experience, interpretation, and treatment of psychiatric symptoms are inevitably shaped by society, culture, and other beliefs (such as religion or spirituality), as well as biology and medicine.
- Psychiatry is a surprisingly good subject to re-examine from a cultural standpoint and offers particular opportunities to link anthropological theory to a broader set of issues. Often, mental health professionals work at the very edges of human experience.
- A range of factors are relevant, to varying degrees, in the relationships between culture, diagnosis, and management in psychiatry, including ethnicity, race, racism, migration, life events, acculturation, and cultural identity.
- Psychiatry should be cautious about accepting all of the roles that society seeks to assign it, and should explicitly acknowledge the degree to which it is shaped by culture and society – and the ways in which a thoughtful psychiatry can interact with both, for the benefit of all.
- Two particular demands made of psychiatry require added thought and attention: society's demand that psychiatry become a general repository of ill-defined 'risk' (even when such risk is not linked with mental illness) and the growing demand for psychiatric medication even when it is not indicated ('a pill for every ill').
- Misuse of psychiatric diagnoses, practices, treatments, and institutions is a long-standing problem which requires careful reflection, remediation, and prevention for the future.
- Key steps include teaching and modelling professionalism within psychiatry; deepening awareness of cultural factors; addressing sexism, ageism, racism, and discrimination; and realising psychiatry's potential to act as a vehicle for empowerment, especially for people who experience several kinds of discrimination and marginalisation at the same time.

References

Bartlett A. Sexual diversity and UK psychiatry and mental health. In: Ikkos G, Bouras N (eds), *Mind, State and Society: Social History of Psychiatry and Mental Health in Britain 1960–2010* (pp. 336–47). Cambridge: Cambridge University Press, 2021 (https://doi.org/10.1017/9781911623793.036).

Bhattacharya R, Gupta S, Bhugra D. Globalization and psychiatry. In: Morgan C, Bhugra D (eds), *Principles of Social Psychiatry* (Second Edn) (pp. 141–53). Chichester: Wiley-Blackwell/John Wiley and Sons, Ltd., 2010.

Bhugra D. Conclusions: religion, mental illness and mental health – the way forward. In: Bhugra D (ed.), *Psychiatry and Religion: Context, Consensus and Controversies* (pp. 230–2). London and New York: Routledge, 1996.

Bhugra D, Gupta S. Culture and its influence on diagnosis and management. In: Morgan C, Bhugra D (eds), *Principles of Social Psychiatry* (Second Edn) (pp. 117–31). Chichester: Wiley-Blackwell/John Wiley and Sons, Ltd., 2010a.

Bhugra D, Gupta S. Medical professionalism in psychiatry. *Advances in Psychiatric Treatment* 2010b; 16: 10–13 (https://doi.org/10.1192/apt.bp.108.005892).

Bhugra D, Gupta S, Smyth G, Webber M. Stakeholders' expectations of psychiatric professionalism. In: Bhugra D, Malik A, Ikkos G (eds), *Psychiatry's Contract with Society: Concepts, Controversies, and Consequences* (pp. 59–71). Oxford: Oxford University Press, 2011.

Borman E. Changing professionalism. In: Bhugra D, Malik A, Ikkos G (eds), *Psychiatry's Contract with Society: Concepts, Controversies, and Consequences* (pp. 209–20). Oxford: Oxford University Press, 2011.

Burns T. *Our Necessary Shadow: The Nature and Meaning of Psychiatry*. London: Allen Lane, 2013.

Busfield J. Sexism and psychiatry. *Sociology* 1989; 23: 343–64 (https://doi.org/10.1177/0038038589023003002).

Connors MH, Large MM. Calibrating violence risk assessments for uncertainty. *General Psychiatry* 2023; 36: e100921 (https://doi.org/10.1136/gpsych-2022-100921).

Cruess SR, Cruess RL. Medicine's social contract with society: its nature, evolution, and present state. In: Bhugra D, Malik A, Ikkos G (eds), *Psychiatry's Contract with Society: Concepts, Controversies, and Consequences* (pp. 123–46). Oxford: Oxford University Press, 2011a.

Cruess RL, Cruess SR. Teaching professionalism. In: Bhugra D, Malik A, Ikkos G (eds), *Psychiatry's Contract with Society: Concepts, Controversies, and Consequences* (pp. 103–22). Oxford: Oxford University Press, 2011b.

Gulati G, Dunne CP, Kelly BD. Violence risk assessment in psychiatry: nobody can predict the future. *BMJ Opinion*, 17 November 2020 (https://blogs.bmj.com/bmj/2020/11/17/violence-risk-assessment-in-psychiatry-nobody-can-predict-the-future/) (accessed 18 October 2023).

Hall I, Deahl M. Are psychiatrists sexist? A study of bias in the assessment of psychiatric emergencies. *Psychiatric Bulletin* 1995; 19: 538–40 (https://doi.org/10.1192/pb.19.9.538). (Link to license: http://creativecommons.org/licenses/by/4.0/) (accessed 21 October 2023).

Hinton DE, Simon NM. Toward a cultural neuroscience of anxiety disorders: the multiplex model. In: Kirmayer LJ, Lemelson R, Cummings CA (eds), *Re-Visioning Psychiatry: Cultural Phenomenology, Critical Neuroscience, and Global Mental Health* (pp. 343–74). Cambridge: Cambridge University Press, 2015.

Holmes CA, Warelow P. Implementing psychiatry as risk management: *DSM-IV* as a postmodern taxonomy. *Health, Risk & Society* 1999; 1: 167–78 (https://doi.org/10.1080/13698579908407016).

Ikkos G. Psychiatry, professionalism, and society: a note on past and present. In: Bhugra D, Malik A, Ikkos G (eds), *Psychiatry's Contract with Society: Concepts, Controversies, and Consequences* (pp. 9–22). Oxford: Oxford University Press, 2011.

Ikkos G, Bouras N, Tyrer P. Madness and society in Britain. *BJPsych Bulletin* 2023; 47: 152–6 (https://doi.org/10.1192/bjb.2022.45). (Link to license: https://creativecommons.org/licenses/by/4.0/) (accessed 19 October 2023).

Jones K. Society looks at the psychiatrist. *British Journal of Psychiatry* 1978; 132: 321–2 (https://doi.org/10.1192/bjp.132.4.321).

Joseph D, Bhui K. Race, state and mind. In: Ikkos G, Bouras N (eds), *Mind, State and Society: Social History of Psychiatry and Mental Health in Britain 1960–2010* (pp. 348–60). Cambridge: Cambridge University Press, 2021 (https://doi.org/10.1017/9781911623793.037).

Kelly BD. Homosexuality and Irish psychiatry: medicine, law and the changing face of Ireland. *Irish Journal of Psychological Medicine* 2017; 34: 209–15 (https://doi.org/10.1017/ipm.2015.72).

Kelly BD. *In Search of Madness: A Psychiatrist's Travels Through the History of Mental Illness.* Dublin: Gill Books, 2022.

Kelly BD. *Asylum: Inside Grangegorman.* Dublin: Royal Irish Academy, 2023.

Kleinman A. *Patients and Healers in the Context of Culture: An Exploration of the Borderland between Anthropology, Medicine, and Psychiatry.* Berkeley, Los Angeles, and London: University of California Press, 1980.

Kleinman A. *Rethinking Psychiatry: From Cultural Category to Personal Experience.* New York: The Free Press, 1988.

Lemelson R, Tucker A. Afflictions: psychopathology and recovery in cultural context. In: Kirmayer LJ, Lemelson R, Cummings CA (eds), *Re-Visioning Psychiatry: Cultural Phenomenology, Critical Neuroscience, and Global Mental Health* (pp. 483–514). Cambridge: Cambridge University Press, 2015.

Li S, Xi Z, Barnett P, Saunders R, Shafran R, Pilling S. Efficacy of culturally adapted interventions for common mental disorders in people of Chinese descent: a systematic review and meta-analysis. *Lancet Psychiatry* 2023; 10: 426–40 (https://doi.org/10.1016/s2215-0366(23)00118-9). (Link to license: https://creativecommons.org/licenses/by/4.0/) (accessed 20 October 2023).

Lydall G, Malik A. Training and professionalism. In: Bhugra D, Malik A, Ikkos G (eds), *Psychiatry's Contract with Society: Concepts, Controversies, and Consequences* (pp. 73–88). Oxford: Oxford University Press, 2011.

Mars B, Heron J, Kessler D, Davies NM, Martin RM, Thomas KH, Gunnell D. Influences on antidepressant prescribing trends in the UK: 1995–2011. *Social Psychiatry and Psychiatric Epidemiology* 2017; 52: 193–200 (https://doi.org/10.1007/s00127-016-1306-4). (Link to license: https://creativecommons.org/licenses/by/4.0/) (accessed 18 October 2023).

Marsella AJ, Sartorius N, Jablensky A, Fenton FR. Cross-cultural studies of depressive disorders: an overview. In: Kleinman A, Good B (eds), *Culture and Depression: Studies in the Anthropology and Cross-Cultural Psychiatry of Affect and Disorder* (pp. 299–324). Berkeley, Los Angeles, and London: University of California Press, 1985.

Organisation for Economic Co-operation and Development. *Health at a Glance 2021: OECD Indicators.* Paris: OECD Publishing, 2021 (https://doi.org/10.1787/ae3016b9 -en). (Link to license: https://www.oecd.org/termsandconditions/) (accessed 7 November 2023).

Organisation for Economic Co-operation and Development. *Health at a Glance 2023: OECD Indicators.* Paris: OECD Publishing, 2023 (https://doi.org/10.1787/7a7afb35 -en). (Link to license: https://www.oecd.org/termsandconditions/) (accessed 7 November 2023).

Poole R, Robinson CA, Breaking out of the citadel: social theory and psychiatry. *BJPsych Bulletin* 2023; 47: 146–9 (https://doi.org/10.1192/bjb.2022.17). (Link to license: https://creativecommons.org/licenses/by/4.0/) (accessed 21 October 2023).

Robertson M, Walter G. Psychiatric ethics and the 'new professionalism'. In: Bhugra D, Malik A, Ikkos G (eds), *Psychiatry's Contract with Society: Concepts, Controversies, and Consequences* (pp. 221–39). Oxford: Oxford University Press, 2011.

Rose N. *Our Psychiatric Future: The Politics of Mental Health.* Cambridge and Medford, MA: Polity Press, 2019.

Royal College of Psychiatrists. *Equal Opportunities.* London: Royal College of Psychiatrists, 2023 (https://www.rcpsych.ac.uk/about-us/work-for-us/our-partners/equal-opportunities) (accessed 21 October 2023).

Shorter E. *How Everyone Became Depressed: The Rise and Fall of the Nervous Breakdown.* Oxford: Oxford University Press, 2013.

Van Voren R. Political abuse of psychiatry - an historical overview. *Schizophrenia Bulletin* 2010; 36: 33–5 (https://doi.org/10.1093/schbul/sbp119).

8   Self-Harm and Suicide

Chapter Content Advisory

This chapter discusses issues such as self-harm, suicide, depression, mental illness, and related matters in direct terms, in order to demystify, delineate, and understand them better. For this reason, certain readers might find certain sections distressing. If you are concerned about any of these matters from a personal perspective or in relation to family, friends, or colleagues, please contact a registered health care provider immediately, and follow their advice.

Brad was 15 years old when he started to harm himself. An intelligent high-achieving boy, Brad had always done well in school and had many friends until the age of 14. He enjoyed sport and was especially good at football. For many years, Brad played on the school football team and always looked forward to training on Friday evenings. Brad would spend time at his friend Liam's house before training and after matches. Brad and Liam were inseparable: they went to school together, played together, and their families went on vacation together.

When Brad became 14, things began to change. Over time, Brad became reluctant to attend football training and sometimes skipped matches. The team coach noticed this and mentioned it to Brad's parents. They agreed that this was likely just a phase and would pass. But Brad also spent less time with Liam and started avoiding the 'pizza parties' he used to enjoy with his friends at the weekends. At home, Brad was silent and withdrawn. He scarcely spoke a word to his older brother, and spent all his time in his room on his phone.

Brad's parents were worried, but they assumed that this was a teenage phase. Many teenagers become more solitary, appear preoccupied, and communicate less with their families for periods of time. Liam, too, was concerned about his friend Brad, but soon began to spend time with other friends and other teammates at the football club.

Soon, Brad rarely went out, except to school, and, even then, he attended reluctantly. His grades deteriorated rapidly, even in history, which had been his favourite subject. Brad stopped going to football and spent most of his time alone.

One day, when Brad's mother was tidying Brad's room, she found two boxes of matches at the bottom of a drawer. Brad's mother thought this was strange:

DOI: 10.4324/9781003378495-9

why did Brad have matches in his room? He did not smoke cigarettes or light candles. Brad's mother took the matches away and said nothing to Brad that day. She did not want to upset or embarrass Brad. Besides, Brad was very moody and would probably fly into a rage if his mother mentioned the matches.

But Brad's mother was worried and discussed it with Brad's father. They spoke about it together, and the next day they asked Brad about the matches. Brad became angry. He said that he was 15 years old and could live his own life. He said that his mother was not allowed into his bedroom ever again. Brad stormed upstairs and slammed his bedroom door. Brad's parents were disappointed, but not surprised: this was the response they expected.

Several hours later, Brad came back downstairs. He was very upset, sobbing uncontrollably. Brad told his mother that he used the matches to burn himself. Brad rolled up his sleeves and showed his mother multiple small burns on his upper arms. Some of the burns were old and some were quite new. Brad said he burnt himself where nobody could see the burns. He said he could not go to football training anymore because his friends would see the burns on his arms in the changing rooms. Brad was very upset.

Brad's parents were shocked and distressed. 'Why do you do this?', his mother asked. Brad replied: 'I don't know. I just feel tense. I wish I could stop, but I don't think I can. I get so tense'.

Brad's mother had never seen anything like this before and was deeply confused. 'Why do you do this?', she kept asking. 'I just feel tense', Brad kept replying. Soon, they were both in tears, both deeply upset, and both with no idea what to do next.

Introduction

Deliberate self-harm is common. Suicide is less common, but is also a constant feature of all societies for which there is recorded history. Both non-fatal deliberate self-harm and suicide are public health problems of great magnitude and both merit close attention. Both deliberate self-harm and suicide involve deep suffering at the level of the individual, their family, the community, and society as a whole.

Brad's experience of deliberate self-harm is not uncommon, and neither are the experiences and responses of his parents. Brad feels upset, tense, and alone. He lacks the emotional and psychological skills to manage his feelings, which seem overwhelming to him. He is surprised and confused by his own behaviour and feels ashamed when his parents find out. If he cannot explain this behaviour to himself, how can he explain it to them? Is he mentally ill?

Brad's parents are also in a difficult, distressing position. They are baffled by Brad's behaviour and struggle to understand why he burns himself. They want to help, but their initial reactions are confusion and helplessness. This experience is entirely new to them, so they struggle to react in the level-headed, supportive way that they might wish to. They do not know what to do next, or where to turn. Who can help? And how?

Against this background, this chapter examines issues relating to 'Self-Harm and Suicide'. It starts by exploring definitions of self-harm and suicide, and then looks at suicide in the history of psychiatry, with particular reference to the views and writings of leading asylum doctors of the nineteenth century. Global rates of suicide are discussed, along with consideration of trends over recent decades, including the impact of the Covid-19 pandemic on rates of suicide.

This chapter pays particular attention to the (very limited) value of 'risk assessment' in individual cases of mental illness or psychological distress, and the use of evidence-based approaches to suicide prevention, focussing especially on public health measures and the broader social context in which self-harm and suicide occur and are managed. Issues relating to suicide and the law are explored, including the decriminalisation of suicide and attempted suicide in various jurisdictions (e.g., in India's Mental Healthcare Act, 2017), the use of 'risk' of suicide in mental health legislation (commonly as part of criteria for admission or treatment without consent), and some of the issues surrounding physician-assisted suicide (PAS), which is a topic that commands increasing attention around the world. The chapter concludes with a consideration of useful directions for future research and service developments in this area.

But, first, how are deliberate self-harm and suicide defined?

Definitions of Self-Harm and Suicide

Suicide is intentional self-killing, while deliberate self-harm is the intentional infliction of non-fatal harm on oneself. The latter includes a wide variety of methods such as self-cutting and self-burning (Kelly, 2017).

The definitions of deliberate self-harm and suicide are the subjects of ongoing debate. Many people would agree that intentionally cutting one's wrists constitutes deliberate self-harm, but what about other, less clear forms of self-harm, such as smoking cigarettes? There is widespread awareness that smoking reduces life expectancy owing to smoking related diseases such as cancer and heart disease. But does this mean that smoking can be accurately or usefully regarded as a form of deliberate self-harm? Or is it better seen as an addictive or medical condition, like a physical illness, over which the person has some, but limited, control?

There are also questions about the definition of suicide. For example, if a person routinely uses illegal drugs and is aware that their level of drug use is such that they could easily die of an 'accidental' overdose, does that mean that if they are found dead following drug use, the death is a form of suicide? Or is their death an accident? Or is it the result of an illness, such as dependence on alcohol or other substances, and thus similar to a death from pneumonia? Or is it a combination of all of these?

In this scenario, it is useful to consider the concept of a 'sub-intended' death. This might occur when a person might not identify a single moment when they decide to end their life, but rather make a series of choices which indicate, at the very least, significant ambivalence about living and dying; e.g., routine excessive use of alcohol or drugs, despite knowing the risks of self-harm or death. This can be compounded by a diagnosed condition (such as a dependence disorder) and a degree of accidental or excessive use of substances on any given occasion.

In this way, a death that results from a person knowingly taking risks that might result in death can be considered a 'sub-intended' death; i.e. a death which is attributable to a combination of personal behaviour, an addictive condition, or other diagnosis, and additional circumstances, as indicated in each case. Many deaths fit this category, especially among persons with substance misuse conditions who lose hope and lose sight of reasons to live, owing to their condition, without ever having a fully articulated, fully conscious desire to die.

Regardless of precise definitions, self-harm and suicide are major public health issues and merit attention at all levels: individual, family, community, and society (Knipe et al., 2022). In the United States, the National Institute of Mental Health (NIMH), in common with similar organisations across other jurisdictions, provides clear information to the public about risk factors for suicide:

People of all genders, ages, and ethnicities can be at risk. Suicidal behavior is complex, and there is no single cause. The main risk factors for suicide are:

- Depression, other mental disorders, or substance use disorder.
- Chronic pain.
- Personal history of suicide attempts.
- Family history of a mental disorder or substance use.
- Family history of suicide.
- Exposure to family violence, including physical or sexual abuse.
- Presence of guns or other firearms in the home.
- Having recently been released from prison or jail.

(National Institute of Mental Health, 2023)

Looking at the scientific literature more broadly, general risk factors for nonfatal deliberate self-harm include female gender, younger age, poor social support, major life events, poverty, being divorced, being unemployed, mental illness, and a history of previous deliberate self-harm (Kelly, 2017). Risk factors for suicide include male gender, poor social support, major life events, family history of suicide, chronic painful illness, mental illness, and a history of previous deliberate self-harm. Availability of means is also significant for both deliberate self-harm and suicide (see below).

In terms of mental illness, suicide is associated with major depressive disorder (long-term risk of suicide: 10%–15%), bipolar affective disorder (10%–20%), schizophrenia (10%), and alcohol dependence syndrome (15%) (Williams, 1997). In addition, individuals who engage in deliberate self-harm have a 30-fold increased risk of completed suicide over the following four years (Cooper et al., 2005). Other contextual factors also matter, as the NIMH points out:

> For people with suicidal thoughts, exposure, either directly or indirectly, to others' suicidal behavior, such as that of family members, peers, or celebrities can also be a risk factor [...] Stressful life events (such as the loss of a loved one, legal troubles, or financial difficulties) and interpersonal stressors (such as shame, harassment, bullying, discrimination, or relationship troubles) may contribute to suicide risk, especially when they occur along with suicide risk factors.
>
> (National Institute of Mental Health, 2023)

Overall, then, there are risk factors for deliberate self-harm and suicide at the level of the individual, in the context of their family and social circle, and against the backdrop of their socio-economic situation, as well as the events of day-to-day life. This makes it even more important that we look after each other in the changing, challenging, and often overwhelming circumstances in which so many people find themselves. As the NIMH points out, 'family and friends are often the first to recognise the warning signs of suicide, and they can take the first step toward helping a loved one find mental health treatment' (National Institute of Mental Health, 2023).

Self-Harm and Suicide in the History of Psychiatry

Self-harm and suicide have featured in ancient societies, traditional literatures, and religious texts since the beginning of recorded history (Williams, 1997). Social and religious responses shifted considerably over time, resulting in increased medicalisation of self-harm and suicide, especially in the twentieth century (Alvarez, 1974). The emergence of the discipline of psychiatry within the profession of medicine during the nineteenth century laid the groundwork for this shift, as is reflected in the writings of various prominent asylum doctors on the subject of suicide.

In 1853, James Foulis Duncan (1812–1895), a leading Irish asylum doctor and (later) president of the Medico-Psychological Association (1875), wrote extensively about suicide in his book, *Popular Errors on the Subject of Insanity Examined and Exposed* (Duncan, 1853). Using the language of the times, Duncan argued that suicide could be the result of a 'delusion', such 'as when the individual fancies that he has received a divine commission to offer himself up as a voluntary sacrifice for the benefit of others':

It may in other instances proceed from the derangement of natural conscience, leading the individual to look upon that with satisfaction, or at least without remorse, which in health he would be ready to denounce [...] It may still further emanate from a depressed condition of the moral feelings, rendering the individual to a great degree unconscious of what he is doing; and lastly, it may be the result of a perverted condition of the instinctive principle of self-preservation, and then it is perpetrated suddenly under the influence of a momentary impulse, and without apparent premeditation.

(Duncan, 1853; p. 86)

Duncan located the impulse to self-harm very much within the individual, consistent with increased medicalisation of suicide at this time. He drew particular attention to

persons whose consciences have been awakened to a sense of guilt arising from irregularities in their past life, and who think that they have committed the unpardonable sin, or that they are delivered over to a condition of hopeless despair.

(p. 87)

He urged caution, however, at presuming that everyone who died by suicide was necessarily mentally ill: 'Is the mere act of self-destruction of itself a proof that the person who committed it was insane at the time? Medical authorities are divided on this point' (p. 93). They remain so divided today.

Five years after Duncan's book, in 1858, two leading English asylum doctors, John Charles Bucknill and Daniel H. Tuke, elaborated on the types of 'conditions of the mind' that were linked with suicide, in their classic *Manual of Psychological Medicine: Containing the History, Nosology, Description, Statistics, Diagnosis, Pathology, and Treatment of Insanity, With an Appendix of Cases* (Bucknill & Tuke, 1858; p. 202). For Bucknill and Tuke, again in the language of the times, psychological or psychiatric conditions affected different people in different ways:

of two patients, equally a prey to melancholia, the one will attempt to terminate his existence, while the other, so far from contemplating, will recoil with horror from, the act. By the latter, the natural desire to retain life may be possessed in much greater force than by the former; or there may survive, in one, religious convictions antagonistic to the execution of the act of suicide, which may either never have been present in the other, or have been paralyzed by disease. Other motives than those now referred to, may prompt self-destruction. Thus, the act may be intimately associated with delusional forms of insanity; or again, it may be instantly committed, in consequence of any one of the feelings receiving a shock.

(Bucknill and Tuke, 1858; p. 202)

Given this variability in risk and behaviour across patients who were 'equally a prey to melancholia', it was clear that constant vigilance was needed. Thomas Clouston, another well-known asylum doctor, addressed this matter in his 1883 book, *Clinical Lectures on Mental Diseases*:

> The question of the patient being suicidal should never in any case of melancholia be left unconsidered, and the risk of his becoming suicidal should never in any case be left unprovided for [...] When a man takes away his own life, or even when a serious attempt is made, it is so distressing to everyone connected with the patient, so hurtful to his prospects, and so damaging to the reputation and foresight of the doctor in charge, and so in the teeth of the radical medical principle to obviate the tendency to death, that no pains should be spared to guard against its occurrence.
>
> (Clouston, 1883; p. 112)

As psychiatry developed during the remainder of the nineteenth century and the long twentieth century, responses to deliberate self-harm and suicide shifted to reflect both the evolving discipline of psychiatry and broader social changes, which have always influenced psychiatry profoundly (Kelly, 2022). The role of social risk factors became especially apparent: poor social support, major life events, poverty, getting divorced, and being unemployed. The availability of means (e.g., tablets to take overdoses) was also found to be significant, along with sociocultural interpretations of deliberate self-harm and suicide, and the behaviour of others.

There was also, from the outset, clear recognition of the phenomenon of 'copycat' suicides. As long ago as 1853, Duncan referred to 'those cases of suicide that seem to have their origin in the principle of imitation':

> It is a well-ascertained fact that when one case of self-destruction happens, especially when it takes place in a large town, and excites an unusual degree of attention, several others are sure to follow, presenting precisely similar circumstances.
>
> (Duncan, 1853; p. 89)

This matter remains relevant today, as one element within the complex set of risk factors for deliberate self-harm and suicide that have evolved and become apparent over the past two centuries.

Global Rates of Suicide

Given the diversity of personal, medical, social, and other risk factors associated with self-harm and suicide, it is not surprising that rates change over time. What is interesting, however, is the magnitude of the shift over recent decades (which is substantial), the direction of the change (which is positive), and its distribution around the world (which is uneven). This merits close attention if we are to understand the challenges presented by suicide today and the best ways to address them.

In 2019, Naghavi on behalf of the Global Burden of Disease Self-Harm Collaborators used 'estimates from the Global Burden of Disease Study 2016 to describe patterns of suicide mortality globally, regionally, and for 195 countries and territories by age, sex, and socio-demographic index, and to describe temporal trends between 1990 and 2016' (Naghavi on behalf of the Global Burden of Disease Self-Harm Collaborators, 2019; p. 1). This group found that there were an estimated 817,000 deaths from suicide globally in 2016, accounting for approximately 1.49% of total deaths that year. This is an enormous number of deaths which confirms suicide as a public health problem of the greatest magnitude.

Looking at trends over time, however, data showed that 'the age standardised mortality rate for suicide decreased by 32.7% (27.2% to 36.6%) worldwide between 1990 and 2016' (p. 1). This is an extraordinarily important statistic and one which offers real hope for the future. While a one-third decline in the suicide rate is not nearly enough, it shows that positive change is possible. If the rate can decline by one third, surely it can decline by another third? Or more? Nobody is born wanting to die by suicide, and even one suicide is one too many.

Notwithstanding the positive trend and progress to date, then, there is clearly still more work to be done. Naghavi on behalf of the Global Burden of Disease Self-Harm Collaborators is clear on this point:

> When ranking leading causes by age standardised mortality rate, this study found that suicide deaths were in the leading 10 causes of death across eastern Europe, central Europe, high income Asia Pacific, Australasia, and high income North America.
>
> (Naghavi on behalf of the Global Burden of Disease Self-Harm Collaborators, 2019; p. 11)

They also note that the decline in the suicide mortality rate is not universal: men still have higher rates of suicide than women at all time-points (except among those aged 15 to 19 years), and the greatest decline in rates is seen in women, rather than men, thus potentially widening the gender gap. In addition, much of the global decline to date is attributable to falls in suicide mortality in China and India, rather than certain other countries:

> Taken as a whole, these patterns reflect a complex interplay of factors, specific to regions and nations, including sociodemographic, sociocultural, and religious factors; levels of economic development, unemployment and economic events; distribution of risk factors, such as exposure to violence or use

of alcohol and drugs; choices of and access to means of suicide; and patterns of mental illness [...] as well as culturally specific relations with suicide. Moreover, although the decrease in suicide mortality has been substantial during the period 1990 to 2016, if current trends continue, only 3% of 118 countries will attain the Sustainable Development Goals target to reduce suicide mortality by one third between 2015 and 2030.

> (Naghavi on behalf of the Global Burden of
> Disease Self-Harm Collaborators, 2019; p. 11;
> citations omitted)

These international variations highlight regions and issues that need particular attention, but the global decline in the suicide mortality rate is still an enormously positive development overall. It provides clear evidence of progress rather than deterioration in at least one important indicator of mental health. The declining trend does not support the idea of an overall 'crisis' in mental health (Council of Economic Advisors, 2022; see also Chapter 1 of this book: 'Why Does Psychiatry Exist?'). There is, of course, still substantial work to be done, and global statistics mean little to those who are suicidal or bereaved by suicide, but there are reasons for optimism (Kelly, 2023a).

Since these data were published in 2019, the world experienced one of the largest public health emergencies of recent decades: the Covid-19 pandemic. Covid-19 brought enormous physical and mental suffering, and the loss of millions of lives, but there was also more resilience than many people might have anticipated in such difficult circumstances. There were certainly mental health problems during the pandemic, and some people suffered ongoing symptoms from Covid-19, but there was no surge of serious mental illness after the outbreak (Kelly, 2023b). So, how did the pandemic affect suicide rates?

In 2023, one 'systematic review with meta-analysis' examined 'suicide before and during the Covid-19 pandemic', and 'identified 51, 55, and 25 samples for suicidal ideation, attempt, and death by suicide' (Yan et al., 2023; p. 1). This group found that 'the prevalence of suicidal ideation increased significantly' and 'suicide attempts were more prevalent during the pandemic', but there was no significant change in rates of death owing to suicide. In other words, there was increased distress among some people, but this did not translate into increased rates of suicide during Covid-19.

This is broadly consistent with another systematic review and meta-analysis of 137 studies of mental health symptoms before and during the pandemic, which reported no overall negative change in terms of general mental health and anxiety symptoms, although there was a slight worsening of depressive symptoms, and women were more affected than men (Sun et al., 2023). Writing about this study in the *Guardian*, Hall noted the consistency in overall findings about suicide, and also the fact that some subgroups of the population were more affected than others:

The researchers at McGill said their findings were consistent with the largest study on suicide during the pandemic – which found no increase – and applied to most groups, including different ages, sexes, genders and whether people had pre-existing conditions. Three-quarters of the research focused on adults, mostly from middle- and high-income countries.

However, they acknowledged that women had experienced worsening anxiety, depression or general mental health symptoms during the pandemic, possibly due to juggling more family responsibilities, or because more work in health or social care, or, in some cases, due to domestic abuse.

(Hall, 2023)

In 2023, the Organisation for Economic Co-operation and Development (OECD) provided a similarly nuanced account of the mental health effects of the pandemic:

OECD analysis has shown that population mental health went up and down over the course of the pandemic – typically worsening during periods when infection and death rates were high, or when stringent containment measures were in place. Available data point to some recovery in population mental health as the pandemic situation improved, but also suggest that mental ill-health remains elevated [...] Persistently high levels of mental distress 'beyond' the pandemic could reflect the confluence of multiple crises: the cost-of-living crisis, climate crisis and geopolitical tensions.

Shocks such as pandemics, severe weather events and financial crises can also heighten the risk of suicidal behaviour. While complex social and cultural factors affect suicidal behaviour, mental ill-health increases the risk of dying by suicide. Rates of death by suicide currently vary almost six-fold across OECD countries, and are over three times higher for men than women.

(Organisation for Economic Co-operation and
Development, 2023; p. 80)

Overall, evidence to date indicates that the Covid-19 pandemic increased rates of distress and suicidal ideation, but not rates of completed suicide. As the OECD points out, other factors inevitably influence suicide rates: gender, social circumstances, cultural factors, environmental concerns, and various other matters. But, as best as can be established, Covid-19 did not increase rates of suicide.

Assessing Risk of Self-Harm and Suicide

Notwithstanding the declining rate of suicide over recent decades, self-harm and suicide remain public health challenges of the greatest magnitude. They are also acute challenges at the level of individual patient care, so a great deal of effort has been devoted to identifying risk factors for self-harm and suicide (as outlined above). Similar attention has been devoted to trying to predict the risk of given individuals engaging in deliberate self-harm or dying by suicide, especially if they have signs of mental illness or have expressed suicidal ideation in the past.

Overall, however, research in this field indicates that it is not possible to predict suicide at the level of the individual, at least not in an actuarial or statistical way (Kelly, 2017; Hawton et al., 2022). While certain people can be regarded as low-risk or high-risk at certain times, based on general risk factors, it is still not possible to predict who will die by suicide and who will not. Assessing and understanding risk factors can help to inform care and shape therapeutic relationships, but it does not provide a mathematical evaluation of risk. Suicide cannot be predicted, even in apparently high-risk circumstances.

Recent research strongly supports this position. In 2019, one systematic review and simulation of prediction models for suicide attempts and deaths found that the accuracy of suicide prediction models for 'predicting a future event is near 0' (Belsher et al., 2019; p. 642). There are many reasons for this. In statistical terms, suicide is a rare event, which means that risk assessment methods inevitably have low positive predictive values (Knipe et al., 2022). This is true even in apparently high-risk groups: one follow-up survey found that fewer than 1 in 200 people who experience suicidal thoughts go on to complete suicide (Gunnell et al., 2004).

In addition, risk factors for self-harm and suicide are widely distributed across populations, so the vast majority of people with such risk factors will not die by suicide. As a result, the 'population paradox' means that the absolute number of people who die by suicide is greater in the 'low-risk' group, because a greater proportion of the population are classified as 'low risk'. In short, prediction is impossible, even in apparently high-risk groups and even using risk assessment tools.

There are also potential harms from inaccurate or inappropriate risk assessment, including possible alienation of patients, restriction of care based on apparent low-risk status, and impairment of therapeutic relationships. It is conceivable that some of these factors could increase distress and maybe even increase the risk of suicide in the long term, rather than help reduce it. So-called 'risk assessment' might itself present a risk.

Given that deliberate self-harm is more common than suicide, it is statistically possible that prediction models will perform better for self-harm than for suicide. One 2022 study examined the use of clinician assessment, patient self-report, and electronic health records (EHRs) 'to predict suicide attempts within 1 and 6 months of presentation at an emergency department (ED) for psychiatric problems' (Nock et al., 2022; p. 1). Findings suggested 'that the ability to identify patients at high risk of suicide attempt after an ED visit for psychiatric problems improved using a combination of patient self-reports and EHR data' (p. 2). More specifically:

In the best 1-month model, 30.7% (positive predicted value) of the patients classified as having highest risk (top 25% of the sample) made a suicide attempt within 1 month of their ED visit, accounting for 64.8% (sensitivity) of all 1-month attempts. In the best 6-month model, 46.0% (positive predicted value) of the patients classified at highest risk made a suicide attempt within 6 months of their ED visit, accounting for 50.2% (sensitivity) of all 6-month attempts.

(Nock et al., 2022; p. 1)

Research is ongoing in this area, with interesting work on the topics of machine learning to identify suicide risk among text-based crisis counselling encounters (Broadbent et al., 2023) and the development of a clinical prediction rule for suicide in severe mental illness (Senior et al., 2020) and a clinical prediction score to evaluate the risk of death by suicide following self-harm presentations to health care (Fazel et al., 2023), among other initiatives.

At the present time, however, it remains the case that it is not possible to predict self-harm or suicide at the level of the individual. Moreover, risk can change rapidly in response to myriad factors that are unpredictable, unknown, and possibly unknowable. The element of impulsivity in much suicidal behaviour adds further to the difficulty with prediction.

This is not a new conclusion. In 1883, Thomas Clouston made similar points in his book, *Clinical Lectures on Mental Diseases*:

No tendency to suicide exists at all in many melancholics from beginning to end of their disease, but it does exist in some form or other, in wish, intention, or act in four out of every five of all the cases, and we can never tell when it is to develop in any patient. The intention and the act may come on suddenly, by suggestion from without or within, or by the sight of opportunity or means of self-destruction.

(Clouston, 1883; p. 112)

One hundred and forty years later, the NIMH emphasised the difficulty with prediction in a similar fashion, along with the need for a flexible response as circumstances evolve and presentations change:

Most people who have risk factors will not attempt suicide, and it is difficult to tell who will act on suicidal thoughts. Although risk factors for suicide are important to keep in mind, someone who is actively showing warning signs of suicide may be at higher risk for danger and in need [of] immediate attention.

(National Institute of Mental Health, 2023)

Overall, it is impossible to predict which patients will die by suicide and which will not. Even following meticulous psychiatric evaluation, 'risk assessment', treatment, effective communication with family, and close follow-up, it is still entirely possible that any given person will engage in deliberate self-harm or suicide (Kelly, 2017). All of these assessments and services should be provided, and they might both alleviate distress and reduce the risk of self-harm and suicide. But it remains the case that the outcome cannot be predicted for any given person: even with the highest standard of assessment, treatment, and care on any given day, deliberate self-harm or suicide can still occur on that same day, and cannot be predicted.

Evidence-Based Approaches to Suicide Prevention

So, if suicide cannot be predicted in individual cases, can it be prevented? A great deal of time and effort have been rightly devoted to preventing suicide, given that it remains an intensely individual tragedy as well as a substantial public health problem. The fact that rates are declining globally indicates that positive change is possible.

Against this background, the issue of preventing self-harm and suicide can be considered at three levels: the political level (e.g., re-shaping the landscape of risk for psychological distress, mental illness, and suicide), the population level (e.g., restricting access to means of deliberate self-harm and suicide for the entire population), and the individual level (e.g., seeking to alleviate distress, treat mental illness, and reduce the likelihood or severity of self-harm). While there are connections across the three levels, it is useful to consider each in turn.

First, at the broadest political level, it is necessary to address the root causes of much (but not all) psychological distress, mental illness, deliberate self-harm, and suicide. These root causes include poverty, inequality, injustice, prejudice, and all forms of social exclusion (Kelly, 2022). These problems must be addressed at the political level, locally, nationally, and internationally. Advocating on these themes requires that health care professionals move beyond the world of individual patient care, step outside the clinic, and enter the realms of public advocacy, social activism, and political involvement. Some of the relevant issues are explored in Chapters 9 ('Global Injustice in Mental Health Care') and 10 ('The Future of Psychiatry: Person-Centred Care and System-Level Change') of this book.

Second, restricting access to means of deliberate self-harm and suicide across the entire population can help reduce rates of deliberate self-harm and suicide. Given that it is not possible to predict suicide in individual cases, the strongest evidence to date supports suicide prevention measures that avoid prediction altogether and simply apply to the entire population, regardless of apparent risk. On this basis, restricting access to means of self-harm can prove effective. This might include national bans on the most toxic forms of pesticide in countries where pesticides are commonly used for suicide, or restricting access to fire-arms, in order to reduce risks associated with impulsivity (Knipe et al., 2022).

The effectiveness of population-level interventions stems from the fact that they do not rely on risk assessments at the level of individuals, but apply to everyone in the population. It is important that such measures are tailored to the environments in which they are applied, so as to optimise both acceptability and benefit. The necessity for flexibility in implementation was emphasised in one 'scoping review' of 'facilitators and barriers to implementation of suicide prevention interventions':

> Our results indicate that interventions based on restricting access to the means can benefit from adaptability of the intervention. This means that intervention should in the best-case scenario provide few guiding principles, which can be tailored to the needs of the target environment no matter if it tries to restrict access to certain places, availability of firearms or pesticides. On the other hand, not reflecting the needs and resources of the target group in the intervention can lead to implementation failure.
>
> (Kasal et al., 2023; p. 10)

At the level of the individual, it is important to remain aware of the possibility of self-harm and suicide, to provide open, honest assessments, and deliver care that is responsive, flexible, person-centred, and evidence-based. The NIMH provides a useful list of 'warning signs that someone may be at immediate risk for attempting suicide', including:

- Talking about wanting to die or wanting to kill themselves.
- Talking about feeling empty or hopeless or having no reason to live.
- Talking about feeling trapped or feeling that there are no solutions.
- Feeling unbearable emotional or physical pain.
- Talking about being a burden to others.
- Withdrawing from family and friends.
- Giving away important possessions.
- Saying goodbye to friends and family.
- Putting affairs in order, such as making a will.
- Taking great risks that could lead to death, such as driving extremely fast.
- Talking or thinking about death often (National Institute of Mental Health, 2023).

The NIMH adds that 'other serious warning signs that someone may be at risk for attempting suicide include':

- Displaying extreme mood swings, suddenly changing from very sad to very calm or happy.
- Making a plan or looking for ways to kill themselves, such as searching for lethal methods online, stockpiling pills, or buying a gun.

- Talking about feeling great guilt or shame.
- Using alcohol or drugs more often.
- Acting anxious or agitated.
- Changing eating or sleeping habits.
- Showing rage or talking about seeking revenge (National Institute of Mental Health, 2023).

It is important to use these features as reasons to enquire further into a person's symptoms, rather than using them as a statistical or actuarial method to assess risk, which cannot be reliably assessed at the level of the individual.

In terms of specific interventions, it is vital to establish a strong therapeutic relationship that facilitates disclosure, to suggest involving family or friends in care (as appropriate), and to have clear arrangements for follow-up care and emergency access. Specific therapeutic interventions for self-harm will depend on the individual case and the presence or absence of mental illness. In broad terms, there is evidence to support psychological interventions in certain situations such as dialectical behaviour therapy (DBT) in some people with personality disorders, or brief interventions, although the evidence base is limited (Knipe et al., 2022).

Certain medications for the treatment of particular conditions might also reduce risk in some people, although it is difficult to assemble a complete evidence base because people at apparently high risk of self-harm or suicide are often excluded from clinical trials (Knipe et al., 2022). This is a regrettable problem with the evidence base in psychiatry, which is generally as strong as, or stronger than, the evidence base for treatments in other areas of clinical care, such as cardiovascular medicine (see Chapter 4: 'Treating Symptoms and Disorders').

Despite this methodological issue, there is evidence of potential benefit in terms of reduced suicidal behaviour with certain medications, including, most notably, lithium, which appears to be associated with reduced risk of suicide in people with bipolar disorder and depression. This effect seems to be specific to lithium. As Malhi and colleagues point out, bipolar disorder is a 'serious mental illness that is widely acknowledged as one of the most debilitating and the most likely to result in suicide', and while 'competition has grown within the pharmacological armamentarium for bipolar disorder with newer treatments promoting an image of being safer and easier to prescribe [...] none of these mimics have the additional benefits of preventing suicide' (Malhi et al., 2023; p. 1).

As a result, lithium is, perhaps, the psychiatric medication with the most convincing evidence base for reducing the risk of suicidal behaviour, and this should be considered in prescribing decisions in bipolar disorder. More broadly, individual care should include careful therapeutic risk assessment, formulation, therapeutic risk management, and safety planning, as appropriate to each individual case (Hawton et al., 2022).

Suicide and the Law

This chapter started with the case of Brad, a 15-year-old boy who had been burning his arms with matches for almost a year. When Brad's parents discovered this, it was not clear to them or to Brad what to do. Was he mentally ill? To whom should they turn? Could anything be done? Why was Brad doing this?

We will return to Brad's case at the end of this chapter, which has, so far, considered clinical and therapeutic dimensions of self-harm and suicide; i.e., definitions of deliberate self-harm and suicide, suicide in the history of psychiatry, global rates of suicide over recent decades, the limited value of 'risk assessment', and the use of evidence-based approaches for suicide prevention. But, for Brad and others, are there also legal consequences to their actions, as well as personal and clinical consequences? This is an important issue in many parts of the world and merits close attention.

Three main legal issues arise in relation to deliberate self-harm and suicide: the decriminalisation of suicide and attempted suicide in various countries; the use of 'risk' of self-harm or suicide in mental health legislation as a ground for admission or treatment without consent; and evolving laws governing physician-assisted suicide (PAS) in various jurisdictions, especially in the context of mental illness.

To begin, there is a long history of criminalising attempted suicide in many countries around the world, but developments in science and medicine over the nineteenth and twentieth centuries led to significant changes in attitudes in certain jurisdictions:

> During this period, cognitive and emotional distress were presented as complex phenomena that could also be caused by natural biological factors. Consequently, several countries repealed laws criminalizing suicide, predominantly in Europe and North America.
>
> Advances in attitudes toward human rights, including the Convention on the Rights of Persons with Disabilities, have prompted many other countries to abolish laws that criminalize suicide. Furthermore, the World Health Organization *Mental Health Action Plan 2020-2030*, which calls for human rights oriented policy to tackle suicide, has impelled many countries to commit to decriminalizing suicide.
>
> Despite such breakthroughs, suicide remains criminalized in many countries around the world, particularly in [low- and middle-income countries] in Africa and Southeast Asia which bear the biggest burden of suicide mortality.
>
> (Ochuku et al., 2022; p. 2; citations omitted)

Despite the uneven pace of change, decriminalisation of suicide is progressing. In India, for example, the Mental Healthcare Act, 2017 states that, 'notwithstanding anything contained in section 309 of the Indian Penal Code any person who attempts to commit suicide shall be presumed, unless proved otherwise, to have severe stress and shall not be tried and punished under the said Code' (Section 115(1)). This is a positive development, which will hopefully emphasise health care responses to attempted suicide, rather than criminal proceedings.

The second key legal issue concerns the use of 'risk' of self-harm or suicide in mental health legislation as a ground for admission or treatment without consent. The broader issue of mental health legislation was considered in Chapter 5: 'Treatment Without Consent'. That chapter noted the continued role of 'risk' in criteria for admission and treatment without consent in many jurisdictions, despite our very limited ability to assess risk of harm to self (see above) or others (Large et al., 2024). Future revision of legislation should de-emphasise risk as a criterion for admission and treatment without consent, focussing instead on demonstrated needs and potential benefits of treatment.

The third legal issue concerns laws governing PAS in various jurisdictions, especially in the context of mental illness. A full consideration of this topic is beyond the scope of the present chapter, but it is important to note growing concerns about PAS for mental illness alone, not least because suicidality is a feature of many mental illnesses, and socio-environmental circumstances can be major factors in the onset and progression of such conditions (Gergel, 2024). PAS for mental illness alone also rests uneasily with psychiatry's overall efforts to decrease rates of deliberate self-harm and suicide (Kelly and McLoughlin, 2002).

These concerns, combined with uncertainty about the biological basis and prognosis of many mental illnesses, mean that PAS on the basis of suffering from mental illness is qualitatively different to PAS on the basis of suffering from 'physical' illnesses which have a clearer biological basis and a clearer prognosis. And if PAS is to be provided on the basis of 'unbearable suffering' alone, without requiring any diagnosis, it is unclear why physicians would be involved to begin with. As a result, the provision of PAS for mental illness alone is not advised.

Future Directions for Research and Service Development

This chapter has examined various definitional, clinical, and preventive matters relating to deliberate self-harm and suicide. Throughout all such discussions, it is important to bear in mind the NIMH's reminder that 'suicide is not a normal response to stress':

> **Suicidal thoughts or actions are a sign of extreme distress and should not be ignored.** If these warning signs apply to you or someone you know, get help as soon as possible, particularly if the behavior is new or has increased recently (National Institute of Mental Health, 2023).
>
> (emphasis in the original)

In terms of useful directions for future research and service development, it is helpful to start from a broad, societal perspective. Psychiatry is a social endeavour as well as a medical one, so a wide-angle lens is optimal. From this position, there is a clear need for continued study of the political, social, and economic contexts in which thoughts of self-harm and suicide develop, are interpreted, and are managed. Mental illness is often a factor in these situations, but mental illness does not occur in a vacuum, so it is neither accurate nor helpful to view self-harm and suicide as entirely personal matters (Bharati et al., 2021). Research and interventions need to acknowledge this broader perspective, as well as providing supports at the levels of individuals, families, and communities.

In terms of population measures, Beattie and Devitt note that restricting access to means (as discussed above) and reducing overall alcohol consumption are both likely to help reduce rates of suicide (Beattie and Devitt, 2015). In terms of individual-level care, they note the potential of DBT and lithium for certain patients, as well as the possible roles of follow-up contacts and safety planning interventions. Ochuku and colleagues point to similar 'evidence-based strategies for suicide prevention such as means restriction, improved mental health literacy and access to psychosocial support, and responsible media coverage of suicides' (Ochuku et al., 2022; p. 1). The importance of positive therapeutic relationships cannot be overstated, and the provision of support to families.

Future research could usefully focus on more fine-grained analysis of the underpinnings of the recent decline in suicide rates, the impact of the Covid-19 pandemic (on both mental health and rates of self-harm and suicide), and the precise ways in which evidence-based approaches to prevention are best devised. For example, which are the most impactful models of means restriction, and in what ways should these vary from country to country? At the level of the individual, to what extent do follow-up contacts and safety planning interventions help, and do particular models work better than others? What are the roles for technology? And what is the role of artificial intelligence (AI), if it is judiciously deployed?

In terms of legislative change, future research might usefully interrogate legal and regulatory responses to suicide and self-harm across jurisdictions, with comparative legal analysis of both national legislation and international standard-setting. Can one set of standards be recommended for every legal system around the world, regardless of historical, cultural, and legal backgrounds? Legislative change is often slow, and sometimes wisely so.

The use of 'risk' of self-harm or suicide in mental health legislation as part of criteria for admission or treatment without consent is a particular cause for concern, as is the provision of PAS for mental illness alone. Regarding the latter, further research might conceivably help establish how to systematically and reliably differentiate a desire to die that stems from mental illness from a desire to die that does not. For now, however, such a distinction can be essentially impossible to make, and legal provisions often fail to reflect the complexity, ambiguity, and changeability of clinical assessments in these situations.

Brad, the 15-year-old boy whom we met at the start of this chapter, had been burning his arms with matches for almost a year. When his parents found out, they were deeply upset. They spoke to Brad about it, but none of them knew what to do next. Brad's mother phoned her sister, who suggested that Brad should see his general practitioner (family doctor). The doctor spoke with Brad and his mother, and listened when Brad tried to explain why he burnt himself. 'Does it relieve the tension?', the doctor asked. Brad was honest: 'Burning my arms takes away some of the tension for a few minutes, but then it comes back. I know that it makes me feel worse in the end. I am so ashamed.'

The doctor referred Brad to see a child and adolescent psychiatrist, who discussed the situation in detail with Brad and his parents. Brad was quite embarrassed and asked to see the psychiatrist on his own, without his parents, even though he was not yet 16. Brad's parents agreed to this, and Brad discussed his problems privately with the psychiatrist. Brad was worried about schoolwork and about his friends. 'My friends all seem so confident', he said. 'Am I the only one who is anxious, tense, and burning their arms? Have you ever seen anything like this before? Am I out of control? What should I do now?'

The psychiatrist listened to Brad's concerns and reassured Brad that he was not alone. The psychiatrist told Brad that other people experience similar problems, but people often do not talk about it. Brad understood this: he didn't really want to talk about it either, so why would anyone else? That made sense.

The psychiatrist recommended that Brad attend a series of appointments with a qualified psychotherapist, focussing on dealing with difficult emotions, tolerating distress, and developing better coping mechanisms. Brad asked: 'Am I mentally ill?' The psychiatrist told Brad that he was not mentally ill, but needed support, treatment, and follow-up. Brad's parents asked: 'Will Brad continue to self-harm?' They really wanted to ask: 'Is it likely that Brad will die by suicide?' They were terrified.

The psychiatrist reassured both Brad and his parents. Brad showed good insight into his problems and was willing to reach out for help. This was very positive, as was the fact that Brad had a supportive family – even if Brad still slammed his bedroom door sometimes. While Brad's self-harm placed him at higher risk of suicide compared to someone who did not self-harm, the most likely outcome was that Brad would improve over time. Psychotherapy would hopefully help Brad to understand his problems, manage his emotions better, develop other coping mechanisms, and stop burning himself. The psychiatrist was steady, pragmatic, and optimistic.

Brad duly attended the psychotherapist for therapy and the psychiatrist for follow-up appointments. Over the following months, Brad stopped burning himself. He still felt the urge to self-harm from time to time, especially when he was under stress. But, with the psychotherapist, Brad identified other, better coping strategies for these situations. Some of these 'coping steps' (as Brad called them) were very simple: standing up, going into another room, or phoning someone. On other occasions, Brad needed to use other coping skills that he learnt for dealing with bigger stresses that might arise. It all took time and effort, but the situation improved substantially, thanks to Brad's hard work, his openness to help, the availability of care, and his family's support.

Brad reached out to his friends again, who were very happy to have him back. He rejoined the football team, and soon looked forward to training. Talking to the psychiatrist six months later, Brad was very critical of himself in the past. He said: 'I don't know what I was thinking when I burnt my arms. Was I thinking at all?' The psychiatrist suggested that Brad should not be so hard on himself. Life is not always easy, the psychiatrist said, and everyone does the best they can. 'It is better to focus on now', she added. 'Now is all we have'. Brad was happy to take this advice.

Key Messages

- Suicide is intentional self-killing, while deliberate self-harm is the intentional infliction of non-fatal harm on oneself. The latter includes a wide variety of methods such as self-cutting and self-burning.
- Self-harm and suicide have featured in ancient societies, traditional literatures, and religious texts since the beginning of recorded history, with increasing medicalisation over time, especially during the twentieth century.
- At a global level, suicide is in decline: between 1990 and 2016, the global, age-standardised mortality rate for suicide decreased by a third.
- Evidence to date indicates that the Covid-19 pandemic increased rates of distress and suicidal ideation, but not rates of completed suicide.
- Despite the identification of certain risk factors for deliberate self-harm and suicide, it remains impossible to predict who will die by suicide and who will not.
- Even with the highest standard of assessment, treatment, and care on any given day, deliberate self-harm or suicide can still occur on that same day, and cannot be predicted.
- Interventions to reduce the occurrence of self-harm and suicide can be considered at three levels: the political level (e.g., re-shaping the landscape of risk for psychological distress, mental illness, and suicide), the population level (e.g., restricting access to means of deliberate self-harm and suicide for the entire population), and the individual level (e.g., seeking to alleviate distress, treat mental illness, and reduce the likelihood or severity of self-harm).
- Lithium in bipolar disorder is the psychiatric medication with the best evidence base to indicate that it diminishes the occurrence of suicidal behaviour.

- Three main legal issues arise in relation to deliberate self-harm and suicide: decriminalisation of suicide and attempted suicide; the use of 'risk' of self-harm or suicide in mental health legislation as a ground for admission or treatment without consent; and evolving laws governing physician-assisted suicide (PAS) in various jurisdictions, especially in the context of mental illness.
- Future service development could usefully focus on optimal models of evidence-based interventions to reduce rates of self-harm and suicide; e.g., means restriction, access to specific treatments, and responsible media coverage.
- Further research could helpfully examine the broad social and political contexts of self-harm and suicide, improved means of prevention, and the role of legislation and regulatory frameworks in both preventing and responding to self-harm and suicide across jurisdictions.

References

Alvarez A. *The Savage God: A Study of Suicide.* Harmondsworth: Penguin Books Ltd., 1974.

Beattie D, Devitt P. *Suicide: A Modern Obsession.* Dublin: Liberties Press, 2015.

Belsher BE, Smolenski DJ, Pruitt LD, Bush NE, Beech EH, Workman DE, Morgan RL, Evatt DP, Tucker J, Skopp NA. Prediction models for suicide attempts and deaths: a systematic review and simulation. *JAMA Psychiatry* 2019; 76: 642–51 (https://doi.org/10.1001/jamapsychiatry.2019.0174).

Bharati K, Lobo L, Shah J. *Revisiting Suicide From a Socio-Psychological Lens.* London and New York: Routledge, 2021.

Broadbent M, Medina Grespan M, Axford K, Zhang X, Srikumar V, Kious B, Imel Z. A machine learning approach to identifying suicide risk among text-based crisis counseling encounters. *Frontiers in Psychiatry* 2023; 14: 1110527 (https://doi.org/10.3389/fpsyt.2023.1110527). (Link to licence: https://creativecommons.org/licenses/by/4.0/) (accessed 7 November 2023).

Bucknill JC, Tuke DH. *A Manual of Psychological Medicine: Containing the History, Nosology, Description, Statistics, Diagnosis, Pathology, and Treatment of Insanity, With an Appendix of Cases.* Philadelphia: Blanchard and Lea, 1858.

Clouston TS. *Clinical Lectures on Mental Diseases.* London: J. A. Churchill, 1883.

Cooper J, Kapur N, Webb R, Lawlor M, Guthrie E, Mackway-Jones K, Appleby L. Suicide after deliberate self-harm: a 4-year cohort study. *American Journal of Psychiatry* 2005; 162: 297–303 (https://doi.org/10.1176/appi.ajp.162.2.297).

Council of Economic Advisors. *Reducing the Economic Burden of Unmet Mental Health Needs.* Washington, DC: The White House, 2022 (https://www.whitehouse.gov/cea/written-materials/2022/05/31/reducing-the-economic-burden-of-unmet-mental-health-needs/). (Link to licence: https://creativecommons.org/licenses/by/3.0/us/) (accessed 7 November 2023).

Duncan JF. *Popular Errors on the Subject of Insanity Examined and Exposed.* Dublin: James McGlashan, 1853.

Fazel S, Vazquez-Montes MDLA, Molero Y, Runeson B, D'Onofrio BM, Larsson H, Lichtenstein P, Walker J, Sharpe M, Fanshawe TR. Risk of death by suicide following self-harm presentations to healthcare: development and validation of a multivariable clinical prediction rule (OxSATS). *BMJ Mental Health* 2023; 26: e300673 (https://doi .org/10.1136/bmjment-2023-300673). (Link to licence: https://creativecommons.org/ licenses/by/4.0/) (accessed 7 November 2023).

Gergel TL. The future of mental health law: the need for deeper examination and broader scope. In: Kelly BD, Donnelly M (eds), *Routledge Handbook of Mental Health Law* (pp. 704–26). London and New York: Routledge, 2024.

Gunnell D, Harbord R, Singleton N, Jenkins R, Lewis G. Factors influencing the development and amelioration of suicidal thoughts in the general population: cohort study. *British Journal of Psychiatry* 2004; 185: 385–93 (https://doi.org/10.1192/bjp .185.5.385).

Hall R. Covid's effect on mental health not as great as first thought, study suggests. *Guardian*, 8 March 2023 (https://www.theguardian.com/society/2023/mar/08/ covid-effect-mental-health-study-mcgill-university) (accessed 5 November 2023) (Courtesy of Guardian News & Media Ltd.).

Hawton K, Lascelles K, Pitman A, Gilbert S, Silverman M. Assessment of suicide risk in mental health practice: shifting from prediction to therapeutic assessment, formulation, and risk management. *Lancet Psychiatry* 2022; 9: 922–8 (https://doi.org /10.1016/S2215-0366(22)00232-2).

Kasal A, Táborská R, Juríková L, Grabenhofer-Eggerth A, Pichler M, Gruber B, Tomášková H, Niederkrotenthaler T. Facilitators and barriers to implementation of suicide prevention interventions: scoping review. *Cambridge Prisms: Global Mental Health* 2023; 10: e15 (https://doi.org/10.1017/gmh.2023.9). (Link to licence: https:// creativecommons.org/licenses/by/4.0/) (accessed 7 November 2023).

Kelly BD. *Mental Health in Ireland: The Complete Guide for Patients, Families,* Health Care Professionals and Everyone Who Wants to Be Well. Dublin: The Liffey Press, 2017.

Kelly BD. *In Search of Madness: A Psychiatrist's Travels Through the History of Mental Illness.* Dublin: Gill Books, 2022.

Kelly BD. Hope on mental health. *Economist*, 4 November 2023a.

Kelly BD. *Resilience: Lessons from Sir William Wilde on Life After Covid.* Dublin: Eastwood Books, 2023b.

Kelly BD, McLoughlin DM. Euthanasia, assisted suicide and psychiatry: a Pandora's box. *British Journal of Psychiatry* 2002; 181: 278–9 (https://doi.org/10.1192/bjp.181 .4.278).

Knipe D, Padmanathan P, Newton-Howes G, Chan LF, Kapur N. Suicide and self-harm. *Lancet* 2022; 399: 1903–16 (https://doi.org/10.1016/S0140-6736(22)00173-8).

Large M, Callaghan S, Ryan CJ. Risk of harm and involuntary psychiatric treatment. In: Kelly BD, Donnelly M (eds), *Routledge Handbook of Mental Health Law* (pp. 342–55). London and New York: Routledge, 2024.

Malhi GS, Bell E, Jadidi M, Gitlin M, Bauer M. Countering the declining use of lithium therapy: a call to arms. *International Journal of Bipolar Disorders* 2023; 11: 30 (https:// doi.org/10.1186/s40345-023-00310-x). (Link to licence: https://creativecommons.org /licenses/by/4.0/) (accessed 7 November 2023).

Naghavi M, on behalf of the Global Burden of Disease Self-Harm Collaborators. Global, regional, and national burden of suicide mortality 1990 to 2016: systematic analysis for the Global Burden of Disease Study 2016. *BMJ* 2019; 364: l94 (https://doi.org /10.1136/bmj.l94). (Link to licence: https://creativecommons.org/licenses/by/4.0/) (accessed 7 November 2023).

National Institute of Mental Health. *Suicide Prevention.* Bethesda, MD: National Institute of Mental Health, 2023 (https://www.nimh.nih.gov/health/topics/suicide-prevention #part_9890). (Link to Copyright Policy: https://www.nimh.nih.gov/site-info/policies #part_2718) (accessed 10 November 2023).

Nock MK, Millner AJ, Ross EL, Kennedy CJ, Al-Suwaidi M, Barak-Corren Y, Castro VM, Castro-Ramirez F, Lauricella T, Murman N, Petukhova M, Bird SA, Reis B, Smoller JW, Kessler RC. Prediction of suicide attempts using clinician assessment, patient self-report, and electronic health records. *JAMA Network Open* 2022; 5: e2144373 (https://doi.org/10.1001/jamanetworkopen.2021.44373). (Links to licence: https://jamanetwork.com/pages/cc-by-license-permissions; https://creativecommons .org/share-your-work/cclicenses/; https://creativecommons.org/licenses/by/4.0/) (accessed 7 November 2023).

Ochuku BK, Johnson NE, Osborn TL, Wasanga CM, Ndetei DM. Centering decriminalization of suicide in low- and middle-income countries on effective suicide prevention strategies. *Frontiers in Psychiatry* 2022; 13: 1034206 (https://doi.org/10 .3389/fpsyt.2022.1034206). (Link to licence: https://creativecommons.org/licenses/ by/4.0/) (accessed 13 November 2023).

Organisation for Economic Co-operation and Development. *Health at a Glance 2023: OECD Indicators.* Paris: OECD Publishing, 2023 (https://doi.org/10.1787/7a7afb35 -en). (Link to license: https://www.oecd.org/termsandconditions/) (accessed 7 November 2023).

Senior M, Burghart M, Yu R, Kormilitzin A, Liu Q, Vaci N, Nevado-Holgado A, Pandit S, Zlodre J, Fazel S. Identifying predictors of suicide in severe mental illness: a feasibility study of a clinical prediction rule (Oxford Mental Illness and Suicide Tool or OxMIS). *Frontiers in Psychiatry* 2020; 11: 268 (https://doi.org/10.3389/fpsyt.2020 .00268). (Link to licence: https://creativecommons.org/licenses/by/4.0/) (accessed 7 November 2023).

Sun Y, Wu Y, Fan S, Dal Santo T, Li L, Jiang X, Li K, Wang Y, Tasleem A, Krishnan A, He C, Bonardi O, Boruff JT, Rice DB, Markham S, Levis B, Azar M, Thombs-Vite I, Neupane D, Agic B, Fahim C, Martin MS, Sockalingam S, Turecki G, Benedetti A, Thombs BD. Comparison of mental health symptoms before and during the covid-19 pandemic: evidence from a systematic review and meta-analysis of 134 cohorts. *BMJ* 2023; 380: e074224 (https://doi.org/10.1136/bmj-2022-074224).

Williams M. *Suicide* and Attempted Suicide: Understanding the Cry of Pain. London: Penguin Books Ltd., 1997.

Yan Y, Hou J, Li Q, Yu NX. Suicide before and during the COVID-19 pandemic: a systematic review with meta-analysis. *International Journal of Environmental Research and Public Health* 2023; 20: 3346 (https://doi.org/10.3390/ijerph20043346). (Link to licence: https://creativecommons.org/licenses/by/4.0/) (accessed 7 November 2023).

9 Global Injustice in Mental Health Care

Carl was 16 years of age when he first showed signs of serious mental illness. Carl's father had a diagnosis of schizophrenia, but died by suicide before Carl was born. Carl's mother was addicted to drugs, so Carl was brought up in a series of foster homes. Carl was physically abused as a child in two of these placements. As a result, Carl did not do well at school. He was suspended on several occasions. He left school permanently at the age of 16.

Carl was first arrested for possession of cannabis when he was 16. He was released without charge, but was arrested numerous times over the following years for similar offences. Carl was twice convicted of possessing drugs. He was also convicted of robbery, but not sent to prison. He was fined and assigned a probation officer, with whom he did not cooperate.

Carl tried to find work, but his lack of education and criminal record made that impossible. Carl signed up for social welfare payments, but found that this was not enough for his growing drug habit. Carl now used cannabis daily and took cocaine at weekends. Finding it difficult to rent an apartment or a room anywhere, Carl moved in with a group of other people who smoked cannabis. They lived together in a squat – an abandoned house that they broke into and simply stayed in.

Around two months after Carl moved into this arrangement, he began to feel paranoid. He felt that the people with whom he lived were talking about him behind his back, stealing his money, and planning to harm him. He was not clear why this was happening, but he was certain that he was in danger. One night, after everyone went to sleep, Carl set the house on fire.

The fire went out quickly and nobody was hurt, but a passer-by who saw the flames called the fire brigade. Both a fire brigade and an ambulance arrived a few minutes later. The paramedics from the ambulance spoke with Carl and saw that he was not burnt. When they asked how the fire began, Carl was honest: 'I started it because these people are planning to harm me. They might kill me. I don't know them. They are dangerous to me'.

The paramedics asked Carl if he took drugs and Carl said he smoked cannabis, but insisted that cannabis had nothing to do with it. 'There's a plot', he said. 'I don't know who is behind it, but my life is in danger'. Carl added that he

DOI: 10.4324/9781003378495-10

sometimes heard 'the man' talking to him, even when there was nobody there. 'The man' told Carl to 'watch his back'.

After some discussion, the paramedics persuaded Carl to come to the Emergency Department at the hospital for assessment. Carl got into the ambulance, but did not stay in the Emergency Department to be assessed. He left the hospital before being seen and went to the city centre where he bought cocaine. Later that night, Carl was arrested in a disturbed state outside a bar, shouting that people were trying to kill him and that the only safe place for him was prison. Eventually, the police arrested him and placed him in a cell in the police station while they tried to figure out what to do next.

The next morning, Carl appeared in Court, charged with disturbing the peace and attempted arson. The judge recognised Carl because he had appeared in her courtroom many times previously. While she had never sent Carl to prison before, she was concerned that his offending behaviour was escalating. He had placed lives at risk. Also, Carl had never paid his fines in the past and had not engaged with the probation officer. With great reluctance, the judge sent Carl to a remand prison to await a full Court hearing. She instructed that he be provided with a free solicitor and medical care as needed, including psychiatric assessment.

Introduction

Carl's case is a common one: a mixture of social disadvantage, childhood trauma, substance misuse, symptoms of mental illness, and offending behaviour. His story can be told in very different ways, depending on the background of the person telling it. There is a clear social dimension: poverty, social exclusion, and imprisonment. The story can also be told using the terminology of psychology: adverse childhood circumstances, experiences of trauma, and limited opportunity to develop adaptive coping skills. Carl's trajectory also has a psychiatric dimension, with symptoms of paranoia and thought disorder following substance misuse.

Too often, these approaches – sociological, psychological, and medical – are seen as different aspects or separate components of a person's story. This is misleading. They are better seen as different languages which can be used to describe the same thing: one human being's experience of themselves and the world. For some people, the language of sociology makes most sense, prioritising social, economic, and political interpretations of circumstances and events. For others, the language of psychology is most attractive, constructing meaning and creating a valuable feeling of understanding. And, for other people, the language of medicine proves the most useful: symptoms, illnesses, disorders, conditions, evidence, and treatments.

Against this background, this chapter seeks to blend these approaches, foregrounding social considerations in its examination of 'Global Injustice in Mental

Health Care'. The chapter starts by using evidence from the World Health Organization (WHO) and other sources to demonstrate and describe global inequity in mental health care. Particular attention is given to the relationships between mental illness and poverty, unemployment, homelessness, imprisonment, reduced rates of marriage, and issues relating to migration. The concept of 'structural violence' is used to explore the political, economic, and social circumstances that shape the landscape of risk for mental illness, the likelihood of receiving care, and contrasting outcomes for people with mental illness around the world. The chapter starts with evidence on this topic, summarises responses at international level, emphasises the centrality of dignity, and concludes with an outspoken manifesto for culturally informed change.

Global Inequity in Mental Health Care

Levels of self-reported well-being vary greatly around the globe. The *World Happiness Report 2023*, published by the Sustainable Development Solutions Network, reported average levels of happiness in 137 countries around the world over a three-year period from 2020 to 2022 (Helliwell et al., 2023). Happiness was rated from zero to ten, with a higher score indicating greater happiness. The happiest country in the world was Finland (with a score of 7.8 out of 10), followed by Denmark (7.6), Iceland (7.5), Israel (7.5), and the Netherlands (7.4). The least happy country surveyed was Afghanistan (1.9 out of 10), followed by Lebanon (2.4), Sierra Leone (3.1), Zimbabwe (3.2), and the Democratic Republic of Congo (3.2). Ireland was in 14th place (6.9 out of 10), the United States in 15th place (6.9), and the United Kingdom in 19th place (6.8).

Happiness surveys have many methodological limitations including differing understandings of happiness between individuals, contrasting cultural contexts in different countries, and the fleeting nature of happiness and life satisfaction in many people's lives. Despite these limitations, the headline findings from most studies of happiness and well-being are remarkably consistent over time: happiness tends to be higher in countries that are wealthy, stable, and peaceful, and lower in countries that are poor, unstable, and troubled by conflict and socioeconomic challenges. This is especially true in countries that do not enjoy the opportunity to re-build their social infrastructure between periods of challenge, instability, and war. These circumstances erode happiness and well-being.

In terms of the provision of mental health care, similar differences between countries are apparent around the globe. In low- and middle-income countries, up to 85% of people with severe mental illness receive no treatment whatsoever (Insel et al., 2015). This is directly attributable to a lack of resources for the relevant services and the low political priority accorded to mental health in many regions. The WHO points out that mental health conditions 'cause 1 in 5 years lived with disability':

Two of the most common mental health conditions, depression and anxiety, cost the global economy US$ 1 trillion each year. Despite these figures, the global median of government health expenditure that goes to mental health is less than 2%.

(World Health Organization, 2023)

These figures vary around the world but remain generally insufficient. Moitra and colleagues, in 'a systematic review and Bayesian meta-regression analysis' of 'the global gap in treatment coverage for major depressive disorder in 84 countries from 2000–2019', highlight these differences in no uncertain terms, although coverage is remarkably patchy even in high-income settings:

Treatment coverage for health service use ranged from 51% [95% UI (uncertainty intervals) 20%, 82%] in high-income locations to 20% [95% UI 1%, 53%] in low- and lower middle-income locations. Treatment coverage for mental health service use ranged from 33% [95% UI 8%, 66%] in high-income locations to 8% [95% UI <1%, 36%] in low- and lower middle-income countries. Minimally adequate treatment (MAT) rates ranged from 23% [95% UI 2%, 55%] in high-income countries to 3% [95% UI <1%, 25%]) in low- and lower middle-income countries.

(Moitra et al., 2022; p. 2)

Elsewhere, Moitra and colleagues point out that, 'despite the high prevalence of mental health conditions worldwide, treatment coverage remains low and varies by setting and population':

Furthermore, data on treatment coverage is not routinely collected despite it being part of international priorities such as the targets set by the World Health Organization Mental Health Action plan [World Health Organization, 2021]. There are sparse data on treatment coverage from many parts of Sub-Saharan Africa and Asia that comprise nearly three quarters of the world's population [Moitra et al., 2022]. This continues to hold true particularly for major depressive disorder [MDD]. Analyses of treatment coverage data from 84 countries estimated mental health treatment coverage for MDD to be 33% in high-income countries and only 8% in [low- and middle-income countries] [Moitra et al., 2022]. There has been little literature in recent years on treatment coverage for severe mental disorders (SMDs) such as schizophrenia. Recent analyses estimate treatment coverage for schizophrenia to be 9.4% in Ukraine, 19% in the Philippines, and 10% in Ethiopia [Kemp et al., 2022; Alem et al., 2009].

(Moitra et al., 2023; p. 304)

Even in high-income countries, there are demonstrable variations in the provision of different types and levels of care for mental illness. In 2020, Eurostat reported dramatic variations in hospital bed numbers for psychiatric care across European Union (EU) member states (Eurostat, 2020). This survey found that Belgium had the most psychiatric beds per capita, at 135 psychiatric beds per 100,000 inhabitants, followed by Germany (128) and Latvia (122). Italy had the lowest (9 psychiatric beds per 100,000 inhabitants), followed by Cyprus (18) and Ireland (34). The EU average was 73 psychiatric beds per 100,000 population, but the differences between countries were substantial.

International comparisons of bed numbers are always challenging because different countries count psychiatric beds differently and have contrasting histories in the development of models of care. It is even more challenging to compare community-based services across borders, because outpatient care takes different forms and is accessed in different ways in various countries. In addition, most cross-national comparisons of mental health services to date tend to look at features of psychiatric care that are prioritised in high-income countries, such as inpatient beds, admissions, and outpatient clinics. These comparisons do not capture other forms of care that might be more culturally or locally appropriate than the specific parameters of multi-disciplinary care that are currently privileged in high-income countries. For these and other reasons, cross-national comparisons of levels of mental healthcare are both complex and contested (Applbaum, 2015).

Even with these caveats, however, the variations described across all of these studies are considerable. These differences are unlikely to be entirely attributable to differing service models or challenges with cross-national comparisons. Overall, findings indicate that the nature and levels of care provided for mental illness vary dramatically around the world. More care is generally provided in high-income countries (albeit with considerable variations between countries), but levels of care are generally inadequate in all regions of the world.

Social Exclusion and Mental Illness

There are many definitions of the term 'social exclusion' (Boardman et al., 2023). For the purpose of the present discussion, social exclusion is regarded as including (but not limited to) the processes whereby many people with mental illness and their families are partially or fully excluded from full and equal participation in the societies in which they live. Particular attention is given to the relationships between mental illness and poverty, unemployment, homelessness, imprisonment, reduced rates of marriage, and certain issues relating to migration, especially refugee status.

The association between mental illness and poverty is a long-standing one. Psychiatric epidemiologists were among the first to describe this link and it has been a strong feature of the literature since then (Muntaner et al., 2008). This relationship is bi-directional: people who are poor are more likely to suffer from serious mental illness, and serious mental illness impairs future income and prospects for financial well-being. These associations are often related to other indicators of social exclusion which are discussed here, including unemployment, homelessness, and imprisonment, which often co-occur in different combinations for different people at various points in their lives.

People with mental illness are at increased risk of unemployment compared to people without mental illness (Boardman & Rinaldi, 2021). Again, there are bi-directional aspects to this relationship: while conditions such as schizophrenia impair employment prospects for the future, unemployment itself is associated with higher rates of anxiety, depression, and alcohol and substance misuse. Bio-psycho-social approaches to treatment could usefully focus more on supporting a return to training and employment, especially for people with enduring mental health problems. Traditionally, mental health services have not accorded sufficient weight to this goal as part of overall treatment plans.

In addition to poverty and unemployment (and often as a result of them), people with mental illness have increased rates of homelessness, with resultant high levels of psychiatric morbidity among homeless populations (Timms, 2021). While there have been some responses to this situation in certain areas, the factors driving homelessness remain largely unaddressed. These include a lack of accommodation options for many people with serious mental illness when they are discharged from acute psychiatric inpatient care. In that circumstance, patients are sometimes discharged to the streets once their episode of illness is partially resolved, owing to the pressure for inpatient psychiatric care for people in more acute stages of illness and the absence of appropriate hostel beds in the community for those discharged.

This, in turn, can increase the risk of imprisonment of people with mental illness, often for minor offences which would not lead to the imprisonment of someone who is mentally well and has a fixed address (Kelly, 2005). While many people with mental illness are fully responsible for their actions, mental illness can and should be considered in certain cases. Long-standing challenges in this area are centred on difficult interactions between criminal law and psychiatry, which Peay describes as 'problematic bedfellows' (Peay, 2024; p. 268). At the system level, it is well established that there is an inverse relationship between psychiatric hospital beds and prison places, with reciprocal time trends demonstrated in many countries (O'Neill et al., 2021). Torrey notes that, as mentally ill homeless persons became a subject of increasing national concern in the US during the 1980s, the number of mentally ill persons in prisons rose (Torrey, 2014). This remains a problem in many countries today as people with serious mental illness end up in prison even when psychiatric inpatient care would be more appropriate (e.g., Carey, 2023).

These problems stem not only from decisions to reduce bed numbers in psychiatric units and hospitals, but also from a general lack of preventive interventions, broader psychological programmes in primary care, expanded community services, and joined-up social support for people with mental illness and their families (Kelly, 2023). Many countries have seen an increased focus on lifestyle measures to support mental well-being over recent decades, but there is also a need to acknowledge the lived realities of severe mental illness. There are effective treatments for conditions such as schizophrenia, provided multidisciplinary services are available and accessible to those who need them (see Chapter 4: 'Treating Symptoms and Disorders'). If these services and supports are not available, problems such as unemployment, homelessness, and imprisonment intensify and can lead to downward social spirals among many people with mental illness.

Other factors can also contribute to this situation, including, on occasion, legislation that fails to protect the rights of people with mental illness and can even discriminate against them. For example, many people with mental illness have a lower likelihood of ever marrying and a higher likelihood of divorce compared to people without mental illness (Breslau et al., 2011). This is especially the case among people with certain conditions such as major depression and alcohol abuse. The reasons for this are likely complex, but it is noteworthy that, in 2016, one study of domestic laws in 193 countries found that 37% of countries explicitly prohibited marriage by persons with mental health problems (Bhugra et al., 2016). In 21 countries (11% of those surveyed), the presence of mental health problems could render a marriage void or could be considered as grounds for nullity of marriage. Such laws are inconsistent with human rights and further diminish social inclusion among many people with mental illness.

Finally, there are various links between mental illness and migration. While this is a very broad topic that is beyond the scope of the present chapter, it merits mention in the context of social exclusion. The first point to note is that many people who migrate or become refugees show extraordinary resilience in the face of deeply challenging circumstances (Hughes & Katona, 2021). There are, however, also associations between refugee status and increased risk of mental illness, including (but not limited to) post-traumatic stress disorder. For refugees, basic needs must be met, in addition to addressing mental health issues. This involves providing psychosocial support that is culturally appropriate, as well as tailored mental health care for the full diversity of psychological and psychiatric problems that can develop. Social inclusion is a key part of this process and merits greater consideration at the levels of both policy and individual care.

Overall, there are significant relationships between mental illness and poverty, unemployment, homelessness, imprisonment, reduced rates of marriage, and issues relating to migration, especially the experiences of refugees. Taken together, these factors increase the risk of social exclusion and incremental distancing of people with mental illness and their families from full and equal participation in the societies in which they live.

Structural Violence and Mental Illness

Carl, the young man whom we met at the start of this chapter, experienced substance misuse problems, mental illness, social challenges (including homelessness), and eventual imprisonment. All of these experiences contributed to social exclusion and added further to the difficulties in Carl's life. This common combination of experiences reflects a set of arrangements and processes in society that routinely fail to meet the needs of people with mental illness and various other problems. In fact, a great many of these societal arrangements and structures seem to actively work *against* people with conditions such as schizophrenia and other enduring mental illnesses, leading to negative social outcomes for all concerned: the person, their family, their community, and society in general.

These matters have come to the fore over recent decades owing to the emergence of empirical evidence about the social determinants of mental health, along with the limited progress of biomedical technology in delivering new treatments for many common mental illnesses (Poole & Robinson, 2021). Psychiatry has always had a strong social dimension, but this aspect of the discipline is, perhaps, more engaged today than it has ever been in the past.

It can be useful to look at experiences such as those of Carl using the concept of 'structural violence'. Structural violence is a term that encompasses forces such as poverty, racism, socio-economic inequality, and discrimination which inevitably have an influence on people's health (Farmer, 1999). The term 'structural violence' finds its origins in the Liberation Theology of Latin America, but the concept has been applied to medical and public health issues over recent decades, including the epidemic of tuberculosis in prisons in the former Soviet Union and the spread of HIV/AIDS in Haiti (Kelly, 2005). For these and similar health problems, it is argued that the spread and population impact of such conditions are related, in significant part, to the social, economic, and political forces that shape the landscape of risk for developing the conditions in the first place, the contexts in which health care is provided (or not provided), and the likelihood that recovery does or does not occur.

As Carl's case history demonstrates, the concept of structural violence can also be used to explore the social, economic, and political forces that shape the landscape of risk for mental illness and substance misuse, the likelihood of receiving care, and contrasting outcomes for people with mental illness in different circumstances. Schizophrenia provides a good example of how these factors can decisively shape a person's experience of the condition and its impact on their life, notwithstanding evidence of a substantial (if poorly understood) biological basis for the illness. Social factors matter profoundly too.

To begin, people from lower socio-economic groups have an earlier age at first presentation with schizophrenia, and longer durations of untreated illness, both of which are associated with poorer outcomes (Kelly, 2005). People with schizophrenia are also at increased risk of homelessness and imprisonment, both of which increase the disability and stigma associated with mental illness, deepen social exclusion, and impede long-term recovery. In addition, as discussed, migration is associated with increased rates of certain mental illnesses, including schizophrenia, and this relationship seems to be mediated by psychosocial factors, including difficulties building social capital in smaller migrant groups.

Against this background, it is clear that social, economic, and societal factors combine with the stigma that is wrongly associated with mental illness to constitute a form of structural violence. This limits meaningful access to psychiatric and social services for many people and amplifies the effects of schizophrenia in their lives. As a consequence of these overarching social, economic, and political arrangements and processes, many people with schizophrenia are systematically excluded from full participation in social and civic life, and have longer, more difficult experiences of illness. In the most challenging cases, they are constrained to live lives that are shaped by exclusion, stigma, isolation, homelessness, and denial of rights – problems which are either created or greatly magnified by pernicious forms of structural violence that impact them disproportionately.

Addressing these issues is a complex, urgent matter. Increased recognition of the social determinants of mental health and illness is crucial, along with the incorporation of such considerations into evolving aetiological models of mental illness. In the more immediate term, the enhancement of the individual agency of people with mental illness is likely to be key to any solution (Kelly, 2006), as well as the empowerment of their families, whose interests are often ignored completely. Legislative reform can help with certain aspects of this process but must be combined with service developments and grassroots community initiatives that are appropriate to their cultural settings (Kelly, 2012). Many of these matters are considered later in this chapter, as part of a manifesto for change.

Finally, it is possible that social exclusion and structural violence were both intensified in recent years owing to the Covid-19 pandemic. Bhattacharya and colleagues performed a 'qualitative inquiry' into 'social injustice in the neoliberal pandemic era for homeless persons with mental illness' in India (Bhattacharya et al., 2021). They concluded that 'the pandemic and the resulting challenges across societies highlighted the existing social injustices in a neoliberal world for historically marginalised populations like homeless persons with mental illness (HPMI)':

The nationwide lockdown in India to resist the spread of the virus posed a unique challenge to this vulnerable population [...] Critical insights from the study bring out experiences of HPMI during COVID-19 as a victim of structural violence, highlighting their exclusion and victimization due to the existing marginalized status, living closer to the edge as a consequence of the lockdown, lack of awareness of the gravity of the pandemic situation. The experiences of the stakeholders, on the other hand, pointed out the role of community members and social workers in partially mitigating the challenges. This study indicates that to mitigate the aftermaths, stakeholders, including community members, need to work together for rebuilding and enhancing the strength and resilience of the marginalized populations like HPMI, who are historically victims of social injustice in the neoliberal pandemic era.

(Bhattacharya et al., 2021; p. 1)

Responses to Global Injustice in Mental Health Care

So far in this chapter, we have explored the case of Carl, a young man with substance misuse problems, mental illness, and social challenges (including homelessness). Carl was eventually imprisoned after being charged with disturbing the peace and attempted arson. The judge took this course of action with great reluctance but felt there was no other option at that point. She instructed that Carl be provided with a free solicitor and medical care as needed, including psychiatric assessment, while in prison awaiting trial.

Despite these caveats, imprisonment is still an extremely negative outcome for Carl. It deepens his social exclusion and adds further to the difficulties he is likely to face in the future. Also, prison is toxic for people with mental illness, not least because delivery of care is complex in custodial settings. Follow-up treatment and support are also difficult to coordinate effectively in many jurisdictions.

After considering Carl's case (to which we will return later), this chapter then looked at evidence from the WHO and other sources to demonstrate and describe global inequity in mental health care, which is substantial. Care is more likely to be available in high-income countries, but there is also considerable variation within high-income countries in terms of the level and nature of support provided. Particular attention was devoted to the relationships between mental illness and poverty, unemployment, homelessness, imprisonment, reduced rates of marriage, and issues relating to migration. The concept of 'structural violence' was evoked to describe the political, economic, and social circumstances that shape the landscape of risk for mental illness, the likelihood of receiving care, and contrasting outcomes for people with mental illness in different circumstances around the world.

Carl was a clear victim of structural violence at several levels and in various ways over the course of his life. Following a challenging early childhood, Carl experienced physical abuse in two foster homes. His schooling was disrupted, and he drifted into drug misuse during his teenage years. This led to criminal activity, conviction in court, and consequent difficulty finding work. These circumstances intensified Carl's drug misuse and contributed directly to his homelessness. Against this background, and with a family history of schizophrenia and drug misuse, Carl became paranoid, believing that the people with whom he lived were talking about him behind his back, stealing his money, and planning to harm him. This fuelled further criminal activity: Carl set the house on fire, was arrested by the police, and ultimately ended up in prison.

At every step along the way, Carl's trajectory presented needs and challenges to systems of accommodation, education, treatment for drug misuse, mental health care, and criminal justice. And at every step, those systems were either inadequate or inappropriate to Carl's requirements. As a person with mental illness and substance misuse, prevailing social and political arrangements not only failed to support Carl in the ways that he needed, but actually amplified his problems, deepened his social exclusion, magnified his mental illness, and ultimately imprisoned him. Like all citizens, Carl bears primary responsibility for his actions and decisions, but systems of public care and social support also bear responsibility for theirs – and all were proven inadequate in the case of Carl.

So, what can be done? Carl's case is not uncommon. Prisons all over the world are filled with people like Carl. While Carl remains responsible for his own life and actions, it should be possible for social supports and mental health services to provide more, better, earlier support for Carl, and help him to reduce the likelihood of adverse outcomes, such as criminal activity, imprisonment, and probable early death.

The first step is to acknowledge that, despite the (unclear) biological basis of many mental illnesses, social circumstances still play a substantial role in shaping the risk of mental illness, the likelihood of treatment, and ultimate outcomes. Biology does not necessarily trump social circumstances; biology and social conditions are intimately linked, and both act together to produce illness, suffering, and – hopefully – recovery.

At the international level, the UN and WHO clearly recognise the role of the social environment in these circumstances. In 2006, the UN's Convention on the Rights of Persons with Disabilities (CRPD) made this point in Article 1, which placed 'full and effective participation in society on an equal basis with others' at the heart of its description of 'persons with disabilities':

The purpose of the present Convention is to promote, protect and ensure the full and equal enjoyment of all human rights and fundamental freedoms by all persons with disabilities, and to promote respect for their inherent dignity. Persons with disabilities include those who have long-term physical, mental, intellectual or sensory impairments which in interaction with various barriers may hinder their full and effective participation in society on an equal basis with others.

(United Nations, 2006; Article 1)

Consistent with this, the 'general principles' of the CRPD include 'full and effective participation and inclusion in society' and 'equality of opportunity' (Article 3). Article 28 confirms a right to an 'adequate standard of living and social protection':

> States Parties recognize the right of persons with disabilities to an adequate standard of living for themselves and their families, including adequate food, clothing and housing, and to the continuous improvement of living conditions, and shall take appropriate steps to safeguard and promote the realization of this right without discrimination on the basis of disability.

The WHO also recognises the role of the social environment in mental illness. In 2022, the WHO published its *World Mental Health Report: Transforming Mental Health for All*, which identified three key routes to transformation (World Health Organization, 2022). These included:

- Deepening the value and commitment that we accord to mental health as individuals, communities, and governments; and matching that value with greater commitment, engagement, and investment by all stakeholders, in all sectors.
- Reshaping the physical, social, and economic features of environments (e.g., homes, schools, workplaces, and the wider community) so as to better protect mental health, seek to prevent mental health conditions, and give everyone equal opportunity to thrive and reach the highest attainable standard of mental health and well-being.
- Strengthening mental health care so that the full range of mental health needs can be met through community-based networks of affordable, accessible, and quality services and support.

Dignity

Statements of rights, policy recommendations, and the publications of international organisations such as the UN and WHO are important tools for addressing the injustices experienced by people with mental illness. They provide directions for national legislation, suggest content for local policies, and prompt various initiatives to provide treatment and support, and address social exclusion. Before considering further steps that might be taken at national or local levels, however, it is helpful to reflect on a key value that lies at the heart of most of the pronouncements of international bodies and that underpins many codes of medical ethics (e.g., Medical Council, 2024). This is the principle of dignity.

The CRPD starts by 'recalling the principles proclaimed in the Charter of the United Nations which recognise the inherent dignity and worth and the equal and inalienable rights of all members of the human family as the foundation of freedom, justice and peace in the world' (United Nations, 2006; Preamble). The CRPD goes on to state that 'the principles of the present Convention shall [include] respect for inherent dignity, individual autonomy including the freedom to make one's own choices, and independence of persons' (Article 3).

But what is dignity? How is it defined? And can the concept of dignity be used to address the social and other injustices experienced by people with mental illness and their families?

The Oxford English Reference Dictionary defines dignity as the state of being worthy of respect or honour (Pearsall & Trumble, 1996). In practice, however, dignity can be difficult to define precisely (Seedhouse & Gallagher, 2002), and the concept is not without its critics. Pinker notes that dignity can be a subjective concept, can be ambiguous, and is something that we often voluntarily relinquish in certain circumstances (Pinker, 2008). The same can be said of all values, however, including autonomy, and these still play important roles in moral and ethical reasoning. Against this background, dignity has enough substance and meaning to merit consideration, interrogation, and judicious application, provided this is done mindfully and with an awareness of the conceptual limitations of all such principles (not just dignity).

In a detailed consideration of dignity in bioethics and biolaw, Beyleveld and Brownsword outlined useful conceptualisations of 'dignity as empowerment' and 'dignity as constraint' (Beyleveld and Brownsword, 2001; p. 11). The idea of dignity as empowerment centres on individual dignity as the key foundation for human rights, consistent with various declarations of rights, including the CRPD. According to this conceptualisation, dignity reinforces claims to self-determination rather than limiting free choice. Most people readily identify with this idea of dignity.

Beyleveld and Brownsword also argued that a conception of 'dignity as constraint' was evident in some thinking about limits to be placed on biomedicine, consistent with a position that biomedical practice should not be driven entirely by individual choice, but by a shared concept of dignity that extends beyond individuals (Beyleveld & Brownsword, 2001; p. 29). In other words, dignity can reflect an objective value that reaches further than the individual such that, if a person inadvertently violates this value, human dignity is compromised irrespective of whether or not the person has knowingly agreed to perform the act in question (Kelly, 2016a). This is an objective dimension of dignity, in addition to the subjective one.

If a person with severe mental illness lacks sufficient understanding of their situation, they may violate this shared, objective idea of dignity, potentially resulting in catastrophic loss of personal dignity, and subsequent admission and treatment without consent under mental health legislation, or arrest and imprisonment (Kelly, 2024). This objective dimension of dignity is notably important for people who (usually temporarily) lack the understanding or mental capacity to protect subjective dignity or to recognise its loss, to varying degrees (Feldman, 2002). These people still possess intrinsic human dignity by virtue of the simple fact of being human. In these circumstances, there is a powerful moral and, ideally, legal duty to protect and restore the dignity of each person by having regard for their dignity, rights, and welfare when making decisions that relate to them (Kelly, 2014).

Psychiatry can play an important role in this task, by providing safe, effective, compassionate treatments in a context that protects rights and promotes dignity, sometimes including admission and treatment without consent when all other options have failed. Too often, however, models of care can fail to protect dignity and sometimes even erode it. The psychiatric literature contains remarkably little explicit reference to patient dignity or ways in which psychiatry can improve or undermine it. Key themes in the limited literature to date include coercion, powerlessness, care environments, relationships with staff, impact of involuntary treatment, and paradoxes (Plunkett & Kelly, 2021).

More research is needed on this topic, not least because, when patients' experiences of dignity are studied, results are not always as expected. One study of psychiatry inpatients found that patients with higher levels of perceived coercion reported less self-rated dignity, but there was no significant difference in self-rated dignity between voluntary and involuntary patients (Plunkett et al., 2022). Patients with higher levels of insight reported lower dignity, but dignity was not significantly associated with age, gender, ethnicity, diagnosis, or length of stay in hospital.

Protecting dignity is an important function of psychiatry. In clinical settings, this means that dignity preservation should be a precondition for safety and a design priority for healing in all therapeutic spaces (Plunkett & Kelly, 2024). In the community more broadly, according priority to dignity means mental health professionals working to protect rights and promote dignity by providing effective care, advocating for service reforms, and campaigning against injustice in various ways. These matters are considered next, in the final section of this chapter which presents a manifesto for change.

Manifesto for Change

In light of the prevalence of global injustice and inequity in mental health care, and strong relationships between mental illness and poverty, unemployment, homelessness, imprisonment, reduced rates of marriage, and issues relating to migration, what can be done to address so many matters? Combating structural violence can be deeply challenging, given its embeddedness in prevailing political, economic, and social circumstances. Statements of rights and policies at the international level are helpful, but protecting dignity requires *actions* at the levels of individuals, communities, countries, and the planet as a whole. Everyone is involved, often at several levels, and frequently at the same time. So, what can we *do?*

At the level of the individual patient, psychiatrists and other mental health professionals can usefully continue to provide compassionate, person-centred care, especially in light of the strong evidence base to support various psychiatric interventions (see Chapter 4 of this book: 'Treating Symptoms and Disorders'). We also need to acknowledge the challenges of providing care in the absence of certainty about the biological basis of the conditions being treated, and a reliance on history and symptoms rather than biological tests for diagnosis. This is not necessarily a problem. Apparent certainty in other areas of medicine is often an illusion. The uncertainties within psychiatry can prompt ongoing reflection and humility within the discipline, which has treatments that can work extremely well, but which also involves dealing with uncertainty on a day-to-day basis (Barron, 2019). We can work constructively with this uncertainty if we do so honestly, in open partnership with patients and their families.

Community based initiatives outside formal mental health services are also important and should be supported, especially when they accord closely with local cultures. In Zimbabwe, the *Guardian* reported on one initiative that involves grandmothers, who are 'trained but unqualified health workers', taking turns on a park bench to hear people's stories:

> They listen to the battered wife who has attempted suicide twice, the man who hates women after he became infected with HIV, the unemployed single mother driven to despair by the struggle of raising four children.
> The benches are a safe place for people struggling with depression, which in the Shona language is called *kufungisisa*, 'thinking too much'.
> It is a world away from conventional approaches to mental healthcare, but the Friendship Bench project has changed the lives of an estimated 27,000 Zimbabweans suffering from depression and other mental disorders.
>
> (Mberi, 2017)

At the level of countries, it is evident from the happiness data at the start of this chapter that well-being flourishes in countries that are wealthy, stable, and peaceful (Helliwell et al., 2023). Countries that are poor, unstable, and troubled by conflict and socioeconomic challenges are less likely to report high levels of happiness. Conflict and war are especially corrosive owing to mass traumatisation and the displacement of large groups of people. As Moitra and colleagues point out, 'international conflict and instability in the last few years have harmed the mental health of displaced populations' (Moitra et al., 2023; p. 305). All sides suffer the psychological and psychiatric ill-effects of conflict (Kelly, 2022a). This creates a strong incentive for mental health professionals to work for peace in conflict zones in order to minimise impact on mental health (among other reasons).

At the level of national politics, it is clear that mental health services have always been deeply influenced by prevailing political ideologies. Most recently, Scull argues that deinstitutionalisation was a neoliberal policy, consciously selected and pursued over many decades (Scull, 2021). If community care is implemented properly, it is likely to cost just as much as the hospital care that preceded it (McCrone, 2021). The merit of community care is not that it is cheaper than hospital care or more in line with neoliberal values, but that it sets some people free. You cannot put a price on that.

Even so, while the idea of care in the community has a great deal to recommend it, policies of deinstitutionalisation do not provide much guidance for times when community care is inadequate. What is the right move at that point? We have seen that psychiatric bed numbers vary considerably, even within the EU (Eurostat, 2020). Should there be a partial return to more inpatient care, in light of some of the demonstrated deficiencies of community care? A swing back to institutions would be an error (Gilhooley & Kelly, 2018). Political, economic, and cultural contexts change constantly (Cohen et al., 2008), so positive reforms are always possible. Mental health professionals can usefully advocate for better, more community care for mental illness, inpatient beds when needed, expanded social support, reform of criminal justice systems, improved legislation (Gostin et al., 2019), and programmes to prevent and address homelessness among people with enduring conditions (Timms, 2021).

At the international level, bodies such as the UN and WHO are active in the area of mental health care and policy, but require engagement from mental health professionals if their statements and initiatives are to be relevant, effective, and clinically informed (Kelly, 2024). More broadly still, the issue of sustainability has become central to initiatives and advancements in global mental health. Mental health is a global public good which is relevant to sustainable development in every country and (as we have seen) is strongly linked with social and environmental conditions (Patel et al., 2018). Future research could usefully focus more on not only the biology and burden of mental disorders, but also the interactions between social, economic, and environmental determinants (Pedersen, 2015). Current initiatives could helpfully take greater account of their sustainability and the ways in which good mental health is linked with good planetary health at a time of climate crisis.

Taking this broader view of psychiatry and mental health care requires courage, humility, and a willingness to work with incremental change. Creating a global mental health agenda raises inevitable issues about differing understandings of psychological distress around the world, and this adds complexity to the desire to alleviate suffering today, as well as build sustainable health systems for the future (Kirmayer, 2015). These considerations do not always rest easily with each other, but that should not result in paralysis: some progress is better than none (Kelly, 2022b). Similarly in mental health legislation, the desire to protect specific individual rights should be balanced appropriately with rights to treatment and care, and should be weighed against potential paradoxical negative outcomes, such as loss of life (Treffert, 1973). This kind of complexity can fuel and inform progress, rather than impede it.

In the end, a great deal of progress depends not only on the provision of care to individual patients and support for their families, but also on social and political action to improve systems of health and social care in general. The time for professional political neutrality is gone, especially in light of growing awareness of links between psychiatric suffering, political economy, and sustainability (Ikkos, 2023). While there are many examples of good care around the world, the nature and quality of services still vary considerably (Kelly, 2016b). As we have discussed, particular groups suffer more from both mental illness and discrimination: people who are homeless, prisoners, and many migrants, especially refugees.

The solutions to these problems are as much political as they are medical. If political will exists, mental health services will be improved, discrimination can be addressed, and sustainable mental health systems can flourish. To make change happen, we need to not only provide the best care possible, but also campaign for better services, advocate loudly, register to vote, and ensure politicians and decision-makers promote all of the rights of people with mental illness and their families. This includes the right to treatment as well as the right to liberty, social rights as well as economic ones. Political action is vital: *aux barricades!*

Carl, the young man whom we met at the start of this chapter, had a combination of social disadvantage, childhood trauma, substance misuse, mental illness, and offending behaviour. He finally ended up in prison, where he remained paranoid, believing that people were trying to kill him. He also heard the voice of 'the man', warning of danger. This was Carl's first time in prison and the other prisoners were cruel to him, taking his food and taunting him constantly.

Carl saw the psychiatrist in prison and asked if he could go to the hospital. The psychiatrist spoke at length with Carl and felt that he had a psychotic illness, caused or worsened by drug use. Schizophrenia was a real possibility in light of Carl's symptoms and family history, although it was difficult to be certain with so much drug use. The psychiatrist placed Carl on a waiting list for the hospital and, in the meantime, recommended antipsychotic medication for likely schizophrenia. Carl was also offered counselling, which he declined.

After three weeks in prison, Carl's psychotic symptoms diminished, owing to both his reduced access to cannabis and the antipsychotic medication. After another two weeks, Carl was released from prison. A social worker found him a room to rent. Carl stayed there for two months. He stopped taking the antipsychotic medication. He kept away from cannabis, but three weeks later his paranoid symptoms returned. Carl developed the belief that his new housemates were trying to kill him. He left the house and slept on the street for three nights. Again, he believed his life was in danger.

The next day, Carl went back to Court to see if the judge would send him to prison, but because he was not charged with anything, he was asked to leave the Court. The policeman there advised him to go to the hospital. Carl left the Court and went to the hospital, but there was a long waiting time in the Emergency Department. Carl left the hospital and slept on the street that night. In the early morning, wet and hungry, Carl broke into a house and stole money. The police were called, and they found Carl unconscious in the street behind the house, having taken a large quantity of drugs.

Carl was brought to hospital in a coma. He tested positive for cannabis and cocaine. He never regained consciousness and died three days later.

Key Messages

- Different countries report varying levels of happiness and well-being, contrasting provision of mental health care, and different numbers of psychiatric beds, with significant divergences even between high-income countries, where provision is generally greater.
- All around the globe, serious mental illness is often associated with societal injustice, social exclusion, poverty, unemployment, homelessness, imprisonment, reduced rates of marriage, and various issues relating to migration, especially refugee status.
- The concept of 'structural violence' can help to describe, explain, and understand the adverse political, economic, and social circumstances that shape the landscape of risk for mental illness, the likelihood of receiving care, and contrasting outcomes. The Covid-19 pandemic likely deepened social exclusion and injustice in many places.
- Protecting dignity is an important function of psychiatry. In clinical settings, this means that dignity preservation should be a precondition for safety and a design priority for healing spaces. In the community, this means providing effective care, advocating for service reforms, and campaigning against injustice.
- Addressing injustice and promoting dignity require actions at the levels of individuals, communities, countries, and the planet as a whole.
- At the level of the individual, mental health professionals can usefully continue to provide compassionate, person-centred, evidence-based care, especially in light of the strong evidence base to support various psychiatric interventions (even in the face of uncertainty). Culturally appropriate community-based initiatives outside formal mental health services are also important and should be supported.
- At the level of countries, there is a strong incentive for mental health professionals to work for peace in conflict zones (in order to minimise impact on mental health) as well as advocate for better, more community care for mental

illness everywhere, inpatient beds when needed, expanded social support, reform of criminal justice systems, improved legislation, and programmes to prevent and address homelessness.

- At the international level, organisations such as the United Nations and World Health Organization are active in mental health care and policy, and require engagement from mental health professionals if their statements and initiatives are to be relevant, effective, and clinically informed.
- In the area of mental health legislation, the desire to protect specific individual rights should be balanced appropriately with rights to treatment and care, and should be weighed against potential paradoxical negative outcomes, such as loss of life.
- There is growing awareness of links between psychiatric suffering, political economy, and sustainability. The solutions to these challenges are as much political as they are medical. It is time to step beyond the clinic and take political action to improve mental health and social care, and to achieve greater justice by working assertively on these issues in partnership with people with mental illness and their families.

References

Alem A, Kebede D, Fekadu A, Shibre T, Fekadu D, Beyero T, Medhin G, Negash A, Kullgren G. Clinical course and outcome of schizophrenia in a predominantly treatment-naive cohort in rural Ethiopia. *Schizophrenia Bulletin* 2009; 35: 646–54 (https://doi.org/10.1093/schbul/sbn029).

Applbaum K. Solving global mental health as a delivery problem: toward a critical epistemology of the solution. In: Kirmayer LJ, Lemelson R, Cummings CA (eds), *Re-Visioning Psychiatry: Cultural Phenomenology, Critical Neuroscience, and Global Mental Health* (pp. 544–74). Cambridge: Cambridge University Press, 2015.

Barron D. Psychiatry's inevitable hubris (blog). *Scientific American*, 8 May 2019 (https://blogs.scientificamerican.com/observations/psychiatrys-inevitable-hubris/) (accessed 22 December 2023).

Beyleveld D, Brownsword R. *Human Dignity in Bioethics and Biolaw.* Oxford: Oxford University Press, 2001.

Bhattacharya P, Khemka GC, Roy L, Roy SD. Social injustice in the neoliberal pandemic era for homeless persons with mental illness: a qualitative inquiry from India. *Frontiers in Psychiatry* 2021; 12: 635715 (http://dx.doi.org/10.3389/fpsyt.2021.635715). (Link to licence: https://creativecommons.org/licenses/by/4.0/) (accessed 21 December 2023).

Bhugra D, Pathare S, Nardodkar R, Gosavi C, Ng R, Torales J, Ventriglio A. Legislative provisions related to marriage and divorce of persons with mental health problems: a global review. *International Review of Psychiatry* 2016; 28: 386–92 (http://dx.doi.org/10.1080/09540261.2016.1210577).

Boardman J, Killaspy H, Mezey G. *Social Inclusion and Mental Health: Understanding Poverty, Inequality and Social Exclusion* (Second Edn). Cambridge: Cambridge University Press, 2023.

Boardman J, Rinaldi M. Work, unemployment and mental health. In: Ikkos G, Bouras N (eds), *Mind, State and Society: Social History of Psychiatry and Mental Health in Britain 1960–2010* (pp. 326–35). Cambridge: Cambridge University Press, 2021 (https://doi.org/10.1017/9781911623793.035).

Breslau J, Miller E, Jin R, Sampson NA, Alonso J, Andrade LH, Bromet EJ, de Girolamo G, Demyttenaere K, Fayyad J, Fukao A, Gălăon M, Gureje O, He Y, Hinkov HR, Hu C, Kovess-Masfety V, Matschinger H, Medina-Mora ME, Ormel J, Posada-Villa J, Sagar R, Scott KM, Kessler RC. A multinational study of mental disorders, marriage, and divorce. *Acta Psychiatrica Scandinavica* 2011; 124: 474–86 (http://dx.doi.org/10.1111/j.1600-0447.2011.01712.x).

Carey S. Prisons are not for the mentally ill – we desperately need more psychiatric beds. *Irish Independent*, 2 December 2023 (https://www.independent.ie/opinion/comment/sarah-carey-prisons-are-not-for-the-mentally-ill-we-desperately-need-more-psychiatric-hospital-beds/a606903541.html) (accessed 21 December 2023).

Cohen CI, Timimi S, Thompson KS. A new psychiatry? In: Cohen CI, Timimi S (eds), *Liberatory Psychiatry: Philosophy, Politics, and Mental Health* (pp. 275–85). Cambridge: Cambridge University Press, 2008.

Eurostat. *Mental Health Care - Psychiatric Hospital Beds.* Luxembourg: Eurostat, 2020 (https://ec.europa.eu/eurostat/web/products-eurostat-news/-/edn-20201009-1#) (accessed 20 December 2023).

Farmer P. Pathologies of power: rethinking health and human rights. *American Journal of Public Health* 1999; 89: 1486–96 (https://doi.org/10.2105/ajph.89.10.1486).

Feldman D. *Civil Liberties and Human Rights in England and Wales* (Second Edn). Oxford: Oxford University Press, 2002.

Gilhooley J, Kelly BD. Return of the asylum. *British Journal of Psychiatry* 2018; 212: 69–70 (http://dx.doi.org/10.1192/bjp.2017.19).

Gostin LO, Monahan JT, Kaldor J, DeBartolo M, Friedman EA, Gottschalk K, Kim SC, Alwan A, Binagwaho A, Burci GL, Cabal L, DeLand K, Evans TG, Goosby E, Hossain S, Koh H, Ooms G, Roses Periago M, Uprimny R, Yamin AE. The legal determinants of health: harnessing the power of law for global health and sustainable development. *Lancet* 2019; 393: 1857–910 (http://dx.doi.org/10.1016/S0140-6736(19)30233-8).

Helliwell JF, Layard R, Sachs JD, De Neve J-E, Aknin LB, Wang S. (eds.). *World Happiness Report 2023.* New York: Sustainable Development Solutions Network, 2023 (http://worldhappiness.report/) (accessed 20 December 2023).

Hughes P, Katona C. Refugees, asylum and mental health in the UK. In: Ikkos G, Bouras N (eds), *Mind, State and Society: Social History of Psychiatry and Mental Health in Britain 1960–2010* (pp. 361–72). Cambridge: Cambridge University Press, 2021 (https://doi.org/10.1017/9781911623793.038).

Ikkos G. Book review: *Social Inclusion and Mental Health: Understanding Poverty, Inequality and Social Exclusion. British Journal of Psychiatry* 2023; 223: 494 (https://doi.org/10.1192/bjp.2023.73).

Insel TR, Collins PY, Hyman SE. Darkness invisible: the hidden global costs of mental illness. *Foreign Affairs* 2015; 94: 127–35 (https://www.foreignaffairs.com/articles/africa/darkness-invisible) (accessed 20 December 2023).

Kelly BD. Structural violence and schizophrenia. *Social Science and Medicine* 2005; 61: 721–30 (http://dx.doi.org/10.1016/j.socscimed.2004.12.020).

Kelly BD. The power gap: freedom, power and mental illness. *Social Science and Medicine* 2006; 63: 2118–28 (http://dx.doi.org/10.1016/j.socscimed.2006.05.015).

Kelly BD. Mental illness and structural violence. *Irish Medical Journal* 2012; 105: 30 (https://archive.imj.ie/ViewArticleDetails.aspx?ArticleID=8440) (accessed 21 December 2023).

Kelly BD. Dignity, human rights and the limits of mental health legislation. *Irish Journal of Psychological Medicine* 2014; 31: 75–81 (http://dx.doi.org/10.1017/ipm.2014.22).

Kelly BD. *Dignity, Mental Health and Human Rights: Coercion and the Law.* London and New York: Routledge, 2016a.

Kelly BD. Political action is central to addressing mental health crisis. *Observer*, 9 October 2016b (https://www.theguardian.com/theobserver/2016/oct/08/political-action-central-address-mental-health-crisis) (accessed 22 December 2023) (Courtesy of Guardian News & Media Ltd.).

Kelly BD. Trauma and displacement in Ukraine: the challenge to medicine and politics. *QJM* 2022a; 115: 269–70 (http://dx.doi.org/10.1093/qjmed/hcac090).

Kelly BD. *In Search of Madness: A Psychiatrist's Travels Through the History of Mental Illness.* Dublin: Gill Books, 2022b.

Kelly BD. TDs must keep promise to improve nation's mental health in Sláintecare plan. *Irish Independent*, 4 December 2023 (https://www.independent.ie/opinion/letters/letters-government-tds-must-be-held-to-promise-to-improve-nations-mental-health-as-part-of-slaintecare/a480383140.html) (accessed 22 December 2023).

Kelly BD. The right to mental health care in mental health legislation. In: Kelly BD, Donnelly M (eds), *Routledge Handbook of Mental Health Law* (pp. 384–402). London and New York: Routledge, 2024.

Kemp CG, Concepcion T, Ahmed HU, Anwar N, Baingana F, Bennett IM, Bruni A, Chisholm D, Dawani H, Erazo M, Hossain SW, January J, Ladyk-Bryzghalova A, Momotaz H, Munongo E, Oliveira E Souza R, Sala G, Schafer A, Sukhovii O, Taboada L, Van Ommeren M, Vander Stoep A, Vergara J, Waters C, Kestel D, Collins PY. Baseline situational analysis in Bangladesh, Jordan, Paraguay, the Philippines, Ukraine, and Zimbabwe for the WHO Special Initiative for Mental Health: Universal Health Coverage for Mental Health. *PLoS One* 2022; 17: e0265570 (https://doi.org/10.1371/journal.pone.0265570).

Kirmayer LJ. Re-visioning psychiatry: toward an ecology of mind in health and illness. In: Kirmayer LJ, Lemelson R, Cummings CA (eds), *Re-Visioning Psychiatry: Cultural Phenomenology, Critical Neuroscience, and Global Mental Health* (pp. 622–60). Cambridge: Cambridge University Press, 2015.

Mberi R. Harare's park bench grandmas: 'I speak to them and feel a load is lifted off my heart'. *Guardian*, 14 April 2017 (https://www.theguardian.com/global-development/2017/apr/14/harare-friendship-bench-grandmothers-mental-health-zimbabwe) (accessed 22 December 2023) (Courtesy of Guardian News & Media Ltd.). See also: (https://www.friendshipbenchzimbabwe.org/) (accessed 22 December 2023).

McCrone P. Mental health policy and economics in Britain. In: Ikkos G, Bouras N (eds), *Mind, State and Society: Social History of Psychiatry and Mental Health in Britain 1960–2010* (pp. 103–10). Cambridge: Cambridge University Press, 2021 (https://doi.org/10.1017/9781911623793.013).

Medical Council. *Guide to Professional Conduct and Ethics for Registered Medical Practitioners* (Nineth Edn). Dublin: Medical Council, 2024 (https://www.medicalcouncil

.ie/news-and-publications/publications/guide-to-professional-conduct-and-ethics-for
-registered-medical-practitioners-2024.pdf) (accessed 22 December 2023).

Moitra M, Owens S, Hailemariam M, Wilson KS, Mensa-Kwao A, Gonese G, Kamamia
CK, White B, Young DM, Collins PY. Global mental health: where we are and where
we are going. *Current Psychiatry Reports* 2023; 25: 301–11 (https://doi.org/10.1007
/s11920-023-01426-8). (Link to licence: https://creativecommons.org/licenses/by/4
.0/) (accessed 20 December 2023).

Moitra M, Santomauro D, Collins PY, Vos T, Whiteford H, Saxena S, Ferrari AJ.
The global gap in treatment coverage for major depressive disorder in 84 countries
from 2000-2019: a systematic review and Bayesian meta-regression analysis. *PLoS
Medicine* 2022; 19: e1003901 (https://doi.org/10.1371/journal.pmed.1003901). (Link
to licence: https://creativecommons.org/licenses/by/4.0/) (accessed 20 December
2023).

Muntaner C, Borrell C, Chung H. Class exploitation and psychiatric disorders: from
status syndrome to capitalist syndrome. In: Cohen CI, Timimi S (eds), *Liberatory
Psychiatry: Philosophy, Politics, and Mental Health* (pp. 131–46). Cambridge:
Cambridge University Press, 2008.

O'Neill CJ, Kelly BD, Kennedy HG. A 25-year dynamic ecological analysis of
psychiatric hospital admissions and prison committals: Penrose's hypothesis updated.
Irish Journal of Psychological Medicine 2021; 38: 182–5 (https://doi.org/10.1017/
ipm.2018.40).

Patel V, Saxena S, Lund C, Thornicroft G, Baingana F, Bolton P, Chisholm D, Collins PY,
Cooper JL, Eaton J, Herrman H, Herzallah MM, Huang Y, Jordans MJD, Kleinman A,
Medina-Mora ME, Morgan E, Niaz U, Omigbodun O, Prince M, Rahman A, Saraceno
B, Sarkar BK, De Silva M, Singh I, Stein DJ, Sunkel C, Unützer J. The *Lancet*
Commission on global mental health and sustainable development. *Lancet* 2018; 392:
1553–98 (http://dx.doi.org/10.1016/S0140-6736(18)31612-X).

Peay J. Mental illness and criminal law: irreconcilable bedfellows? In: Kelly BD,
Donnelly M (eds), *Routledge Handbook of Mental Health Law* (pp. 255–71). London
and New York: Routledge, 2024.

Pearsall J, Trumble B (eds.). *The Oxford English Reference Dictionary* (Second Edn).
Oxford and New York: Oxford University Press, 1996.

Pedersen D. Social inequalities and mental health outcomes - toward a new architecture
for global mental health. In: Kirmayer LJ, Lemelson R, Cummings CA (eds),
*Re-Visioning Psychiatry: Cultural Phenomenology, Critical Neuroscience, and
Global Mental Health* (pp. 613–21). Cambridge: Cambridge University Press, 2015.

Pinker S. The stupidity of dignity. *New Republic* 2008; 238: 28–31 (https://newrepublic
.com/article/64674/the-stupidity-dignity) (accessed 22 December 2023).

Plunkett R, Kelly BD. Dignity: the elephant in the room in psychiatric inpatient care?
A systematic review and thematic synthesis. *International Journal of Law and
Psychiatry* 2021; 75: 101672 (http://dx.doi.org/10.1016/j.ijlp.2021.101672).

Plunkett R, Kelly BD. Should dignity preservation be a precondition for safety and a
design priority for healing in inpatient psychiatry spaces? *AMA Journal of Ethics*
2024; 26: E205–11.

Plunkett R, O'Callaghan AK, Kelly BD. Dignity, coercion and involuntary psychiatric
care: a study of involuntary and voluntary psychiatry inpatients in Dublin. *International
Journal of Psychiatry in Clinical Practice* 2022; 26: 269–76 (http://dx.doi.org/10
.1080/13651501.2021.2022162).

Poole R, Robinson C. Social theory, psychiatry and mental health services. In: Ikkos G, Bouras N (eds), *Mind, State and Society: Social History of Psychiatry and Mental Health in Britain 1960–2010* (pp. 32–40). Cambridge: Cambridge University Press, 2021 (https://doi.org/10.1017/9781911623793.006).

Scull A. UK deinstitutionalisation: neoliberal values and mental health. In: Ikkos G, Bouras N (eds), *Mind, State and Society: Social History of Psychiatry and Mental Health in Britain 1960–2010* (pp. 306–13). Cambridge: Cambridge University Press, 2021 (https://doi.org/10.1017/9781911623793.033).

Seedhouse D, Gallagher A. Undignifying institutions. *Journal of Medical Ethics* 2002; 28: 368–72 (http://dx.doi.org/10.1136/jme.28.6.368).

Timms P. Homelessness and mental health. In: Ikkos G, Bouras N (eds), *Mind, State and Society: Social History of Psychiatry and Mental Health in Britain 1960–2010* (pp. 251–61). Cambridge: Cambridge University Press, 2021 (https://doi.org/10.1017/9781911623793.028).

Torrey EF. *American Psychosis: How the Federal Government Destroyed the Mental Illness Treatment System.* Oxford: Oxford University Press, 2014.

Treffert DA. 'Dying with their rights on'. *American Journal of Psychiatry* 1973; 130: 1041 (https://doi.org/10.1176/ajp.130.9.1041).

United Nations. *Convention on the Rights of Persons with Disabilities.* New York: United Nations, 2006 (https://social.desa.un.org/issues/disability/crpd/convention-on-the-rights-of-persons-with-disabilities-crpd) (accessed 21 December 2023).

World Health Organization. *World Mental Health Atlas 2020.* Geneva: World Health Organization, 2021 (https://www.who.int/publications/i/item/9789240036703) (accessed 20 December 2023).

World Health Organization. *World Mental Health Report: Transforming Mental Health for All.* Geneva: World Health Organization, 2022 (https://www.who.int/publications/i/item/9789240049338). (Licence: CC BY-NC-SA 3.0 IGO https://creativecommons.org/licenses/by-nc-sa/3.0/igo/) (accessed 21 December 2023).

World Health Organization. *Mental Health.* Geneva: World Health Organization, 2023 (https://www.who.int/health-topics/mental-health#tab=tab_2) (accessed 20 December 2023).

10 The Future of Psychiatry

Person-Centred Care and System-Level Change

Hua was a happy child. She did well in school and had many friends. Hua especially enjoyed ballet classes which she attended with her friend, Xiu. Xiu lived next door and, like Hua, did well at school. Hua was an only child and her parents were thoughtful and supportive. Hua had many cousins, whom she saw from time to time.

When Hua was 15, her behaviour began to change. Hua became more interested in ballet, arriving at practice early and staying late afterwards. Her teacher was pleased at first, but then suggested that perhaps Hua did not need to spend so much time in the ballet studio. Hua was a good dancer, and her teacher was worried that maybe Hua was overdoing it. Hua told Xia that she would stop spending so long at ballet class, but would do extra practice at home instead.

A few months later, Hua's parents noticed that Hua had taken up running. Hua went for a run every morning. At first, Hua's run would take 20 minutes, but soon Hua was running for almost an hour each morning. Hua would get up an hour early, so that she could have her run and still be at school on time. Hua's parents suggested to Hua that maybe she was running too much, but Hua said that running gave her energy.

At school, Hua continued to achieve good results, but Xia noticed that Hua did not eat her lunch at school. Hua's mother gave Hua sandwiches to bring to school for lunch, but Xia saw Hua throw the sandwiches in the bin. Xia also noticed that, beneath the loose clothing that Hua was now wearing, Hua had lost weight. Hua was always slim, but now she was even thinner. Xia mentioned this to Hua, who said she hadn't noticed any change, but did not want to gain 'any more weight'. Xia said that there was no need to worry about gaining weight, in light of all the ballet and exercise, but Hua said: 'I don't want to be fat'.

The following week, Hua's father was passing the bathroom door when he heard the sound of someone vomiting. When Hua came out of the bathroom, he asked Hua if she was alright. Hua said she was fine. Hua's father spoke to Hua's mother, who shared his concern. Together, they spoke to Hua, asking her if everything was alright. Hua denied that there was any problem or that she had been vomiting. Hua said she was fine.

Hua's parents were worried. Hua was losing weight, exercising too much, and making herself vomit after eating. She ate very little food at home, saying

DOI: 10.4324/9781003378495-11

that she ate at school. But, as Xia knew, Hua was not eating at school. Hua's parents did not know what to do. Hua denied that there was a problem, saying that she just enjoyed exercising a lot. Hua's parents hoped that this was a teen-age phase that would pass.

One day, Hua's mother went to use the family computer and found that Hua had forgotten to close down the webpage she had been reading. The webpage presented a list of ways to lose extreme amounts of weight, including avoiding meals, exercising excessively, and self-induced vomiting. These were all the behaviours that Hua had demonstrated over the previous months. Hua's mother was enormously distressed. She rushed downstairs and said to Hua's father: 'I think Hua has an eating disorder'. Hua's father did not know what she meant but, looking at the webpage, he recognised Hua's behaviour. Clearly something needed to be done. But what?

Introduction

Disordered eating has been a feature of the history of humanity since earliest times. In the nineteenth century, asylum doctors noted various relationships between problems with eating and mental illness. In 1871, George Fielding Blandford (1829–1911), a relatively enlightened practitioner, wrote, in the language of the times, that 'a patient's eating and drinking may arrest our attention':

> He [sic] may eat voraciously, or very little, or absolutely nothing [...] I inquire closely into the eating and drinking of the patient, and constantly find that, whatever may be the proportions of the latter, the former is in defect [...] Thus, for lack of nourishment the brain becomes more and more exhausted, just at the time that it ought to have an extra supply. Regularity in meals, by which I mean the eating an adequate quantity at regular intervals, and not allowing a very long period, even at night, to elapse without food, often does much good.
>
> (Blandford, 1871; pp. 163, 184)

The idea of 'anorexia nervosa' as a specific mental illness emerged more clearly over the subsequent century. Today, the condition can still prove deeply challenging to manage, but advances in treatment, particularly for adolescents, support the benefits of specialised, family-based interventions (Zipfel et al., 2015). Adults with anorexia nervosa also have a realistic chance of substantial improvement or recovery, especially with a combination of anorexia nervosa-specific psychotherapy and re-nourishment, if they can access treatment in a timely fashion.

The development of ideas about anorexia nervosa reflect many of the areas explored in earlier chapters of this book, including the core therapeutic purposes of psychiatry (Chapter 1: 'Why Does Psychiatry Exist?'), the development of the discipline of psychiatry within medicine (Chapter 2: 'The History of Psychiatry'), the strengths and limitations of diagnostic practices over time (Chapter 3: 'Diagnosing Mental Illness'), the nature and outcomes of interventions for mental illness (Chapter 4: 'Treating Symptoms and Disorders'), the role of consent in care, and treatment in the absence of consent (Chapter 5: 'Treatment Without Consent'), the limited progress in biomedical research into many mental illnesses to date (Chapter 6: 'Neuroscience and Psychiatry'), the impact of culture and social forces on all aspects of psychiatry (Chapter 7: 'Psychiatry, Culture, and Society'), patterns of deliberate self-harm and suicide (Chapter 8: 'Self-Harm and Suicide'), and the search for social justice for people with mental illness and their families (Chapter 9: 'Global Injustice in Mental Health Care'). These are all pivotal, contested themes for a discipline that lives in a state of restless transition and constant evolution. Changing attitudes towards disordered eating, and shifting diagnostic practices in this area, constitute just one example of these long-term trends.

Against this background, the current chapter is devoted to 'The Future of Psychiatry: Person-Centred Care and System-Level Change'. This chapter explores specific themes of relevance to psychiatry and mental health care over the decades to come, including the future of diagnosis in psychiatry; the right to mental health care; the future of mental health legislation (including the 'Geneva impasse'); potential roles and risks of artificial intelligence (AI) in mental health care; global mental health policy (including environmental sustainability in the provision and expansion of services); and the overall future of psychiatry both as a discipline within medicine and as a transformative movement to protect and promote the rights of people with mental illness and their families.

These are big issues which are discussed in this chapter and will continue to be explored and debated over many years to come. Here, emphasis is placed on combining compassionate, person-centred, evidence-based care with global pronouncements, national policies, and system-level change in mental health services. The proximate and ultimate aims of these initiatives are to alleviate suffering, enhance social integration, promote rights, and improve mental health. It is logical to start with diagnosis.

The Future of Diagnosis in Psychiatry

In 1988, Irish psychiatrist Anthony Clare previewed an upcoming television series about the human brain in *The Listener*, a BBC publication (Clare, 1988; see also: Kelly & Houston, 2020). In his essay, Clare noted that the science reflected in such a series could help illuminate 'the machinery underlying our mental process, the chemical modulators, the physiological functions [and] anatomical structure':

But the very phenomena which the machinery produces – our innermost beliefs, convictions, preoccupations, desires, fantasies, hopes, fears, loves, and laughs – those elements which make us more than machines still await an equally generous and skilful exposition.

(Clare, 1988; p. 7)

Almost four decades later, Clare might have added 'mental illness' to the list of matters that remain largely unexplained by neuroscience. Despite a great deal of research and a certain amount of progress, common conditions such as depression and schizophrenia remain resolutely unsolved by the biomedical sciences (see Chapter 6: 'Neuroscience and Psychiatry'). While there has been some progress, neuroscience has not delivered nearly enough useful information to transform psychiatry significantly or to present much prospect of substantial change any time soon.

As a result, diagnosis in psychiatry is still based on symptoms, and management is largely empirical. Despite these limitations, and somewhat improbably, psychiatric treatments can be remarkably effective, provided they are used appropriately (see Chapter 4: 'Treating Symptoms and Disorders'). It is an odd situation: even though the origins of most mental illnesses remain obscure, we have treatments that are proven to work and benefit millions of people around the world (Kelly, 2022). We don't know why most of the treatments help, but we know that they do, at least as much as in other areas of medicine, and sometimes more so.

Despite its manifest limitations, the formulation and re-formulation of diagnostic categories will likely remain central to psychiatry over the decades to come (see Chapter 3: 'Diagnosing Mental Illness'). Provided diagnoses are held lightly in individual clinical encounters and are not over-burdened with meaning or significance, they can help to link symptoms with treatments, and thus alleviate suffering. Diagnostic systems can also help to guide research about the biological, psychological, and social determinants and correlates of common collections of symptoms, even if the outcomes of biological research will likely show that current diagnostic categories need to be radically re-thought in the future. That would be a welcome development.

Owen and colleagues, in a valuable review of 'genomic findings in schizophrenia and their implications', highlight the challenges that emergent biological findings inevitably present to symptom-based diagnostic systems, as exemplified by research into the genetics of schizophrenia, which is, they point out, 'a highly polygenic condition':

Many specific genes and loci have been implicated that provide a firm basis upon which mechanistic research can proceed. These point to disturbances in neuronal, and particularly synaptic, functions that are not confined to a small number of brain regions and circuits. Genetic findings have also revealed the nature of schizophrenia's close relationship to other conditions, particularly bipolar disorder and childhood neurodevelopmental disorders, and provided an explanation for how common risk alleles persist in the population in the face of reduced fecundity. Current genomic approaches only potentially explain around 40% of heritability, but only a small proportion of this is attributable to robustly identified loci. The extreme polygenicity poses challenges for understanding biological mechanisms. The high degree of pleiotropy points to the need for more transdiagnostic research and the shortcomings of current diagnostic criteria as means of delineating biologically distinct strata.

(Owen et al., 2023; p. 3638)

Over future decades, biological findings will hopefully continue to challenge current diagnostic categories and eventually re-shape them radically. This, in turn, will hopefully assist with the identification of targeted treatments with consequent benefits for patients, families, and psychiatry as a whole. These would be very positive developments.

Stein and colleagues, reviewing the state of psychiatric diagnosis and treatment in *World Psychiatry* in 2022, noted various novel perspectives that recently attained varying levels of prominence in these areas, including clinical neuroscience and personalised pharmacotherapy; new statistical approaches to nosology, assessment, and research; the advents of deinstitutionalisation and care in the community; the strengthening of evidence-based psychotherapy; digital phenotyping and digital therapies; and the emergence of global mental health and task-sharing approaches to care (Stein et al., 2022). They note that while each of these developments offers genuine hope for the years ahead, each presents only a partial view of the whole. The authors conclude that while there has been progress in recent times, future advancement is likely to be incremental and iterative, rather than a paradigm shift. This is especially true of diagnosis in psychiatry, which evolves continuously.

Increasingly meaningful and useful diagnosis will undoubtedly lie at the heart of much future change in mental health care. Robust, systematic evidence is essential in this process, ensuring that revised categorical or dimensional approaches to diagnosis are rooted in reality, rather than theory. Thornicroft emphasises the importance of involving people with experience of mental illness in future revisions of diagnostic categories (Thornicroft, 2022). If undertaken mindfully, this process can help psychiatric diagnosis to become more accurate, accessible, and appropriate, and hopefully guide towards more effective, person-centred treatments in the future.

The Right to Mental Health Care

If improved diagnosis can lead to better care, should such care be framed as a human right, in order to optimise access? If so, how can we harness the power of this right?

Since the advent of the United Nations' (UN) Convention on the Rights of Persons with Disabilities (CRPD) (United Nations, 2006), it is possible to spend an infinite amount of time interpreting and re-interpreting ambiguously phrased UN and World Health Organization (WHO) statements about rights, chiefly by reference to other equally ambiguous UN and WHO pronouncements. But does such activity enhance the liberty enjoyed by people with mental illness, or deliver any identifiable benefit? Are other approaches more suited to health and social care, approaches which are deeply aware of human rights, but find their fundamental roots in politics, service development, evidence of benefit, or an ethics of interpersonal care?

Most discussions of rights in psychiatry tend to focus on the right to liberty in the context of admission and treatment without consent (see Chapter 5: 'Treatment Without Consent'). This is understandable, given the gravity of the issues involved in these circumstances. It is, however, also useful to look at the other human rights outlined in statements such as the Universal Declaration of Human Rights (UDHR), which was adopted by the UN General Assembly in 1948 (United Nations, 1948).

The UDHR stated that the 'recognition of the inherent dignity and of the equal and inalienable rights of all members of the human family is the foundation of freedom, justice and peace in the world' (Preamble). As we noted earlier in this book, the UN emphasised that 'all human beings are born free and equal in dignity and rights. They are endowed with reason and conscience and should act towards one another in a spirit of brotherhood' (Article 1). These rights apply to everyone, 'without distinction of any kind, such as race, colour, sex, language, religion, political or other opinion, national or social origin, property, birth or other status' (Article 2).

Among the specific rights outlined, the UDHR referred to 'health and well-being':

> Everyone has the right to a standard of living adequate for the health and well-being of himself [sic] and of his family, including food, clothing, housing and medical care and necessary social services, and the right to security in the event of unemployment, sickness, disability, widowhood, old age or other lack of livelihood in circumstances beyond his control.
>
> (Article 25(1))

How can such a right be realised, given that countries are at different stages of development, have contrasting understandings of health and well-being, and will attain these ideals progressively, unevenly, and slowly, if at all? Realising a 'right to health' is not a simple matter, but it is a vital one (Tobin, 2012; Wolff, 2012).

Eighteen years after the UDHR, in 1966, two separate covenants were adapted by the UN General Assembly, providing further detail about different kinds of rights: the *International Covenant on Civil and Political Rights* (United Nations, 1966a) and the *International Covenant on Economic, Social and Cultural Rights* (United Nations, 1966b). According to this paradigm, civil and political rights were to be realised immediately, while social and cultural rights were to be realised progressively. The *International Covenant on Economic, Social and Cultural Rights* recognised 'the right of everyone to the enjoyment of the highest attainable standard of physical and mental health' (Article 12), consistent with the UDHR.

The inclusion of 'mental health' in this definition is important. The fact that this right is not realised by many people with mental illness today underscores the importance of viewing mental health care as both a human right and a moral entitlement (Flaskerud, 2009). There is also a strong *ethical* argument in favour of a right to mental health care, in light of the clear benefit it would convey to both individuals and society (Green, 2000), including people whose mental illness impairs their understanding of their need for care and support (Lamb, 1990).

In 2000, the UN Committee on Economic, Social and Cultural Rights (CESCR) sought to clarify the 'right to health' in more detail, arguing that this right includes 'both freedoms and entitlements':

> The right to health is not to be understood as a right to be *healthy*. The right to health contains both freedoms and entitlements. The freedoms include the right to control one's health and body, including sexual and reproductive freedom, and the right to be free from interference, such as the right to be free from torture, non-consensual medical treatment and experimentation. By contrast, the entitlements include the right to a system of health protection which provides equality of opportunity for people to enjoy the highest attainable level of health.
>
> (United Nations Committee on Economic, Social and Cultural Rights, 2000; Paragraph 8)

Psychiatry forms a key part of this 'system of health protection', primarily rooted in outpatient care and support, supplemented by voluntary inpatient treatment when needed, but also including admission and treatment without consent in accordance with national legislation when all other interventions have failed (Kelly, 2024a). There is also a right to, or at least a reasonable expectation of, preventive care. Herring argues in favour of a right to be protected from dying by suicide (Herring, 2022).

In 2006, the CRPD articulated the right to health specifically in the context of 'persons with disabilities', stating 'that persons with disabilities have the right to the enjoyment of the highest attainable standard of health without discrimination on the basis of disability' (United Nations, 2006; Article 25). The CRPD adds that 'States Parties shall take all appropriate measures to ensure access for persons with disabilities to health services that are gender-sensitive, including health-related rehabilitation'.

This right includes access to the full range of mental health treatments and supports, as well as services for physical health. As the Office of the UN High Commissioner for Human Rights (OHCHR) points out, 'there is no health without mental health' (United Nations High Commissioner for Human Rights, 2023). Mental health and physical health are continuous with each other, so equal access to services for both is essential for all.

Despite the value of rights-based approaches to mental health care, simply stating the existence of a 'right to health care' is not sufficient to realise such a right in practice (Glover-Thomas and Chima, 2015). Other activities and approaches are also needed, approaches which are deeply aware of human rights, but find their fundamental roots in an ethics of interpersonal care (see Chapter 1: 'Why Does Psychiatry Exist?'), evidence of benefit (see Chapter 4: 'Treating Symptoms and Disorders'), service development, and political activism (see Chapter 9: 'Global Injustice in Mental Health Care'). Human rights are essential, but they are not nearly enough.

The Future of Mental Health Legislation

Law holds considerable potential for the improvement of physical and mental health in the years ahead. Gostin and colleagues point out that law impacts on global health in several different ways by structuring, sustaining, and mediating certain social determinants of health (Gostin et al., 2019). The law has additional roles in the field of mental health owing to specific aspects of the history of psychiatry, especially the history of 'mental hospitals' (see Chapter 2: 'The History of Psychiatry') and current legislation which permits admission and treatment without consent in certain circumstances, provided various clinical and legal criteria are fulfilled (see Chapter 5: 'Treatment Without Consent').

As a result, mental health legislation will inevitably play a significant role in the future of psychiatry over the decades ahead. The role of legislation in this field is never without controversy. In Chapter 5, we noted the recent 'Geneva impasse' in relation to 'coercive care and human rights', which is outlined by Martin and Gurbai:

> Some within the UN human rights community hold that coercive care can comply with human rights standards, provided that the coercive intervention is a necessary and proportionate means to achieve certain approved aims, and that appropriate legal safeguards are in place. Others have held that coercive care is never justified. Disagreement over this issue has produced an impasse in the UN human rights system.
>
> (Martin and Gurbai, 2019; p. 117)

Martin and Gurbai propose 'distinguishing between the broader class of *nonconsensual* treatment and the narrower subset of such treatment that is aptly described as *coercive*' (p. 119). They also propose several potential steps forward that might help resolve this impasse, all of which merit consideration from stakeholders, regardless of which side of the impasse they find themselves (Kelly, 2024a). Dialogue is essential.

Similarly, McSherry and colleagues explored the 'Geneva impasse' in *BJPsych Open* in 2023, and noted that 'much of the literature on human rights and mental healthcare focusses on whether restrictions on compulsory care are required to meet the requirements of United Nations Conventions' (McSherry et al., 2023; p. 1). They also noted, however, 'an emerging literature identifying measures to promote the right to the enjoyment of the highest attainable standard of mental health':

> Attention is turning to how practical measures such as psychiatric advance directives, different models of supported decision-making and human rights training for mental health service providers, patients, families and carers may assist in promoting human rights.
> There is also a developing literature on the need for states to promote good mental health through appropriate allocation of resources and related 'positive' human rights. The main point of consensus is that coercion in mental healthcare can and should be reduced and the range of voluntary options for support be expanded (McSherry et al., 2023; p. 3).
>
> (citations omitted)

In 2022, the WHO and OHCHR published draft *Guidance on Mental Health, Human Rights, and Legislation* seeking to address many of these issues (World Health Organization and Office of the United Nations High Commissioner for Human Rights, 2022). In their final document, titled *Mental Health, Human Rights, and Legislation: Guidance and Practice*, they provide extensive advice about mental health laws and a 'Checklist for assessing rights-based legislation on mental health' (World Health Organization and Office of the United Nations High Commissioner for Human Rights, 2023; pp. 139–63).

In relation to 'substitute decision-making in mental health services', the WHO and OHCHR state:

> Law can prohibit substitute decision-making in the provision of mental health care and support. This includes repealing the provisions that allow guardians and family members to make decisions for people receiving mental health care or support, as well as eliminating all instances in which the law allows the treating doctor to decide for the person in their 'best interests'.
>
> (World Health Organization and Office of the
United Nations High Commissioner for Human
Rights, 2023; p. 48)

Regarding 'involuntary hospitalisation and treatment', the WHO and OHCHR state:

> To ensure a complete paradigm shift away from coercion in mental health care, legislation can prohibit all involuntary measures and mandate that all services, outpatient or inpatient, implement non-coercive responses.
>
> (World Health Organization and Office of the
> United Nations High Commissioner for Human
> Rights, 2023; p. 66)

It is not clear if the use of the word 'can' in both of these statements means that the WHO and OHCHR are saying that these steps are *possible*, or if the WHO and OHCHR somehow see themselves as in a position to *grant permission* to democratically elected governments to take these steps in national legislation if they wish to do so.

Either way, the WHO and OHCHR go on to present Mexico as an example of a country in which, they say, 'involuntary hospitalisation and treatment are no longer permitted' (p. 67). They also point out, however, that treatment can be provided without consent under certain circumstances in Mexico – emergency circumstances which are remarkably similar to the circumstances in which psychiatric treatment without consent is provided in many jurisdictions at the moment.

Overall, the WHO/OHCHR guidance presents a great deal of useful information in certain areas, but struggles in relation to substitute decision-making and treatment without consent, both of which are mandated by national legislation in many countries which are signatories to the CRPD and various other UN conventions. The emphasis that the WHO and OHCHR place on reducing coercive practices is welcome and important, but their guidance remains curiously divorced from systematic evidence of the effectiveness of many psychiatric interventions (see Chapter 4: 'Treating Symptoms and Disorders'), service-users' acknowledgement of the need for treatment without consent at times (e.g., Gergel et al., 2021), and the nature of modern mental health services in which great efforts are made to avoid coercion which, if it occurs, is rare, legal, and carefully reviewed (Kelly, 2024a). Greater dialogue is needed from both sides of the 'Geneva impasse' if these matters are to be resolved and a collaborative path forward is to be agreed.

Overall, it is clear that legislation will continue to play a significant role in mental health care over future years, even if the precise form of this engagement is likely to evolve (McHale, 2024). Wilson argues in favour of developments that emphasise coercion reduction and increased social support, rather than the abolition of mental health laws (Wilson, 2024). Gergel points to a need for 'deeper examination and broader scope', encompassing issues such as euthanasia and other topics which have traditionally been regarded as lying outside discussions of mental health law (Gergel, 2024).

Clearly, legislation will continue to be one of the crucibles in which the nature of psychiatry will be forged, rights will be protected or delimited, and global mental health will hopefully advance. Legislation is, however, just one factor among many. Other influences include the political priority accorded to mental health services, findings from biological, therapeutic, and social research, and innovations in methods of care delivery. The latter includes, most recently, the emergence of artificial intelligence (AI) in healthcare, which we will consider next.

Roles and Risks of Artificial Intelligence (AI) in Mental Health Care

The advent of so-called AI has prompted an extraordinary period of introspection, speculation, anxiety, and – at times – panic across society in general (Suleyman and Bhaskar, 2023). ChatGPT, an advanced language processing AI developed by OpenAI, has generated particular interest. This application is designed to produce human-like text based on input it receives. It was trained on a large volume of text from multiple sources and is quite extraordinary to use (Kelly, 2024b).

Writing in the *Observer*, Wooldridge described 2023 as 'the year in which artificial intelligence (AI) finally went mainstream. I'm referring, of course, to ChatGPT and its stablemates – large language models':

> Why did ChatGPT take off so spectacularly? First, it is very accessible. Anyone with a web browser can access the most sophisticated AI on the planet. And second, it finally feels like the AI we were promised – it wouldn't be out of place in a movie [...] We've been using AI for a long time without realising it, but finally, we have something that looks like the real deal [...] it really is the beginning of something big.
>
> (Wooldridge, 2023)

Notwithstanding some reasoned, level-headed responses to AI, however, overall reactions have varied greatly. This was to be expected. Every new technology prompts a fresh bout of existential handwringing, as each generation believes that its technology presents vastly greater threats than any technology of the past (Orben, 2020). This was true for the printing press, steam power, radio, television, video, computers, and the Internet.

This cycle is very predictable: anxiety, panic, gradual settling down, and incremental adaptation of new technology. Today, we fear AI, and the cycle is starting again. Soon, more rational appraisals will emerge, followed by a degree of boredom, culminating in a certain amount of change, likely in ways we cannot yet predict.

One of the many ironies is that while AI is certainly artificial, it is far from clear if it is intelligent. AI is, however, a triumph of marketing (Kelly, 2023). Many technology companies appear to be generating a sense of panic based on an odd mix of modest technological progress, waves of apocalyptic hysteria, and canny existential button-pushing. AI tech shares have rocketed in recent times. Nobody ever got rich by assessing technology rationally or underestimating the human propensity to panic.

The truth is that each generation honestly believes that the technological changes it witnesses are not only incrementally bigger than those of the past, but vastly greater to the point of presenting an existential threat to the human race. We have believed this about everything from steam engines to nuclear power, from the printing press to the Internet. We inevitably think that this time is different, more, and worse.

Despite this Sisyphean cycle, our brains remain resolutely unrotted by the telephone, radio, television, video games, the Internet, and AI. Change occurs, but rarely when or how we predict. Perhaps that is what change really means: unpredictable jolts forward from time to time. The truth about technology is usually quite mundane and not tremendously exciting. Change is incremental, and we cope with it. The same will be true this time round, with AI.

Like all new technologies, AI presents real opportunities in many areas of human activity, not least the practice of medicine, including psychiatry. The possibilities range from medical education and research to assisting with certain kinds of care and helping patients to understand diagnosis, treatment, and prognosis. Used wisely, AI can assist with many of these tasks.

Medicine can be an information-heavy endeavour, especially during under-graduate and postgraduate training. If models of AI become more reliable over time, it is likely they will prove to be useful tools for finding and summaris-ing information, although they will still be based on information generated by humans, rather than AI. In addition, AI will not dispense with the need for careful, critical thinking by healthcare professionals. The waves of informa-tion provided by the Internet increased the need for critical thought, rather than diminishing it. AI will do likewise.

For patients and families, the benefits are likely to be significant. Certain models of AI can already provide healthcare information in clear, written for-mats or spoken aloud (for people with poor hearing). They can summarise infor-mation in different ways, translate it, re-state points for greater clarity, make written output larger or smaller (for people with poor vision), and add as much or as little detail as a person might request. The possibilities are vast. Used mind-fully, AI will hopefully help to save time for health care professionals to devote to different tasks that require direct human input.

Careful, critical thought is also vital for patients and families as they explore AI. This caveat is not a disadvantage of AI, but a note about how to use it. With this in mind, it would be wise to emphasise thinking skills in primary and sec-ondary schools and third level, to help ensure that AI and other technologies are used appropriately and well. There is also a need for ethical guidance about AI in healthcare, so the WHO has published two useful documents on *Ethics and*

Governance of Artificial Intelligence for Health: WHO Guidance (World Health Organization, 2021) and *Regulatory Considerations on Artificial Intelligence for Health* (World Health Organization, 2023). Both merit attention and reflection.

Inevitably, the new technology will bring certain changes to society, both positive and negative. Ultimately, however, the potential of AI more than justifies its examination, adaptation, and careful review, especially in medicine, including psychiatry. The existential threat of AI is overstated at present. As matters stand, AI does not show any sign of disproving Bernard Levin's comment in *The Times* in 1978 that 'the silicone chip will transform everything, except everything that matters, and the rest will still be up to us' (Levin, 1978).

Global Mental Health Policy

Regardless of innovations that AI might or might not bring to the delivery of mental health services, an over-arching vision or policy will still be required to direct and coordinate care for people with mental illness and their families. Some likely future directions for global policy were indicated by the WHO in its 2022 *World Mental Health Report: Transforming Mental Health for All* (World Health Organization, 2022). As discussed in Chapter 9 of this book ('Global Injustice in Mental Health Care'), the WHO document recommended deepening the value and commitment accorded to mental health, reshaping environments to better protect mental health, and strengthening mental health care so that the full range of mental health needs can be met through community-based networks of affordable, accessible, and quality services and support.

The WHO also pointed to the need for collaborative action involving individuals, governments, service providers, nongovernmental groups, employers, academics, civil society, and various other stakeholders. They emphasised the importance of making progress on the actions outlined in the document, but noted that not every country would be in a position to achieve everything immediately. Change might be incremental, but it can still occur in the directions outlined – and some positive change is vastly better than none.

In response to this report, Sunkel emphasised the need to build a link between mental health, human rights, and social justice in order to optimise implementation (Sunkel, 2022). Freeman noted that united action is needed for a true transformation of global mental health (Freeman, 2022), while Kestel pointed out that mental health specialists have a key role to play in making change happen (Kestel, 2022). One of those roles is continuing to provide mental health care in a compassionate, person-centred way, but also articulating the strong evidence base for key psychiatric interventions, which are often better supported by systematic evidence than interventions in many other areas of clinical and social care (see Chapter 4: 'Treating Symptoms and Disorders').

In terms of specific treatments, evidence continues to grow confirming the benefits of various therapies, including both medication and non-drug treatments, with the balance between differing approaches varying across the full range of mental illnesses. In schizophrenia and related conditions, for example, the evidence in favour of antipsychotic medication is substantially greater than the evidence supporting non-medication interventions, such as cognitive behaviour therapy (CBT) (Jauhar and Lawrie, 2022). That is not to say that CBT or other psychological approaches cannot help, but rather that the systematic evidence base, as it has evolved, provides more robust support for antipsychotic medication than psychological approaches for this population. In addition, there is overwhelming evidence that antipsychotic use, despite its side effects, is protective against all-cause mortality in schizophrenia, compared to no antipsychotic use (Correll et al., 2022). This is a substantial benefit which is matched by few other interventions in any other area of medicine.

It is important that mental health policy at global, national, and local levels reflects this evolving evidence base for specific interventions and is not fuelled solely by ideology. The evidence evolves continually, so it requires constant attention. Mindfulness-based therapies, for example, are a particular growth area over recent decades. As Strauss and colleagues note in *JAMA Psychiatry*:

> Mindfulness-based cognitive therapy (MBCT) is an in-person group program recommended in national treatment guidelines for depression. Mindfulness involves deliberately bringing nonjudgmental awareness to present-moment experiences (eg, thoughts, feelings, physical sensations, behavioral urges), and this skill can be cultivated through mindfulness practice. In MBCT, daily mindfulness practice supported by verbal guidance and therapist-led discussion is combined with CBT for depression [...] Meta-analyses of RCTs show MBCT is effective for depression, both in terms of reducing the relative risk of relapse for people with a history of recurrent depression and in terms of reducing the severity of symptoms for people experiencing a current episode of depression (Strauss et al., 2023; p. 416).
>
> (citations omitted)

Strauss and colleagues add to this literature with their randomised clinical trial of 'Low-Intensity Guided Help Through Mindfulness (LIGHTMind)'. Clearly, mindfulness-based therapies remain an exciting, developing area of mental health care.

In addition to treatments such as medication and various mainstream psychological approaches, there will always be roles for other treatment options that people prefer for personal reasons. These can involve rediscovering older approaches such as psychoanalysis, which some people find useful (e.g., Connolly, 2023), or linking psychological or psychiatric understandings with religious or spiritual traditions that carry particular weight in some people's lives (e.g., Singh and Sharan, 2023). In mental health care, one size does not fit all, so diversity is the key.

Overall, mental health policy in future years should remain focused on the bio-psycho-social model of care that psychiatry has developed over recent decades, recognising the biological, psychological, and social dimensions of the causation, experience, and alleviation of mental illness, as well as the pathway to long-term recovery. Reductionist approaches, such as the 'psycho-social disability' model, constrict rather than expand this canvas, focus on 'disability' rather than ability and recovery, and fail to embrace the full complexity of the experience of suffering in the human mind and body, located in broader society. We are not just brains; we have bodies, too. And souls.

In addition to further enhancing evidence-based care, there is also a need for mental health policy to take an even broader perspective by deepening its awareness of environmental sustainability in the provision and expansion of services. This taps into the growing awareness of links between the health of body and mind and planetary health. In 2018, the '*Lancet* Commission on global mental health and sustainable development' drew specific attention to the effects of climate change on mental health, and emphasised the need to integrate psychosocial support into humanitarian assistance relating to natural disasters and other sequelae of climate change (Patel et al., 2018).

White and colleagues emphasise the potential for mental health workers to mitigate the mental health impact of climate change in vulnerable populations:

> Mental health professionals including physicians, nurses, physician assistants and other healthcare providers have the opportunity to mitigate the mental health impacts of climate change among vulnerable populations through assessment, preventative education and care. An inclusive and trauma-informed response to climate-related disasters, use of validated measures of mental health, and a long-term therapeutic relationship that extends beyond the immediate consequences of climate change-related events are approaches to successful mental health care in a climate-changing world.
>
> (White et al., 2023; p. 1)

Overall, awareness of climate change is another element in the complex array of factors which are likely to influence mental health policy over the coming decades.

The Future of Psychiatry

Clinical psychiatry is a deeply human endeavour, built on trust, respect, and therapeutic relationships. In 1877, John Millar (1818–1888), a surgeon and asylum proprietor, emphasised the importance of the patient-doctor relationship in his book *Hints on Insanity and Signing Certificates* (Millar, 1877). In the language of the times, Millar wrote:

> When called to attend upon an insane person in the early stages of the disorder, the medical practitioner should bear in mind that his [sic] success with his patient will very much depend upon the impression first produced by his own conduct and demeanour. He should therefore, before visiting him,

make himself thoroughly acquainted with every particular connected with the patient's condition. And, that he may gain his confidence, he must approach and treat him as much like a sane person as possible.

(Millar, 1877; p. 69)

Almost a century and a half later, the therapeutic relationship remains at the heart of the delivery of mental health care. The context and content of care also matter greatly, but human interactions with patients and their families remain central to psychiatry.

So far, the current chapter has identified and considered specific themes that are likely to be relevant to psychiatry and mental health care over the decades to come, including the future of diagnosis; the right to mental health care; the future of mental health legislation (including the 'Geneva impasse'); potential roles and risks of AI in psychiatry; and global mental health policy, including environmental sustainability in the provision and development of services. These topics are highlighted in order to explore the future of psychiatry both as a discipline within medicine and as a transformative movement to protect and promote the rights of people with mental illness and their families.

Overall, the future of psychiatry is predicated on combining compassionate, person-centred, evidence-based care with global pronouncements, national policies, and system-level change, with the aims of alleviating suffering, promoting rights, and improving mental health for all. In 2017, the World Psychiatric Association (WPA) and *Lancet Psychiatry* published the 'WPA-*Lancet Psychiatry* Commission on the Future of Psychiatry', which took a similarly broad view of the challenges ahead, drawing attention to both patient care at the level of the individual and wider issues at the levels of health care systems and society as a whole (Bhugra et al., 2017). The Commission also identified mental health law, digital psychiatry, and psychiatric training as other priority areas.

In terms of treatment at the level of the individual, there is a clear need for enhanced research that optimises current knowledge and expands treatment options in a pragmatic, evidence-based way. We need to fund more clinical trials (to identify new treatments), perform more research about psychological and sociological determinants of mental health and illness (to understand causation better), revitalise public health measures (to assist with prevention and early intervention), and develop ways to deliver meaningful social support to those who need it (Makari, 2023).

While these matters are pressing and require urgent attention, we already have many treatments that work well: medications, psychological therapies, and social interventions (for examples, see Chapter 4: 'Treating Symptoms and Disorders'). As Insel points out, the immediate challenge is to deliver the treatments we have to those who need them (Insel, 2022). This involves scaling up mental health systems and providing interventions and supports which we already know work well for many people.

Part of this task will involve addressing the stigma that is still wrongly associated with mental illness and its treatment, especially the evidence-based use of medication in psychiatry. This will be an iterative process, rather than a one-off intervention. There are many approaches to reducing stigma, some involving being open about personal experiences of mental illness, although this approach is not suitable for everyone (Corrigan, 2022). Reducing self-stigma is often a difficult first step, but it can lead the way to understanding for family, friends, and broader society. Service-providers can help by being open and honest about the merits and demerits of treatments, and providing positive support for people with mental illness and their families.

Psychiatry's bio-psycho-social model offers the best vision for the future owing to its balance of perspectives and inclusive approach to collaboration, intervention, and recovery. In 2022, Bolton pointed to the coherence of the bio-psycho-social model:

> My main contention is that – notwithstanding doubts as to what exactly it is, or indeed whether it is anything – there is a coherent account of it, in terms of both applications to particular health conditions and mechanisms with wide application. There is accumulating evidence from recent decades that psychosocial as well as biological factors are implicated in the aetiology and treatment of a large range of physical as well as mental health conditions.
>
> (Bolton, 2022; p. 228)

Bio-psycho-social psychiatry will work best when it engages with both mechanism and meaning, and promotes research into interactions between biological, psychological, and social determinants of mental illness (McConnell, 2020). There is a long-standing need for psychiatry to re-examine and re-negotiate its social roles, both to avoid the errors of the past (e.g., involvement in eugenics) and to optimise the field's potential for the future (Rose, 2019). This involves greater engagement with concepts such as structural violence (Kelly, 2005), systematic disadvantage, and various other negative social exposures which shape human life and well-being (Rose and Rose, 2023).

Such a shift in emphasis does not mean neglecting treatments and interventions which show strong evidence of effectiveness, but it suggests a parallel need to engage with social, economic, and political circumstances that shape the lives of our patients and their families, as well as the services within which we work and the ways in which we think. Fundamentally, this brings us back to the social and political engagements suggested in Chapter 9 of this book, which was devoted to 'Global Injustice in Mental Health Care' and ways to address it.

Monk-Cunliffe, writing in *BJPsych Bulletin* in 2023, outlines some of the benefits of this approach:

> Population interventions to reduce mental illness would not just benefit our psychiatric patients, they would create a happier, healthier society across the

board. Preventing illness and facilitating healthier lifestyles will also help tackle the climate crisis, which has mental health impacts that affect deprived and marginalised communities more than others and will exacerbate existing socioeconomic inequalities (Zhang et al., 2021). However, despite knowledge of what to do and why, we see that things don't change. To address this we must move beyond the remit of psychiatry and to an even more complicated P: politics.

Many of the changes suggested fall outside the budget of health and into other areas. Government departments work in silos, with education judged by how it improves exam results, not by how it improves health. Policy is short-sighted, limited by the terrifying acceleration of electoral cycles. It's much easier to take a photo next to a new hospital to show voters you've helped them than it is to address social determinants and have someone else reap the rewards at the ballot box 20 years down the line.

(Monk-Cunliffe, 2023; p. 229)

Overall, the future of psychiatry lies in further deepening the already strong evidence base for many psychiatric treatments, inviting critics to examine this systematic evidence for themselves, combining this with knowledge from direct experience of mental illness, and continually re-shaping psychiatry as both a discipline within medicine and a transformative movement to promote the rights of people with mental illness and their families. This involves combining compassionate, person-centred, evidence-based care with broader actions: shaping global pronouncements about health priorities, informing national mental health policies and legislation, and generating system-level change, with the aims of alleviating suffering, promoting rights, enhancing social inclusion, and improving mental health for all.

It is a wildly ambitious agenda, but nothing less will suffice.

Hua, the 15-year-old school girl whom we met at the start of this chapter, was avoiding meals, exercising excessively, self-inducing vomiting, and losing extreme amounts of weight. Eventually, Hua's parents persuaded her to see the family doctor (general practitioner) to 'make sure she was a healthy weight'. The moment Hua walked into the consulting room, the doctor saw that Hua was underweight to the point of endangering her health. The doctor spoke with Hua at length, examined her, weighed her, and measured her height.

The doctor told Hua and her parents that he thought Hua had anorexia nervosa. He explained that this is a condition characterised by significantly low body weight for the person's height, age, and developmental stage. The doctor calculated Hua's 'body mass index' (weight divided by height squared) as 17 kg/m.,[2] which is consistent with anorexia nervosa, especially when considered alongside Hua's persistent pattern of restrictive eating, self-induced vomiting, excessive exercise, preoccupation with body weight, and inaccurate perception of her weight.

Hua was not pleased with this assessment. She became angry. Hua said that the doctor was wrong and that she was, in fact, overweight rather than underweight. Hua asked the doctor for laxatives so that she could be 'thin'. When the doctor said this was not a good idea, Hua walked out of the consulting room and said that her parents could talk to the doctor if they wanted to. Moments later, Hua came back into the room to re-join the conversation, saying that she would listen to the doctor, but that she would decide herself what to do next.

Hua's doctor persuaded Hua to see a psychiatrist, who agreed that Hua had anorexia nervosa. Following a lengthy discussion, the psychiatrist reached an agreement with Hua that she would modify some of her behaviours and attend an outpatient treatment programme for eating disorders. The psychiatrist was part of a multi-disciplinary team that focused on both physical health care and enhanced cognitive behavioural therapy (CBT-E) for eating disorders.

The treatment programme was challenging for both Hua and her family. There was continual negotiation about many aspects of it, but the psychiatrist and their team were experienced in engaging with people with eating disorders. Over time, Hua participated well in the programme (even if she was sometimes ambivalent), and her family offered steady support. After some time, Hua regained a healthy body weight, her self-induced vomiting declined, and she gradually reduced her exercise. Hua remained 'picky' about food, but managed to take a healthy diet most days.

Ultimately, Hua's recovery was slow but definite. There came a time when she looked back on her eating disorder as part of her history, rather than her present. 'I do not understand why I got anorexia nervosa', she told her psychiatrist: 'I recognise that it was part of who I was back then, but that is not who I am now'.

Key Messages

- The future of psychiatry lies in an evolving combination of person-centred care and system-level changes that are compassionate, evidence-based, and developed in partnership with people with mental illness and their families.
- Key issues for the future of psychiatry include the continued development of diagnostic methods; advancing the right to mental health care; shaping the future of mental health legislation in positive ways; managing the roles and risks of artificial intelligence (AI); enhancing global mental health policy (including environmental sustainability); and further developing psychiatry as a discipline within medicine and a transformative movement to promote well-being and protect rights.
- Regarding diagnosis, systematic evidence and patient involvement are essential to ensure that revised categorical or dimensional approaches to diagnosis

are rooted in reality rather than theory, and guide towards more effective, person-centred care.

- Regarding the right to mental health care, it is important to state and protect this right, but other approaches are also needed, approaches which remain deeply aware of human rights, but find their fundamental roots in an ethics of interpersonal care, evidence of benefit, service development, and political activism. Human rights are essential, but they are not enough alone.
- Regarding mental health legislation, it is clear that law will continue to play a significant role in mental health care, even if the precise form of that engagement is likely to evolve, ideally with a focus on protecting rights and reducing coercion, in addition to facilitating much-needed care for people with mental illness and support for their families.
- Regarding AI, it is essential that people with mental illness enjoy the benefits of technological advances on an equal basis with others, and that issues of access, ethics, and evidence of benefit are managed appropriately.
- Regarding global mental health policy, there should be continued focus on the bio-psycho-social model of care, recognising the biological, psychological, and social dimensions of the causation, experience, and alleviation of mental illness, as well as pathways to long-term recovery. The impact of climate change and the need for sustainable services are also key influences on policy.
- The future of psychiatry lies in further deepening the evidence base for psychiatric treatments, inviting critics to examine this systematic evidence for themselves, combining this with knowledge from direct experience of mental illness, and continually re-shaping psychiatry as both a discipline within medicine and a transformative movement to promote the rights of people with mental illness and their families.

References

Bhugra D, Tasman A, Pathare S, Priebe S, Smith S, Torous J, Arbuckle MR, Langford A, Alarcón RD, Chiu HFK, First MB, Kay J, Sunkel C, Thapar A, Udomratn P, Baingana FK, Kestel D, Ng RMK, Patel A, Picker L, McKenzie KJ, Moussaoui D, Muijen M, Bartlett P, Davison S, Exworthy T, Loza N, Rose D, Torales J, Brown M, Christensen H, Firth J, Keshavan M, Li A, Onnela J-P, Wykes T, Elkholy H, Kalra G, Lovett KF, Travis MJ, Ventriglio A. The WPA-*Lancet Psychiatry* Commission on the future of psychiatry. *Lancet Psychiatry* 2017; 4: 775–818 (http://dx.doi.org/10.1016/S2215-0366(17)30333-4).

Blandford GF. *Insanity and its Treatment: Lectures on the Treatment, Medical and Legal, of Insane Patients.* Edinburgh: Oliver and Boyd, 1871.

Bolton D. Looking forward to a decade of the biopsychosocial model. *BJPsych Bulletin* 2022; 46: 228–32 (http://dx.doi.org/10.1192/bjb.2022.34). (Link to license: https://creativecommons.org/licenses/by/4.0/) (accessed 5 January 2024).

Clare A. Brain scan. *The Listener,* 15 September 1988.

Connolly R. On the analyst's couch. *Financial Times,* 13/14 May 2023 (https://www
.ft.com/content/0b7e66f9-085b-46b9-b620-53f480a2ad9a) (accessed 4 January
2024).

Correll CU, Solmi M, Croatto G, Schneider LK, Rohani-Montez SC, Fairley L, Smith N,
Bitter I, Gorwood P, Taipale H, Tiihonen J. Mortality in people with schizophrenia:
a systematic review and meta-analysis of relative risk and aggravating or attenuating
factors. *World Psychiatry* 2022; 21: 248–71 (http://dx.doi.org/10.1002/wps.20994).

Corrigan PW. Coming out proud to erase the stigma of mental illness. *World Psychiatry*
2022; 21: 388–9 (http://dx.doi.org/10.1002/wps.21016).

Flaskerud JH. The 'human right' to mental health care. *Issues in Mental Health Nursing*
2009; 30: 796–7 (https://doi.org/10.3109/01612840903019740).

Freeman M. The world mental health report: transforming mental health for all. *World
Psychiatry* 2022; 21: 391–2 (http://dx.doi.org/10.1002/wps.21018).

Gergel TL. The future of mental health law: the need for deeper examination and broader
scope. In: Kelly BD, Donnelly M (eds), *Routledge Handbook of Mental Health Law*
(pp. 704–26). London and New York: Routledge, 2024.

Gergel T, Das P, Owen G, Stephenson L, Rifkin L, Hindley G, Dawson J, Ruck Keene
A. Reasons for endorsing or rejecting self-binding directives in bipolar disorder: a
qualitative study of survey responses from UK service users. *Lancet Psychiatry* 2021;
8: 599–609 (https://doi.org/10.1016/S2215-0366(21)00115-2).

Glover-Thomas N, Chima SC. A legal 'right' to mental health care? Impediments to
a global vision of mental health care access. *Nigerian Journal of Clinical Practice*
2015; 18: S8–S14 (https://doi.org/10.4103/1119-3077.170822).

Gostin LO, Monahan JT, Kaldor J, DeBartolo M, Friedman EA, Gottschalk K, Kim SC,
Alwan A, Binagwaho A, Burci GL, Cabal L, DeLand K, Evans TG, Goosby E, Hossain
S, Koh H, Ooms G, Roses Periago M, Uprimny R, Yamin AE. The legal determinants
of health: harnessing the power of law for global health and sustainable development.
Lancet 2019; 393: 1857–910 (http://dx.doi.org/10.1016/S0140-6736(19)30233-8).

Green SA. An ethical argument for a right to mental health care. *General Hospital
Psychiatry* 2000; 22: 17–26 (https://doi.org/10.1016/s0163-8343(99)00047-x).

Herring J. *The Right to be Protected from Committing Suicide.* Oxford: Hart Publishing,
2022.

Insel T. *Healing: Our Path from Mental Illness to Mental Health.* New York: Penguin
Press, 2022.

Jauhar S, Lawrie SM. What is the evidence for antipsychotic medication and alternative
psychosocial interventions for people with acute, non-affective psychosis? *Lancet
Psychiatry* 2022; 9: 253–60 (http://dx.doi.org/10.1016/S2215-0366(21)00293-5).

Kelly BD. Structural violence and schizophrenia. *Social Science and Medicine* 2005; 61:
721–30 (http://dx.doi.org/10.1016/j.socscimed.2004.12.020).

Kelly BD. *In Search of Madness: A Psychiatrist's Travels Through the History of Mental
Illness.* Dublin: Gill Books, 2022.

Kelly BD. The existential threat of new technology is just good marketing. *Financial
Times,* 10/11 June 2023 (https://www.ft.com/content/efa84fc1-0461-4552-835c
-6b5d8d56516e) (accessed 4 January 2024).

Kelly BD. AI in medicine - balancing prudence with possibility. *Medical Independent,* 23
January 2024b (https://www.medicalindependent.ie/comment/opinion/ai-in-medicine
-balancing-prudence-with-possibility/) (accessed 24 January 2024).

Kelly BD. The right to mental health care in mental health legislation. In: Kelly BD, Donnelly M (eds), *Routledge Handbook of Mental Health Law* (pp. 384–402). London and New York: Routledge, 2024a.

Kelly BD, Houston M. *Psychiatrist in the Chair: The Official Biography of Anthony Clare.* Newbridge: Merrion Press, 2020.

Kestel D. Transforming mental health for all: a critical role for specialists. *World Psychiatry* 2022; 21: 333–4 (http://dx.doi.org/10.1002/wps.21030).

Lamb HR. Involuntary treatment for the homeless mentally ill. *Notre Dame Journal of Law, Ethics and Public Policy* 1990; 4: 269 80.

Levin B. The questions that machines cannot answer. *Times,* 3 October 1978.

Makari G. What Covid revealed about American psychiatry. *New Yorker,* 13 July 2023 (https://www.newyorker.com/culture/essay/what-covid-revealed-about-american-psychiatry) (accessed 5 January 2024).

Martin W, Gurbai S. Surveying the Geneva impasse: coercive care and human rights. *International Journal of Law and Psychiatry* 2019; 64: 117–28 (http://dx.doi.org/10.1016/j.ijlp.2019.03.001). (Link to license: https://creativecommons.org/licenses/by/4.0/) (accessed 4 January 2024).

McConnell D. Specifying the best conception of the biopsychosocial model. In: Savulescu J, Roache R, Davies W (eds), *Psychiatry Reborn: Biopsychosocial Psychiatry in Modern Medicine* (pp. 381–403). Oxford: Oxford University Press, 2020.

McHale JV. Mental health law: a global future? In: Kelly BD, Donnelly M (eds), *Routledge Handbook of Mental Health Law* (pp. 665–84). London and New York: Routledge, 2024.

McSherry B, Gooding P, Maker Y. Human rights promotion and the 'Geneva impasse' in mental healthcare: scoping review. *BJPsych Open* 2023; 9: e58 (http://dx.doi.org/10.1192/bjo.2023.50). (Link to license: https://creativecommons.org/licenses/by/4.0/) (accessed 4 January 2024).

Millar J. *Hints on Insanity and Signing Certificates.* London: Henry Renshaw, 1877.

Monk-Cunliffe J. How can we overcome health inequalities in psychiatry? *BJPsych Bulletin* 2023; 47: 228–30 (http://dx.doi.org/10.1192/bjb.2023.49). (Link to licence: https://creativecommons.org/licenses/by/4.0/) (accessed 6 January 2024).

Orben A. The Sisyphean cycle of technology panics. *Perspectives on Psychological Science* 2020; 15: 1143–57 (https://doi.org/10.1177/1745691620919372).

Owen MJ, Legge SE, Rees E, Walters JTR, O'Donovan MC. Genomic findings in schizophrenia and their implications. *Molecular Psychiatry* 2023; 28: 3638–47 (http://dx.doi.org/10.1038/s41380-023-02293-8). (Link to licence: https://creativecommons.org/licenses/by/4.0/) (accessed 2 January 2024).

Patel V, Saxena S, Lund C, Thornicroft G, Baingana F, Bolton P, Chisholm D, Collins PY, Cooper JL, Eaton J, Herrman H, Herzallah MM, Huang Y, Jordans MJD, Kleinman A, Medina-Mora ME, Morgan E, Niaz U, Omigbodun O, Prince M, Rahman A, Saraceno B, Sarkar BK, De Silva M, Singh I, Stein DJ, Sunkel C, Unützer J. The *Lancet* Commission on global mental health and sustainable development. *Lancet* 2018; 392: 1553–98 (http://dx.doi.org/10.1016/S0140-6736(18)31612-X).

Rose N. *Our Psychiatric Future: The Politics of Mental Health.* Cambridge: Polity Press, 2019.

Rose D, Rose N. Is 'another' psychiatry possible? *Psychological Medicine* 2023; 53: 46–54 (http://dx.doi.org/10.1017/S003329172200383X).

Singh B, Sharan P. The contagion of mental illness: insights from a Sufi shrine. *Transcultural Psychiatry* 2023; 60: 457–75 (http://dx.doi.org/10.1177/13634615221078131).

Stein DJ, Shoptaw SJ, Vigo DV, Lund C, Cuijpers P, Bantjes J, Sartorius N, Maj M. Psychiatric diagnosis and treatment in the 21st century: paradigm shifts versus incremental integration. *World Psychiatry* 2022; 21: 393–414 (http://dx.doi.org/10.1002/wps.20998).

Strauss C, Bibby-Jones AM, Jones F, Byford S, Heslin M, Parry G, Barkham M, Lea L, Crane R, de Visser R, Arbon A, Rosten C, Cavanagh K. Clinical effectiveness and cost-effectiveness of supported mindfulness-based cognitive therapy self-help compared with supported cognitive behavioral therapy self-help for adults experiencing depression: the Low-Intensity Guided Help Through Mindfulness (LIGHTMind) randomized clinical trial. *JAMA Psychiatry* 2023; 80: 415–24 (http://dx.doi.org/10.1001/jamapsychiatry.2023.0222). (Links to licence: https://jamanetwork.com/pages/cc-by-license-permissions https://creativecommons.org/share-your-work/cclicenses/; https://creativecommons.org/licenses/by/4.0/) (accessed 6 January 2024).

Suleyman M, Bhaskar M. *The Coming Wave: AI, Power and the Twenty-First Century's Greatest Dilemma.* London: The Bodley Head, 2023.

Sunkel C. A lived experience perspective on the new World Mental Health Report. *World Psychiatry* 2022; 21: 390–1 (http://dx.doi.org/10.1002/wps.21031).

Thornicroft G. Psychiatric diagnosis and treatment in the 21st century: paradigm shifts or power shifts? *World Psychiatry* 2022; 21: 334–5 (http://dx.doi.org/10.1002/wps.21000).

Tobin J. *The Right to Health in International Law.* Oxford: Oxford University Press, 2012.

United Nations. *Universal Declaration of Human Rights.* Paris: United Nations, 1948 (https://www.un.org/en/about-us/universal-declaration-of-human-rights) (accessed 3 January 2024).

United Nations. *International Covenant on Civil and Political Rights.* New York: United Nations, 1966a (https://www.ohchr.org/en/instruments-mechanisms/instruments/international-covenant-civil-and-political-rights) (accessed 4 January 2024).

United Nations. *International Covenant on Economic, Social and Cultural Rights.* New York: United Nations, 1966b (https://www.ohchr.org/en/instruments-mechanisms/instruments/international-covenant-economic-social-and-cultural-rights) (accessed 4 January 2024).

United Nations. *Convention on the Rights of Persons with Disabilities.* New York: United Nations, 2006 (https://social.desa.un.org/issues/disability/crpd/convention-on-the-rights-of-persons-with-disabilities-crpd) (accessed 3 January 2024).

United Nations Committee on Economic, Social and Cultural Rights (CESCR). *CESCR General Comment No. 14: The Right to the Highest Attainable Standard of Health (Art. 12).* Geneva and New York: Office of the United Nations High Commissioner for Human Rights, 2000 (https://digitallibrary.un.org/record/425041) (accessed 4 January 2024).

United Nations High Commissioner for Human Rights. *The Right to Mental Health.* Geneva and New York: Office of the United Nations High Commissioner for Human Rights, 2023 (https://www.ohchr.org/en/special-procedures/sr-health/right-mental-health) (accessed 4 January 2024).

White BP, Breakey S, Brown MJ, Smith JR, Tarbet A, Nicholas PK, Ros AMV. Mental health impacts of climate change among vulnerable populations globally: an integrative review. *Annals of Global Health* 2023; 89: 66 (https://doi.org/10.5334/aogh.4105). (Link to licence: https://creativecommons.org/licenses/by/4.0/) (accessed 5 January 2024).

Wilson K. The future of mental health law: abolition or reform? In: Kelly BD, Donnelly M (eds), *Routledge Handbook of Mental Health Law* (pp. 685–703). London and New York: Routledge, 2024.

Wolff J. *The Human Right to Health*. New York and London: W.W. Norton and Company, 2012.

Wooldridge M. The 10 biggest science stories of 2023 – chosen by scientists: 2. AI finally starting to feel like AI. *Observer*, 24 December 2023 (https://www.theguardian.com/science/2023/dec/23/the-10-biggest-science-stories-of-2023-chosen-by-scientists) (accessed 4 January 2024) (Courtesy of Guardian News & Media Ltd.).

World Health Organization. *Ethics and Governance of Artificial Intelligence for Health: WHO Guidance*. Geneva: World Health Organization, 2021 (https://www.who.int/publications/i/item/9789240029200) (accessed 4 January 2024).

World Health Organization. *World Mental Health Report: Transforming Mental Health for All*. Geneva: World Health Organization, 2022 (https://www.who.int/publications/i/item/9789240049338) (Licence: https://creativecommons.org/licenses/by-nc-sa/3.0/igo/) (accessed 5 January 2024).

World Health Organization. *Regulatory Considerations on Artificial Intelligence for Health*. Geneva: World Health Organization, 2023 (https://iris.who.int/handle/10665/373421) (accessed 4 January 2024).

World Health Organization and Office of the United Nations High Commissioner for Human Rights. *Guidance on Mental Health, Human Rights, and Legislation (Draft)*. Geneva: World Health Organization/Office of the United Nations High Commissioner for Human Rights, 2022 (https://www.ohchr.org/en/calls-for-input/calls-input/draft-guidance-mental-health-human-rights-legislation-who-ohchr) (accessed 4 January 2024).

World Health Organization and Office of the United Nations High Commissioner for Human Rights. *Mental Health, Human Rights, and Legislation: Guidance and Practice*. Geneva: World Health Organization/Office of the United Nations High Commissioner for Human Rights, 2023 (https://www.who.int/publications/i/item/9789240080737). (Link to licence: https://creativecommons.org/licenses/by-nc-sa/3.0/igo/) (accessed 4 January 2024).

Zhang S, Braithwaite I, Bhavsar V, Das-Munshi J. Unequal effects of climate change and pre-existing inequalities on the mental health of global populations. *BJPsych Bulletin* 2021; 45: 230–4 (https://doi.org/10.1192/bjb.2021.26).

Zipfel S, Giel KE, Bulik CM, Hay P, Schmidt U. Anorexia nervosa: aetiology, assessment, and treatment. *Lancet Psychiatry* 2015; 2: 1099–111 (https://doi.org/10.1016/S2215-0366(15)00356-9).

11 Epilogue

Mikhail was 69 when Covid-19 reached his town. Troubled by anxiety all his life, Mikhail's situation became even more challenging during the pandemic. At times, he feared he would not make it out the other side.

Mikhail grew up and lived in the same town for almost all his life. He attended school across the road from his family home and then spent three years working in a nearby city, before returning to his hometown at the age of 20. Mikhail never lived anywhere else since then. 'Where would I go?', he said. 'I like it here'.

Mikhail spent 43 years working in a factory that made wheels for tractors. He moved between manual posts in the factory, but his favourite was at the start of the assembly line. When he was 30, Mikhail was promoted to team leader, but he disliked this position and returned to the assembly line after just a few months. He worked in the factory until he retired at the age of 63. Mikhail was their longest-serving worker ever.

Mikhail suffered from anxiety since an early age. As a child, he was nervous and jumpy, although he still managed to make some friends and complete his school work. As a teenager, Mikhail was awkward and shy, but no more so than many other teenagers. Mikhail met Sofia when he was 21 and they married when he was 23. Apart from Sofia, Mikhail had few friends and mostly kept to himself. The couple had one child, Anastasia.

Mikhail was troubled by anxiety in various ways all through his life. He was content when he was working in his job at the factory, but he struggled if he had to speak in front of a group. He disliked training new employees. Even though Mikhail was one of the factory's most experienced workers, he became anxious if he had to demonstrate anything in front of other people or explain to visitors how the factory operated. Mikhail avoided these situations when he could, worried that he would be embarrassed in front of other people.

Mikhail was also anxious at social gatherings. He avoided these if possible, even gatherings of his own family or Sofia's relatives. Sofia understood Mikhail's concerns, and accepted him as he was, but sometimes his worries annoyed her. Mikhail insisted that he blushed and sweated in social situations, and that other people could see this. Sofia told him that this did not happen, but it was almost impossible to reassure Mikhail. He remained anxious and avoidant no matter

DOI: 10.4324/9781003378495-12

what Sofia said. Mikhail was less uncomfortable when Sofia was with him, but he would still prefer to be at home rather than in company.

Sofia died suddenly the year after Mikhail retired from the factory. Their daughter Anastasia had moved to a distant city, but returned home for three months following her mother's death. After she went back to the city, Mikhail's anxiety worsened. Once he was living alone, Mikhail began to drink alcohol every day, often in the mornings. Soon, he rarely left his house, except to buy food. And he increasingly felt he needed to drink alcohol before going to the shop.

At this point, the Covid-19 pandemic emerged. Mikhail heard about it on the radio and decided that he was at high risk, owing to his age. Mikhail not only adhered to the government's public health restrictions but decided that he needed to be extra careful. He ordered food to be delivered, did not open the front door to anyone (even the postman), and did not go for walks, preferring to sit in his back garden. Mikhail stopped answering the phone, even to Anastasia. Soon, Mikhail had no contact with anyone for weeks on end. He stayed at home in a state of advanced anxiety, utterly disconnected from the world.

Introduction

Mikhail's story was regrettably common during the Covid-19 pandemic that started in 2020 and soon spread around the world. Millions of people died from the direct effects of the virus. For millions of others, the combined effects of biological illness (e.g., viral infection), psychological symptoms (e.g., anxiety), and social disruption (e.g., public health quarantines) presented bio-psycho-social challenges that required specialist interventions and support, not least from bio-psycho-social psychiatry, even in the aftermath of the public health emergency (Kelly, 2023).

Psychiatry has always been shaped by broad, sweeping social forces and the events of history. Today, the discipline continues to exist in a state of constant change owing not least to persisting mysteries about the human mind. While there have been modest advances in the neuroscience of mental illness and its treatment, most common psychiatric illnesses, such as depression and schizophrenia, remain biological conundrums, in need of much more exploration (see Chapter 6: 'Neuroscience and Psychiatry'). For now, the evidence base for key psychiatric treatments, explored in Chapter 4 of this book ('Treating Symptoms and Disorders'), provides a solid basis for current practice and a robust platform for development, even though we do not understand the biological basis of most conditions.

In 2023, the Royal College of Psychiatrists launched a campaign to encourage more people to #ChoosePsychiatry as a career.[1] As part of this initiative, actor and broadcaster Stephen Fry, an honorary fellow of the Royal College of Psychiatrists, pointed out that 'young people preparing for medical careers are realising more and more that the most exciting frontier in medicine is the human mind':

> But its study is more than just an intellectual challenge, it is a pathway to a life in psychiatry - the specialism that fights on the front line in our war against mental illness.
>
> It's vital and rewarding work. I've encountered many doctors who have regretted, later in their careers, that they did not choose psychiatry, but I have never met one who regretted that they did. Because despite what you might think or have heard, psychiatry daily solves problems, saves lives, helps, and heals.
>
> I know I can say with absolute truth that psychiatry saved my life at its lowest moment. I don't believe I would be here today if it were not for the psychiatrist who rescued me. The smartest and most caring minds are needed in this field and – happily – the trend towards choosing psychiatry as a speciality has lately been upward, upward, upward.

This book has been concerned with various specific aspects of psychiatry, ranging from definitions to diagnoses, from the history of the discipline to its future within medicine. This book has also explored psychiatry's evolving role as a broader social movement to protect and promote the human rights of people with mental illness and their families. The key to progressing further along these paths lies in focussing on preventing mental illness when possible, alleviating suffering at all times, and protecting the full range of rights of people with mental illness and their families, including their rights to treatment and support.

The overarching message of this book is that psychiatry offers a reasoned and reasonable path forward, once it is approached and practised with knowledge, awareness, humility, and compassion. The greatest challenge that psychiatry currently faces is global injustice in the distribution of preventive measures, treatment options, social support, and protections for rights. These are political matters as well as medical ones, requiring broad-based, interdisciplinary action to address the challenges presented by mental illness across all communities and in all societies around the world.

With this in mind, this book argues that the evidence-based treatments which psychiatry provides (see Chapter 4: 'Treating Symptoms and Disorders') need to be supplemented by system-level change to address the social exclusion and structural violence experienced by people with mental illness. These topics were explored with particular focus in Chapters 9 ('Global Injustice in Mental Health Care') and 10 ('The Future of Psychiatry: Person-Centred Care and System-Level Change'). These challenges are as urgent and relevant today as they have ever been at any point in the history of psychiatry.

Against this background, Persaud and colleagues propose that a 'Magna Carta' is needed in order to protect the rights of people with mental illness and help address the discrimination they experience in so many spheres of life (Persaud et al., 2021). The Magna Carta is a royal charter of rights that dates from 1215. Various human rights pronouncements explored in earlier chapters of this book articulate many of these rights in the particular context of mental illness (see, for example, Chapter 5: 'Treatment Without Consent'), but further assertion of these rights is urgently needed, along with renewed focus on their realisation in practice.

This task is not unique to psychiatry; it is a central mission across much of medicine. Rudolf Virchow, the great nineteenth-century German pathologist, anthropologist, and politician, said that 'medicine is a social science, and politics nothing but medicine at a larger scale' (Virchow, 1848; MacLeod & McCullough, 1994). This is especially true in psychiatry where failures of social care routinely amplify the impact of mental illness, frustrate efforts at treatment, and result in the social exclusion of people with mental illness and their families. Medicine can play a key role in addressing these matters. Virchow added that physicians are 'the natural attorneys of the poor' and this is as relevant today as it was in the time of Virchow, if not more so (Mackenbach, 2009; FitzPatrick et al., 2021).

To fulfil these social and emancipatory roles, as well as its core therapeutic aims, psychiatry needs not only vision and resources, but trained specialists who are committed to making a difference in the lives of people with mental illness. Recruitment to psychiatry is essential for this task. Hopefully, some medical students will read this book and decide to pursue careers in psychiatry.

In 2023, the Royal College of Psychiatrists' campaign to encourage more people to #ChoosePsychiatry as a career featured not only Stephen Fry, but also Alastair Campbell, the celebrated communicator, writer, and strategist, who, like Fry, is an honorary fellow of the College.[2] Campbell said that whenever he hears 'of a medical student choosing psychiatry, I feel happy knowing that everyone who does choose psychiatry has the chance to make this a better world'.

That is the ultimate aim of psychiatric care and all of medicine: making our world a better place, one person at a time.

Mikhail, the 69-year-old man whom we met at the start of this chapter, suffered from social anxiety for most of his life. He never sought formal treatment for this, preferring to avoid difficult situations and rely on the emotional support of his wife, Sofia. After Sofia died, and Mikhail was living alone, he developed a problem with alcohol. When the Covid-19 pandemic emerged, Mikhail became completely isolated and had no contact with anyone, apart from a weekly food delivery service.

Mikhail's only child, Anastasia, lived in a city that was over 200 kilometres away. When her father stopped answering his phone during the pandemic, Anastasia was distraught. She was not allowed to travel to her father's town, owing to strict Covid-19 travel restrictions. In addition, Anastasia had to work from home and care for her six-year-old son. But Anastasia was profoundly worried that her father might be depressed, physically ill, or even dead, and nobody would know. Like her father, Anastasia was prone to anxiety, but even she realised that the pandemic was a situation in which almost anyone could become extremely anxious. But what could she do?

After some weeks, Anastasia decided to leave her son with a nearby friend and travel to her father's town, even though this violated public health restrictions. Stopped by police as she drove out of the city, Anastasia explained the situation to a stern-looking policeman. She said that she knew she was violating regulations, but she had to check on her father. The policeman listened carefully, thought for a few moments, and then said quietly: 'I would do the same. Go ahead'.

Anastasia found her father in a state of profound anxiety and neglect. His house was a mess, with unwashed dishes everywhere, laundry on the floor, and a dreadful smell. Anastasia was horrified. Too scared of Covid-19 to take Mikhail to the hospital, Anastasia put him in her car and drove him back to her tiny flat in the city. There, she gave Mikhail proper food, helped him clean up, and arranged a video consultation with her general practitioner (family doctor). The doctor advised rest and general care, and mentioned a series of symptoms which, if they occurred, meant Anastasia should bring her father to the hospital, despite the risk of Covid-19. The biggest concern was alcohol withdrawal, but luckily, this did not occur.

In fact, Mikhail did very well. Over a few weeks, Mikhail's physical health recovered and his mood improved. While there was very little space in Anastasia's apartment, Mikhail benefitted hugely from bringing his grandson to the playground and, when school reopened, walking him to school. Mikhail remained anxious about certain social situations, but he had now found a new home in which he was happy.

Given her father's long history of anxiety, Anastasia arranged an appointment for Mikhail to see a psychiatrist. The psychiatrist listened to Mikhail's story and told Mikhail that he likely had social anxiety disorder, complicated by alcohol misuse. The psychiatrist explained that cognitive behaviour therapy can help, and that some people with mixed anxiety and depression benefit from antidepressant medication. She also discussed the role of alcohol in causing or worsening these symptoms. Mikhail understood this part already.

At the end of the consultation, Mikhail asked: 'Do I need medication?' The psychiatrist answered: 'I don't think so. If things change, come back to see me, and we will think of a plan. But no medication for now, anyway'. Then Mikhail asked: 'So, what do I need?' The psychiatrist repeated her advice about anxiety management techniques and avoiding alcohol. Finally, she added: 'There is one more thing, and this is the most important one: keep walking your grandson to school. Then, you will have everything you need'.

Notes

1 https://www.rcpsych.ac.uk/news-and-features/latest-news/detail/2023/10/24/stephen
-fry---alastair-campbell-back----rcpsych-s-award-winning-recruitment-campaign
(accessed 12 January 2024).
2 https://www.rcpsych.ac.uk/news-and-features/latest-news/detail/2023/10/24/stephen
-fry---alastair-campbell-back----rcpsych-s-award-winning-recruitment-campaign
(accessed 12 January 2024).

References

FitzPatrick MEB, Badu-Boateng C, Huntley C, Morgan C. 'Attorneys of the poor': training physicians to tackle health inequalities. *Future Healthcare Journal* 2021; 8: 12–18 (https://doi.org/10.7861/fhj.2020-0242).

Kelly BD. *Resilience: Lessons from Sir William Wilde on Life after Covid.* Dublin: Eastwood Books, 2023.

Mackenbach JP. Politics is nothing but medicine at a larger scale: reflections on public health's biggest idea. *Journal of Epidemiology and Community Health* 2009; 63: 181–4 (https://doi.org/10.1136/jech.2008.077032).

MacLeod SM, McCullough HN. Social science education as a component of medical training. *Social Science and Medicine* 1994; 39: 1367–73 (https://doi.org/10.1016/0277-9536(94)90367-0).

Persaud A, Bhugra D, Das P, Gnanapragasam S, Watson C, Wijesuriya R, Brice T, Clissold E, Castaldelli-Maia JM, Valsraj K, Torales J, Ventriglio A. Magna Carta for individuals living with mental illness. *International Review of Psychiatry* 2021; 33: 75–80 (https://doi.org/10.1080/09540261.2020.1753963).

Virchow R. Der Armenarzt. *Medicinische Reform* 1848; 18: 125–7.

Index

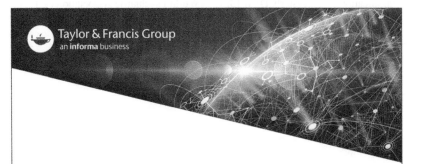

For Product Safety Concerns and Information please contact our EU
representative GPSR@taylorandfrancis.com Taylor & Francis Verlag GmbH,
Kaufingerstraße 24, 80331 München, Germany

Printed and bound by CPI Group (UK) Ltd, Croydon, CR0 4YY
08/06/2025
01897009-0003